Services for People with Learning Disabilities

Services for People with Learning Disabilities explores new developments in provision for people with learning disabilities. An updated version of *Services for the Mentally Handicapped in Britain* (1980), it includes new, additional chapters on current topics such as advocacy and empowerment, and recreation and leisure.

The contributors focus on linking knowledge of user developments with policy and professional practice in both the statutory and non-statutory sectors. They describe the present network of services and explain the NHS and Community Care Act (1990) in terminology accessible to health care professionals and others engaged in this area. The book looks in detail at the concepts underpinning the new legislation, including caremanagement and assessment, quality and inspection, and inter-agency planning. It provides up-to-date information on developments in deinstitutionalisation and community care, residential care, day care, and voluntary and educational services.

With its broad review of the services that are available, *Services for People with Learning Disabilities* will be an invaluable resource for all practitioners in health and community care. It will also give professionals and carers much greater understanding of where changes and improvements are still needed.

Nigel Malin is Reader in Community Care at Sheffield Hallam University.

Services for People with Learning Disabilities

Edited by Nigel Malin

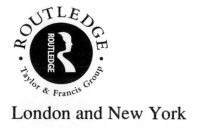

London and New York

First published 1995
by Routledge
11 New Fetter Lane, London EC4P 4EE

Simultaneously published in the USA and Canada
by Routledge
29 West 35th Street, New York, NY 10001

Reprinted 2002

Transferred to Digital Printing 2002

Routledge is an imprint of the Taylor & Francis Group

© 1995 Nigel Malin, selection and editorial matter;
individual chapters, the contributors

Typeset in Times by
Ponting–Green Publishing Services, Chesham, Bucks

Printed and bound in Great Britain by
Biddles Short Run Books, King's Lynn

British Library Cataloguing in Publication Data
A catalogue record for this book is available from the British
Library.

Library of Congress Cataloging in Publication Data
A catalog record for this book has been requested

ISBN 0–415–09937–4 (hbk)
ISBN 0–415–09938–2 (pbk)

Contents

Part II Implementing the Community Care Act

Contributors

Andrew Balchin is currently a Senior Welfare Rights Officer in the Family and Community Services Department of Sheffield City Council. He manages the Benefits Advice Shop and works directly with claimants, providing advice and representation at a wide range of appeal tribunals. Andrew previously worked for the Central London Social Security Advisors Forum and an East London Law Centre. He is a member of the local Child Poverty Action Group, campaigns against the Child Support Act and is currently undertaking research into anti-poverty strategies as part of an MA course at Sheffield Hallam University.

John Brown is Director of Studies for the MA in Services for People with Learning Disabilities at the Department of Social Policy and Social Work, University of York. Since the late 1970s he has had responsibility for a series of externally funded research projects into various aspects of staff training in learning disabilities. He is also Director of Studies for a postgraduate Diploma in Health Services Management for hospital consultants run in partnership with Yorkshire Regional Health Authority.

John Hattersley was Principal Clinical Pyschologist at Lea Hospital, Kidderminster, between 1976 and 1986. From 1980 to 1986 he held various Principal and Top Grade posts in clinical psychology, notably in Southampton and Sheffield. In 1986 he became Unit General Manager for Sheffield Learning Disability Services; and from 1989 to 1991 he was Unit General Manager for Sheffield Mental Health Services. During his five years as Unit General Manager within large provider units he became highly skilled in resource allocation and prioritisation between high-budget community mental health programmes. In 1991 he became Director of the School of Health and Community Studies at Sheffield Hallam University.

Professor James Hogg is Chair of Profound Disabilities, University of Dundee, and Director of the White Top Research Unit, Dundee University. He has a dual appointment with Tayside Regional Council Social Work Department as Director of the White Top Centre, a day, respite and resource service for adults with profound learning disabilities. He is author and editor of several books concerned with learning and disability, particularly on profound disability and on ageing and learning disability.

Bob Hudson is a Visiting Fellow in Community Care Studies at the University of Durham and a Senior Lecturer in Social Policy at New College Durham. He has taught professionals and managers from health and social care settings for many years and has published widely in the academic press. Currently he is engaged in a range of projects related to the health and community care reforms. His new book, *Making Sense of Markets in Health and Social Care* was published in 1994.

Glenys Jones trained as a teacher and taught children in mainstream schools. She then worked as a Research Officer on three different research projects, funded by the Department of Education and the Department of Health, studying the educational provision for children with special needs and evaluating assessment services for children with learning disabilities. Following this, She worked for five years as an educational psychologist. For the last six years, she has worked full-time as Research Officer on a study into the provision and approaches for children and adults with autism funded jointly by the Department of Health and the Department for Education.

Dr Nigel Malin is Reader in Community Care at Sheffield Hallam University. His research interests relate to linking policy with professional practice, service planning and design of services for people with learning disabilities. As editor of two books, *Reassessing Community Care* (Croom Helm, 1987) and *Implementing Community Care* (Open University Press, 1994) he has for the past twenty years conducted research on residential and community day services, training and workforce planning, case registers, staff attitudes and behaviour, and been a teacher and supervisor both in general social policy and policy relating to professional health and welfare programmes.

Jill Manthorpe is Lecturer in Community Care in the Department of Social Policy and Professional Studies at the University of Hull. She has particular interest in the relationships between health and social services and private, voluntary and family networks. She acts as an Independent Chair of Individual Programme Plan meetings in Humberside and is a non-executive director of the Hull and Holderness Community Health NHS Trust. She has published recently on multi-disciplinary education, grandparenting, informal care, ethnic elders and adult abuse and contributes to training courses for social workers and community nurses.

Dr Paul Martinez taught history at Sheffield University. He developed an interest in welfare rights in a number of different neighbourhood advice centres, became Senior Welfare Rights Officer for Sheffield City Council and managed the Sheffield Benefits Advice Shop for several years. He was a member of the Editorial Board of *The Advisor*, author of numerous articles on welfare benefits and subsequently became Principal Benefits Officer, Sheffield Local Educational Authority. Currently, he is Staff Tutor at The Staff College, the national management development centre for Further and Higher Education, Bristol.

Dr David Race, a researcher, writer, consultant and teacher, has been involved with people with learning disabilities, and services for them, for over twenty years. He has studied services in Hong Kong, the US, Canada and Sweden, and been involved in various forms of training and evaluation, both in the UK and abroad, around social valorisation issues. He is currently Lecturer at Stockport College, teaching mainly on the BA (Hons) Professional Studies: Learning Difficulties degree.

Dr Ann Richardson is an independent researcher, who has published widely in the broad areas of health and community care. In the field of learning disabilities, she has co-authored two books on the move from the parental home and one report on friendship. Her research on case management was undertaken for the Nuffield Institute for Health, University of Leeds. A contact address is: 39 Glenmore Road, London, NW3 4DA.

Judith Russell is currently Educational Adviser on Disability within Sheffield Hallam University. Previously she worked as Senior Lecturer within the School of Health and Community Studies, teaching on social work courses. She is currently Chair of the Federation of Disability Sports Organisation in Yorkshire and Humberside (an organisation of disabled people) and for fourteen years has been involved in a voluntary capacity in the area of leisure for people with disabilities, particularly learning disabilities.

Dr Oliver Russell is Director of the Norah Fry Research Centre at the University of Bristol. During his training as a child psychiatrist he became aware of the needs of children with learning disabilities. For the past twenty years he has been involved in research and in the development of new approaches to support people with learning disabilities. He also works as a pyschiatrist within a community team and is keen to promote more effective inter-disciplinary collaboration between professionals and carers.

Ken Simons is currently a Research Fellow at the Norah Fry Research Centre, University of Bristol. His previous work includes a project which looked in detail at the relocation of people with learning difficulties from long-stay hospital, and he has recently completed a study of the experiences of people involved in self- or citizen advocacy. His current research is on social services complaints procedures, and innovative approaches to housing for people with learning difficulties.

Professor Ian Sinclair was previously Director of Research at the National Institute of Social Work and is now Professor of Social Work at the

University of York. His recent work has included a study of the use of checklists in the inspection of homes for elderly people and he is currently studying the quality of care in children's homes.

Derek Thomas has since April 1992 been Chief Executive of an independent National Development Team (NDT). From 1987–92, when it was a government agency, he was Director of the NDT and from 1984–7 was District Psychologist, North Manchester Health Authority. Prior to that he worked for 14 years in hospital and community services for people with learning disabilities in Northumberland and the North East. He acted for many years as an adviser to the Rowntree Foundation on its 'mental handicap' programme and as Chair of the Working Group at the King's Fund (*An Ordinary Life*) and as a member (from 1975–8) of the Jay Committee. He recently joined a Department of Health working group on challenging behaviour.

Paul Williams is Lecturer in Social Work at the Department of Community Studies, Reading University, where he teaches and researches on work with people with learning disabilities, community care and anti-discrimination. He is also Director of the Community and Mental Handicap Educational and Research Association which has pioneered teaching in Britain on social role valorisation, advocacy and related topics. He is co-author of a book and certain training materials on self-advocacy by people with learning disabilities.

Acknowledgements

I should like to acknowledge Heather Gibson, Fiona Bailey and Christina Tebbit from Routledge for their advice in orchestrating this book, Elaine Smith for typing chapters and Pauline and Charlotte for their personal support. Further I wish to acknowledge those who created opportunities for the shared training programme on learning disabilities with which I was involved during the 1980s, particularly Tony Thompson, John Agate, Ric Metcalf and Val Reed. I hope the book will be an aid to students and others combing through the morass of service provision, and contribute to wider debate on future developments.

Introduction

A policy overview

Nigel Malin

This book comprises a second edition of *Services for the Mentally Handicapped* (Malin *et al.*, 1980). It includes extra chapters relating to the implications of the National Health Service and Community Care Act (1990) and chapters on advocacy and empowerment, and recreation and leisure services. Otherwise the format is the same as the original: an exploration of main service developments. Some of the arguments presented in the original text are echoed in this edition: people leaving hospital face an uncoordinated patchwork of local resettlement schemes, management and accountability of services at local level remains elusive and disparate, support given to carers far understates acknowledged levels of need, educational and day provision are dominated more by service considerations than planning for individual users.

Since the publication of the first book there have been both contextual and ideological changes in delivery of services. Care in the community has given emphasis sometimes more rhetorical than practical to the deployment of systems of support in ordinary life settings (rather than using residential homes and day centres) and to looking at individual need holistically. In planning, this has been illustrated by efforts to create networks of providers based less on resources of the statutory sector and more on an evolving independent sector. Also, it has become common for users to play an important role in the way services are costed either through making a direct contribution or in being party to contracts drawn up between the user and providers.

Government policy remains that of closing long-stay hospitals for people with learning disabilities but, as Jean Collins' recent research has shown, there are still around 20,000 people in England living in such units and government reliance on local discretion means those opposed to the closure of institutions are able to exploit the difficulties associated with good community services as replacement for institutional provision (Collins, 1993). 'Purchasers (in NHS trusts) are operating under instructions to reduce expenditure. They rarely have the expertise, finance or options available to ensure the service they are buying is what the user wants.' (Ward, 1993).

If legislation on community-based services is to become reality then more effort needs to be made locally to both plan and provide with the needs of users in mind. The emergence of the consumers' movement, People First, was a significant development of the 1980s. Increasing activity among consumers, voluntary groups and, to some degree, academics, has led to a more complex view of community care with the problem redefined not in terms of how best to close hospitals but how the state can structure its policy to respond to the needs of individuals with learning disabilities.

> Even the progressive models of comprehensive community service systems retain(ed) a certain class conception of need . . . reflected in the belief that if we define a range of options, everyone's needs will eventually be met. While it is unrealistic that the range could ever be broad enough to meet everyone's individual needs, in the existing socio-political context, it is a patent absurdity. There is also a lack of flexibility built into the system, particularly in funding mechanisms, which again tend towards broad classes of needs rather than the individualised entitlements. This makes it difficult to respond to changing or complex needs which don't 'fit' the standard classes.
>
> (Stainton, 1992)

Local services still lack teeth for planning at user level (in some ways structures are worse than a decade ago). A report of the Bristol Advocacy Project describes how (understandably) most professionals have a service provider's view of the world assuming that self-advocacy is primarily about commenting on services. As a result they tend to promote service-based models of self-advocacy and it may seem optimistic to expect hard-pressed agencies to fund groups which could well prove to be a thorn in their side (Simons, 1993). It is important to find out what kind of services users want and need. The Community Care Act places faith in community care planning but research has shown that many plans are aspirational and not grounded on studies of need (Wistow *et al.*, 1993); furthermore GPs and purchasers show ignorance about the service needs of people with learning disabilities and of the contributions made by professionals, for example, social workers, occupational therapists and physiotherapists (Langan *et al.*, 1993).

The importance of consulting service users has received a greater emphasis over recent years (Lowe *et al.*, 1987; Brechin and Swain, 1988; Crawley, 1988; Gathercole, 1988; Harper, 1989; Shanly and Rose, 1993.) Such studies have focused on particular forms of provision such as day centres, illustrating the value of friendship networks. Other studies have shown the combination of effects of therapeutic objectives, opportunities created by service design and organisation and the amount and quality of staff performance in establishing better quality residential services (Mansell *et al.*, 1987; Felce, 1988; Landesman, 1988; Felce, 1989; Mansell and Beasley, 1993). Alongside current policies to bring about a shift in responsibility and resources for residential care from health to local authorities and from large institutions to small homely units has been a substantial growth of independent living schemes. A study of such accommodation in four local authority areas indicated that over three-quarters (79.5 per cent) of the 149 schemes surveyed had been opened since 1983, and over half (55.4 per cent) had started up since 1985 (Booth *et al.*, 1988). The implications of relocation have been studied in two major projects (Flynn, 1989; Booth and Simons, 1990) probing both advantages and disadvantages of how people with learning disabilities themselves feel to live independently. The Darenth Park project, a large-scale hospital replacement programme (Korman and Glennerster, 1985; 1990) relocating 660 people in contrast examined the commercial barriers but like another project (Richardson and Higgins, 1992) pointed to organisational, professional and financial constraints in achieving de-institutionalisation to the benefit of residents.

Table I.1 shows over the last ten years a three-fold increase in the number of people with learning disabilities living in private sector accommodation and a general increase in the number of people living in local authority accommodation (from 16,624 to 20,138).

Table I.1 Number of residents supported by local authorities in homes and hostels for people with learning disabilities, by type of home

| As at 31 March | Local authority homes | | | Registered care homes | | | Total supported residents |
	Own homes	Other authorities' homes	Total	Voluntary homes	Private homes	Other accommodation	
1982	11120	394	11514	3424	962	724	16624
1983	11637	412	12085	3538	1053	834	17510
1984	11789	422	12211	3759	1118	836	17924
1985	11870	434	12304	3623	1019	603	17549
1986	12005	329	12334	3039	1103	688	17164
1987	11588	316	11904	3104	1265	746	17019
1988	11770	362	12132	3494	1384	811	17821
1989	11659	393	12052	3723	1610	826	18211
1990	11496	261	11757	4066	1940	726	18489
1991	11302	306	11608	4417	2515	872	19412
1992	11148	321	11469	5138	2678	853	20138

Source: Department of Health Personal Social Services/Local Authority statistics: Residential Accommodation for People with Learning Disabilities – Local Authority supported residents at 31 March 1992/A/T92/11B.

The increase is in the adult age range as opposed to children where there has been a drop in the number cared for from 1,958 to 1,091 over the same period. The number aged 16 to 64 living in all types of local authority accommodation has increased by 28 per cent and those aged 65+ by 67 per cent. The Department of Health has not kept information to illustrate equivalent trends in the use of community care services. Although the rhetoric of community care was couched in terms of 'user choice and control', there was a wide consensus that the proposed shift from residential to 'community' care would be shaped by questions of resources – the overall size of the community care funding 'cake', its distribution between the various agencies concerned in creating the framework for community care to happen, and the power (especially the financial power) of different interest groups to implement their own important agendas (Craig, 1993). The Community Care Act replicated the outline of the White Paper (Department of Health, 1989) but was short on its commitments, mainly confined to user rights to assessment and a care plan. It makes no provision, for example, for authorised representation of people with learning disabilities who may be unable to put their own case nor does it require the local authority to be accountable by giving reasons for not providing a service.

Much of the legislation has been left for agencies to interpret. An intended objective was to solve many of the problems of the past by establishing a new relationship between health and local authorities and between providers and recipients. The Act does not replace existing duties and powers but creates new duties for social services department (SSDs). It links an evaluation of an individual's need for a service to an authority's decision whether to provide for it or not. Section 47 covers assessment and summarises a potential service applicant's new rights as: a right to an assessment and where an assessment is carried out a right to a 'decision' on providing community care services. The assessment right arises 'where it appears to a local authority that any person for whom they may provide . . . community care services may be in need of any such services' (section 47 (1)). The right to a decision arises because the authority 'having regard to the results of (the) assessment, shall then decide whether (the person's) needs call for the provision by them of any . . . services' (section 47 (1) (b)). Where it appears that the person is a 'disabled person' and possibly entitled to services under section 2 of the Chronically Sick and Disabled Persons Act 1970, the authority has also to decide whether to provide such services (section 47 (2)). The absence of prescriptive guidance leaves worries about entitlement, at best ambiguous, at worst confusingly unresolved (Bynoe, 1993). It is not clear whether there is any duty to provide a service once an assessment has shown the need for it as local authorities may still claim that resources remain insufficient to provide for all assessed needs.

This hardly alters entitlements of people with learning disabilities; it places them on a list of local authority priorities left to the discretion of planners and providers. It pays no credit to the contribution that such people are able to make by encouraging work opportunities, friendship or care. The principal changes introduced by the 1990 legislation (with effect from April 1993) are: community care planning, caremanagement and assessment, quality and inspection and extended use of purchasing services from the independent sector.

COMMUNITY CARE PLANNING

The requirement to produce community care plans has served as a catalyst to review and revise joint planning arrangements (Wistow *et al.*, 1991). Most commonly the starting point has been to specify more clearly the remit and responsibilities of different elements in the planning structures, including accountability and relationships between them. Alongside this development authorities needed to give more attention to the need for user, carer and voluntary sector involvement in planning processes (Wistow, 1993). Despite this, service-led approaches have dominated community care planning.

Much of the emphasis has been on reviewing demand for existing services, for example, respite care, residential, day services and specialist provision, improving joint training and refining requirements of the register. Planning demands a proactive approach, examining needs of children and adults living in the community with carers who receive few, if any, services.

CAREMANAGEMENT AND ASSESSMENT

The research on the efficacy of caremanagement is incomplete (Huxley, 1993) yet this process constitutes a centrepiece of how health and social services are expected to deliver the new reforms. The broad measure of agreement about the essential components of caremanagement has been summarised (Challis and Davies, 1986; Kanter, 1989; Hunter, 1990; Thornicroft, 1991; Onyett, 1992; Richardson and Higgins, 1992). Moxley (1989) defines caremanagement as 'a client-level strategy for promoting the co-ordination of human services, opportunities and benefits. The major outcomes of caremanagement are the integration of services and achieving continuity of care' (p.11). The Department of Health Social Services Inspectorate (1991) defines it as 'the process of tailoring services to individual needs' entailing seven stages: publishing information, determining the level of assessment, assessing need, care planning, implementing the care plan, monitoring and reviewing. Richardson and Higgins (1992) discuss in their research how caremanagement may give rise to demands which cannot readily be put into effect – 'individual plans for clients may be devised, based on need, but then become stymied by delay or, indeed, total lack of action' (p. 33). They argue that caremanagement should not be seen as a solution to problems around resources availability and service delivery yet present a strong case for the value of caremanagement based on an illustration of how changes can be brought about simply through defining an individual's needs.

QUALITY AND INSPECTION

The Community Care Act established arm's-length inspection units giving a high profile to inspection within the provision of health and social services. Providers of services to people with learning disabilities have been locked into discussion over the meaning of quality and outcome during the past two decades (such services have provided a trailblazer for other client groups). There are still, however, no legal entitlements to residential and day services in the community, leisure, advocacy or a reasonable income level. In conducting inspection of 'units', for example, residential units, there is much to be gained from a participative approach involving perceptions of users, carers and management on quality standards (Macmillan, 1993). If inspection is to be arm's length as the government wishes, it would be ineffective if it began by alienating views of those at the front-line and if it failed to see a role as facilitator of good staff practice. Beazley (1994) suggests that raising awareness of quality issues focuses the energies of the workforce towards clearer objectives and provides a stimulus for organisational learning and innovation. The current position is to encourage debate on quality but to leave local providers discretion. Legislation has now failed to clarify 'standards' giving no guarantees on personal entitlements to services.

PURCHASING FROM THE INDEPENDENT SECTOR

The government originally proposed that at least 75 per cent of each local authority's total grant was to be spent in the independent sector. This was changed to 64 per cent once it was found that the calculation presupposed a higher transfer element from the Department of Social Security. For these purposes the independent sector was defined as 'meaning not under local authority ownership, management or control' (House of Commons Health Committee, *Third Report*, 1993). The majority of written evidence received during the House of Commons Health Committee's inquiry referred to the shortfall between Income Support and homes' fees (paragraph 66). The problems identified included concerns about the future for residents and their relatives who could no longer afford to top-up payment of residential fees and the future of charities facing financial hardships. Local authorities have made some use of their power to 'top-up' for residents under pension age, although it was illegal for them to do the same for older residents. Some district health authorities also have topped-up people with learning disabilities in independent sector homes who have been discharged from long-stay hospitals.

On the question of unmet need, the Committee recommended that:

> clear guidance be issued urgently to local authorities . . . and, if necessary, legislation introduced to make sure that there are no inhibitions on the ability of social services' departments and health authorities to make a full assessment of unmet needs. It will be difficult to judge in the future whether resources are adequate unless we have a clear indication of the level of need, both met and unmet.
>
> (House of Commons Health Committee, 1993, paragraph 64)

The government response was equivocal claiming that it was up to authorities to set out clearly their priorities and eligibility criteria for services and to collect the evidence they needed for planning purposes (Departments of Health and Social Security, 1993).

If community care is to be realised, then accent is needed on development of the role and function of community-based teams – on evaluating assessment and caremanagement processes relating to those people already living in the community. Investment in this heartland will illuminate needs and responsibilities of those involved in the totality of care: users and carers, services and politicians, the tax-paying public. Frequent derisory reference to the fragmented character of community-based services sometimes serves as an argument against community care. The provision of local services for people with learning disabilities presents, however, a necessary challenge in that it is based on maximising provision of home-based care, requires flexibility and innovation and demands 'fragmentation'. Stabilising fragmentation should become the job of those employed in community settings: carrying out assessments, designing services, securing delivery and identifying costs and responsibilities. The conclusion to the first edition of this book stated:

> There is much interest throughout the country in improving services but while aims may be agreed, methods differ and controversies continue to arise over issues such as staff training, the role of the statutory services, community integration, assessment and teaching. The positions taken by interested groups and individuals reflect their different professional traditions and attitudes, making it more difficult to resolve a problem which rightly requires a multidisciplinary approach but, at the same time, engenders a need to place the client first.
>
> (Malin *et al.*, 1980, p. 235).

The situation has moved on since then, although as regards the last point – placing the client first – the rhetoric has largely preceded practice. More information, more knowledge is required on how people with learning disabilities survive in the community (legislation such as the Disabled Persons Act (1986) and the Community Care Act (1990) provide justification for demanding improved services). The need for resourceful management has never been stronger; not for single track services, but for holistic, integrated services. Within education, health and social services, learning disabilities have remained a low priority and for this reason it is vital that there is robust leadership to disentangle such services from other demands.

The pluralistic concept of caremanagement eschews responsibility for needs-led provision. It is central to the Community Care Act, yet whose needs are being addressed? The power to allocate resources resides in the purchaser of community care and today that is not distinct: the needs-led approach having been upturned by local planning arrangements. What the reforms have achieved is the creation of a role – that of the purchasing agent, which takes clear and unequivocal responsibility for allocation of resources; which must, given excess demand, make overt choices about the rationing of scarce resources and which will, inevitably, be the target of attacks from those who uphold traditional values of universality of access to health and social care. Individual care plans for users with learning disabilities need to become the basis for negotiating better accessed services, better funded services and improved advocacy. This is central to the community care reforms and will change the foundation of the future.

REFERENCES

Beazley, M. (1994) Measuring Service Quality, *in* Malin, N. (ed.) *Implementing Community Care*. Milton Keynes, Open University Press.

Booth, T. and Simons, K. (1990) *Outward Bound: Relocation and Community Care for People with Learning Difficulties*. Milton Keynes, Open University Press.

Booth, T, Phillips, D., Berry, S., Jones, D., Matthews, J., Melotte, C., and Pritlove, J. (1988) Home from Home: a survey of independent living schemes for people with a mental handicap. *Mental Handicap Research*, 2, 2 July, 152–66.

Brechin, A. and Swain, J. (1988) Professional and client relationships: creating a 'working alliance' with people with learning difficulties. *Disability, Handicap and Society*, 3, 213–26.

Bynoe, I. (1993) Rights and Duties. *Community Care*, 25 March, ii–iii.

Challis, D. and Davies, B. (1986) *Casemanagement in Community Care*. Aldershot, Gower.

Collins, J. (1993) *The Resettlement Game, Values into Action*. Wembley, Adept Press.

Craig, G. (1993) *The Community Care Reforms and Local Government Change*, Papers in Social Research No.1. Hull, University of Humberside.

Crawley, B. (1988) *The Growing Voice: A Survey of Self Advocacy Groups in Adult Training Centres and Hospitals in Great Britain*. London, CMH.

Department of Health (1989) *Caring for People (Community Care in the Next Decade and Beyond)*, Cm 849. London, HMSO.

Department of Health Social Services Inspectorate (1991) *Care Management and Assessment: Summary of Practice Guidance*. London, HMSO.

Departments of Health and Social Security (1993) *Government Response to the Third Report from the Health Committee Session 1992–93. Community Care: Funding from April 1993*, Cm 2188. London, HMSO.

Felce, D. (1988) Behavioural and Social Climate in Community Group Residences, *in* Janicki, M. P., Krauss, M. W. and Seltzer, M. (eds) *Community Residences for Persons with Development Disabilities*. Baltimore, Paul H. Brookes.

Felce, D. (1989) *The Andover Project: Staffed Housing for Adults with Severe or Profound Mental Handicaps*. Kidderminster, British Institute of Mental Handicap.

Flynn, M. (1989) *Independent Living for Adults with Mental Handicap*. London, Cassell.

Gathercole, C. (1988) Involving People with Learning Disabilities, *in* Towell, D. (ed.) *An Ordinary Life in Practice*. London, Kings Fund Centre.

Harper, G. (1989) Making Each Day Matter. *Community Living*, 3, 11.

House of Commons Health Committee (1993) *Third Report, Community Care: Funding from April 1993*. London, HMSO.

Hunter, D. (1990) *Case Management in Practice*. Leeds: Nuffield Institute, University of Leeds.

Huxley, P. (1993) Case Management and Care Management in Community Care, *British Journal of Social Work*, 23, 365–81.

Kanter, J. (1989) Clinical Case Management: definition, principles, components. *Hospital and Community Psychiatry*, 40, 361–8.

Korman, N. and Glennerster, H. (1985) *Closing a Hospital – the Darenth Park Project*. London, London School of Economics and Political Science.

Korman, N. and Glennerster, H. (1990) *Hospital Closure*. Milton Keynes, Open University Press.

Landesman, S. (1988) Preventing 'Institutionalisation' in the Community, *in* Janicki, M, Krauss, M. and Seltzer, M. (eds) *Community Residences for Persons with Development Disabilities*. Baltimore, Paul H. Brookes.

Langan, J., Whitfield, M. and Russell, O. (1993) *Community Care and the General Practitioner: Primary Health Care for People with Learning Disabilities*. Bristol, Norah Fry Research Centre.

Lowe, K., De Pavia, S. and Humphreys, S. (1987) *Long Term Evaluation of Services for People with a Mental Handicap in Cardiff: Clients Views*. Cardiff: Mental Handicap in Wales Applied Research Unit.

Macmillan, I. (1993) Quality and Inspection, *in* Malin, N. (ed.) *Community Care for People with Learning Difficulties*, pp. 69–76. Sheffield, Sheffield Hallam University.

Malin, N., Race, D., Jones, G. (1980) *Services for the Mentally Handicapped in Britain*. London, Croom Helm.

Mansell, J. and Beasley, F. (1993) Small Staffed Houses for People with a Severe Learning Disability and Challenging Behaviour. *British Journal of Social Work*, 23, 329–44.

Mansell, J., Felice, D., Jenkins, J., de Kock, V. and Toogood, A. (1987) *Staffed Housing for People with Mental Handicaps*. Tunbridge Wells, Costello.

Moxley, D. (1989) *The Practice of Case Management*. London, Sage.

Onyett, S. (1992) *Case Management in Mental Health*. London, Chapman and Hall.

Richardson, A. and Higgins, R. (1992) *The Limits of Case Management: Lessons from the Wakefield Case Management Project*, Working Paper 5. Nuffield Institute, University of Leeds.

Shanly, A. and Rose, J. (1993) *A Consumer Survey of Adults with Learning Disabilities Currently Doing Work Experience: Their Satisfaction with Work and Wishes for the Future*. Kidderminster, British Institute of Mental Handicap.

Simon, S.K. (1993) *Sticking up for Yourself*. York, Joseph Rowntree Foundation.

Stainton, T. (1992) Big Talk, Small Steps. *Community Living*, July, 16–17.

Thornicroft, G. (1991) The Concept of Case Management for Long-term Mental Illness. *International Review of Psychiatry*, 3, 125–32.

Ward, L. (1993) Two Steps Forward. *Community Care*, 4 Nov., 26–7.

Wistow, G. (1993) Community Care Plans: a strategic overview, *in* Malin, N. (ed.) *Community Care for People with Learning Difficulties*, 6–13. Sheffield, Sheffield Hallam University.

Wistow, G., Leedham, I. and Hardy, B. (1991) Community Care Planning Workshops. *Caring for People*, 8, 14, 16.

Wistow, G., Leedham, I. and Hardy, B. (1993) *Implementing Community Care: Community Care Plans*. London, Department of Health Social Services Inspectorate.

Part I
The service context

1 Classification of people with learning disabilities

David Race

With the first line written on the subject of learning disabilities comes the first problem. For unlike other physiological or biochemical disorders, such as damaged limbs, for which there is general agreement on definitions used for classification, the classification of mental disorder, and specifically that involving people with learning disabilities, has been subject to wide-ranging disagreements among those connected with it. These disagreements, in fact, go beyond classification, and on to causation, prognosis, and the most appropriate method of response by human services. Even the use of the term 'learning disabilities' immediately places the authors in a certain sector of opinion; the use of alternatives such as mental subnormality, mental retard-ation, special needs, developmental disability, mental handicap, or even learning difficulty, would have located them elsewhere. So too, the writing of a book on services, rather than about people with learning disabilities, is seen by some as a political statement, an acceptance of the status quo. However, as Ryan and Thomas (1987) put it: 'The changing definitions of difference constitute the history of mentally handicapped people' and so in an attempt to understand that history it is necessary to trace the definitions and classifications made by both individuals and governments in trying to describe the sort of person that this book defines as having learning disabilities.

The most common confusion still existing in the public mind is the lack of distinction between the two states commonly referred to as 'mental illness' and 'mental handicap'. Matthews (1954) quotes a statute of 1325 (De Praerogativa Regis) which dealt differently with the lands of an 'idiot' and a 'lunatic'. 'Idiots' (i.e. natural fools) were to have their lands protected, their necessities provided for, and their lands passed to the proper heirs on their death. 'Lunatics' (i.e. persons of unsound mind) had their lands protected so that they might be restored to them on their recovery. The difference between the two was thus seen to be one of permanence. The 'idiot' was suffering from an incurable congenital condition, whereas the 'lunatic' was suffering a temporary loss of reason. A more philosophical distinction was made by Locke, when he concluded that,

> In short herein seems to be the difference between Idiots and Madmen, that Madmen put wrong ideas together, and so make wrong propositions, but argue and reason right from them; but Idiots make very few or no propositions and reason scarce at all.
>
> (Locke, 1689)

In other words the essence of the 'idiot' was lack of development or defect of mind, whereas the 'madman' was suffering from a temporary imbalance which still enabled some effective thinking processes to occur.

Tredgold (1952) used an economic analogy, typically negative and chillingly prescient of certain current attitudes. He compared the person who is 'mentally ill' with someone who is temporarily bankrupt and those who are 'mentally defective' with someone who has never possessed a bank account or any money to put in it.

These distinctions seem clear-cut, and there is no doubt that the more extreme cases of learning disability were, and are, easily recognised as such when compared to people with mental health problems. The provision of the fourteenth-century statute covered only the landed few, however, and at the village level no provision, and therefore no classification, was needed for people with learning disabilities. The 'village idiot' was accepted by the community for what he or she was and dealt with at the level appropriate to the times, with all the local variation this entailed. Later, however, along with the poor, the aged and other people unable to find paid employment, people with learning disabilities, other than those of wealthy parents, began to be segregated from their community and put into Poor Law workhouses. These institutions, particularly after the Poor Law Amendment Act of 1834, were specifically designed to act as a deterrent to the 'lazy and shiftless' who were unwilling or unable, for one reason or another, to find work. Since 'work' itself was undergoing its most fundamental change of character at the time, numbers in this group were significant. They included, of course, people with learning disabilities and it was, in many ways, the Industrial Revolution and the workhouse which began the isolation of people with learning disabilities from the public, and from public understanding.

Further details of the development of provision for people with learning disabilities will be given later, but returning to the development of classification, most of the next steps were legal ones. The Lunatic Asylums Act (1853) instructed the justices of every county and borough to provide asylums for the 'pauper lunatics thereof' and stated that a 'lunatic' meant every person of unsound mind 'and every person being an idiot'. This contrasts most confusingly with the working of the Idiots Act (1886) which stated that '"Idiots" or "Imbeciles" do not include lunatics' and that '"Lunatic" does not mean or include idiot or imbecile'. Still further confusion was brought about by the Lunacy Act (1890) which defined a 'lunatic' as 'an idiot or person of unsound mind'. In addition to this lack of distinction between what were, in effect, the most severe and obvious cases of people with learning disabilities and mental health problems, the group known as the 'feeble-minded' then entered the picture. Hitherto this group, now considered to have relatively few learning disabilities, had not been thought to be suffering from any defect but, in the main, to be simply lazy or wicked.

By the last decade of the nineteenth century, however, the concept of feeble-mindedness had developed to such an extent that charitable institutions existed for the 'care and education of the feeble-minded' and in the 1901 census the category of 'feeble-mindedness' was included. This resulted in the reporting of some 13,000 cases.

With the continuing definitional problem, it is scarcely surprising that a Royal Commission, set up in 1904 to make recommendations concerning the care of the 'feeble-minded', requested an extension to its remit to cover all forms of mental disorder, including mental illness. Its report, published in 1908, recommended a general term to cover all these forms of disorder, called 'mental defect'. The terminological confusion was then compounded when this overall category was used synonymously with that applied to a more restricted group, excluding those with mental health problems. The 'mentally deficient' were the class of person classified and dealt with under the Mental Deficiency Act of 1913. This Act provided the first supposedly exact definition of the various grades of 'mental deficiency', which was restricted to that arising 'from birth or from an early age', and its categories were to remain the legal terminology for nearly half a century. It classified 'defectives' under four headings.

1 Idiots – these were persons who were 'so deeply defective in mind from birth or from an early age as to be unable to guard themselves against common physical dangers'.
2 Imbeciles – these were persons who, whilst not as defective as 'idiots' were still incapable of 'managing their own affairs'.
3 Feeble-minded persons – these were persons who were not as 'defective' as 'imbeciles' but required 'care, supervision and control for their own protection or for the protection of others'.
4 Moral defectives – these were persons who 'from an early age display some permanent mental defect coupled with strong vicious or criminal propensities on which punishment has had little or no effect'.

The language of these classifications is a clear indication of how much more of a social and administrative issue, rather than a clinical one, is the situation of people with learning disabilities. All definitions are couched in terms which describe the results of 'defect', rather than any scientific definition of what 'defect' actually is, and all contain descriptive statements which are totally bound up with the contemporary standards and understandings of a particular society. Thus, for example, 'common dangers' in an industrialised western society are very different, then as now, from those found in the remoter parts of the Third World. Even between town and country within a particular society the skills necessary to 'manage one's own affairs' are rather different. The Act was, of course, a product of its time and in particular of the powerful pressures on the government to avoid a 'national degeneracy' resulting from the 'propagation of the unfit'. These fears were given voice by, amongst others, the Eugenics Society. Their prime case was, in Tredgold's words,

> that as soon as a nation reaches that stage of civilisation in which medical knowledge and humanitarian sentiment operate to prolong the existence of the unfit, then it becomes imperative upon that nation to devise such social laws as will ensure that those unfit do not propagate their kind.
>
> (Tredgold, 1909)

The basic impetus was therefore towards segregation, which the Act put into operation, and which will be considered further in Chapter 4. The classification of 'mental defectives', with all its inherent subjectiveness, therefore remained as a potent force.

Although subjective, the definitions do lend themselves to a judgement of social capacity which can be related to the norms of the day, and demand at least individual attention. In contrast, contemporary work elsewhere had just begun to develop the means of applying a 'scientific' classification to the development of the mind which, it was thought, placed individuals in their rightful position in the distribution of intellectual abilities, from where they could never move and by which society could judge their ability. Binet and Simon's series of tests, first published in 1908, and revised in 1911, with their underlying idea of 'mental age' related to chronological age to provide an 'Intelligence Quotient' were quickly added to the prevailing opinions of inherited defect to provide the idea of mental ability as a basic physiological function, unchanging over time, which could be measured scientifically by standardised methods. The implication was therefore that your 'intelligence' was inherited, and no amount of learning or changes in social conditions would affect your position in the cerebral hierarchy.

This criterion for mental ability, and thus for mental disability, found many adherents, especially in the US, where Terman's revision of the Simon/ Binet tests was widely adopted, but debate continued over the nature of 'defect', and the use of purely intellectual criteria for a classification. Tredgold, although one of the foremost proponents of 'national degeneracy' and the need for segregation, maintained his original view that 'social inefficiency', regardless of IQ, should be the means by which 'defectives' should be classified: 'the essential purpose of mind is that of enabling the individual to make a satisfactory and independent adaptation to the ordinary environment of his fellows . . . hence I regard the social as the most logical concept of mental deficiency' (Tredgold, 1952, op.cit.). Pearson, amidst a polemic against American eugenics, also suggested that social inefficiency be the criterion for segregation (Pearson and Jaederholm, 1914; Pearson, 1914) as well as examining some of the theoretical statistical failings of the IQ adherents.

In England, therefore, the accepted classification of 'mental deficiency' was not altered by the new tests from that of the 1913 Act, and the only major change prior to the fifties was the inclusion, in the Mental Deficiency Act of 1927, of the effects of disease or injury as a cause of the 'deficiency'. The later Act therefore added the definition that 'Mental defectiveness means a condition of arrested or incomplete development of mind existing before the age of eighteen years, whether arising from inherent causes or induced by disease or injury' thereby including such causes as encephalitis and meningitis which the definition of the 1913 Act had proscribed.

In the US, no nationally established provision or legal classification existed, but the American Association for the Study of the Feeble-minded (the latter term being then used in the US to cover all levels of learning disabilities) adopted a standard set of IQ levels, with corresponding descriptive terms:

> *Idiots* – were defined as persons with a mental age of not more than thirty-five months or, if a child, an IQ less than twenty-five.
>
> *Imbeciles* – were defined as persons with a mental age of between thirty-six and eighty-three months or, if a child, an IQ between twenty-five and forty-nine.
>
> *Morons* – were defined as persons with a mental age between eighty-four and 143 months inclusive or, if a child, an IQ between fifty and seventy-four.

(AASF, 1921)

IQs and mental ages were measured by the Terman revision of the Binet Scale. The qualitative definitions attached to these groups are essentially similar to the first three categories used in England, i.e. 'Idiots, Imbeciles, and Feeble-minded persons', and thus, to some extent, there was common agreement between the two systems. Both of them, however, suffered over the ensuing thirty to forty years from arbitrariness of application, with over-zealous use of the 'moral defective' category in England being particularly subject to criticism, and the early strict categorisation, and hence segregation, of those with IQs below seventy-five being the most controversial aspect of services in America (Wolfensberger, 1974).

The English position may be summarised by the following quotation from the Wood Report, the report of a committee of experts set up in 1924 to consider the amount and types of special education required for the 'mentally deficient'.

> Let us assume that we could segregate as a separate community, all the families in this country containing mental defectives of the primary amentia type. We should find that we had collected among them a most interesting social group. It would include, as everyone who has extensive practical experience of social service should readily admit, a much larger proportion of insane persons, epileptics, paupers, criminals (especially

recidivists), unemployables, habitual slum dwellers, prostitutes, inebriates and other social inefficients than would contain a group of families not containing mental defectives ... This group comprises practically the lowest ten per cent in the social scale of most communities.

(Mental Deficiency Committee, 1929)

This high moral tone, which in the difficult economic circumstances of the time may have found a ready audience, and again has eerie echoes in the 1990s, justified the classification of many 'social inefficients' as 'defectives', when their IQ levels would not have justified such classification under the American system. It also, of course, had a considerable effect on E.O. Lewis's famous survey, used by the committee, into the incidence of 'mental deficiency' (Lewis, 1929). The author himself states that, 'It was realised at the outset that it would be impossible to include in such a rapid survey many cases of moral deficiency which manifested no intellectual retardation', but goes on to include, in his figures, a large number of 'moral defectives' based solely on assessments of past history of 'immoral' behaviour. This, in turn, led to such people as Burt (1937) arguing for the adoption of IQ testing as the sole means of classifying 'mental deficiency'.

On the other side of the Atlantic however, the IQ definition was under attack for its lack of precision, in that the 'Stanford Revision' (i.e. Terman's) of the Binet Scale, was subject to criticism on this ground. This was heightened by the drastic implication of classification in some states, i.e. sterilisation. In New York State sterilisation did not apply, but the views of Wechsler, who was himself to devise an alternative scale to the Stanford–Binet, on the 'New York State mental hygiene law' are still relevant.

> This law provides that individuals attaining IQs below seventy-five on the 1916 revision of the Stanford-Binet can be classified as mental defectives. As it also states that IQs of adults are to be calculated on a sixteen year basis, actual application of the criterion would automatically classify some twenty per cent of the white and a considerably larger per cent of the adult coloured population of the United States as mental defectives. It is extremely doubtful if those who formulated the provision knew, much less intended, the provision to be as drastic as it would turn out to be if actually applied.
>
> (Wechsler, 1944)

Butler's survey (1951) noted that in 1950 sterilisation laws were still being actively applied in twenty-one of the states to 'mental defectives' defined by their IQ level.

Doll (1941) took the argument of the 'social definition' school a stage further, both by arguing for this concept as the deciding variable, and by devising a scale to 'measure' social competence (Doll, 1953). He defined 'feeble-mindedness' as consisting of:

(1)   Social incompetence, due to
(2)   low degree of intelligence as a result of

(3) incomplete development which is
(4) permanent
(5) obtains at maturity and derives from
(6) constitutional hypoplasia, pathology or dysmetabolism.

(Doll, 1948)

In other words, social incompetence is the criterion, low intelligence merely the cause (and the sole cause according to Doll). Jastak (1949) rejected both the social (Doll) and IQ definitions of 'feeble-mindedness' and suggested that the definition should be determined by performance in a whole series of tests of different mental functions. Further studies, for example by Kingsley and Hyde (1945) and Charles (1953), following up persons earlier considered 'mentally deficient', were finding large numbers to be socially and economically self-sufficient; certainly more people than expected were surviving in society. Cantor (1955) took the point further and argued that 'mental deficiency' is not a once-and-for-all condition whether defined in terms of IQ or social competence and that workers should concentrate on curing rather than classifying. Dexter summed up the growing American opinion about classification as follows:

> In a society like ours which emphasises as an end in itself formal demonstration of skill in the technique of symbolization and co-ordinating meanings, a far higher proportion of mental defectives are likely to be treated as cases of a social problem than would be so treated in a society emphasising some other set of values, for instance the capacity for survival or effective economic contribution.

(Dexter, 1958)

A full review of work on the problems of classification up to the early fifties is found in Sarason (1953) and Sarason and Gladwin (1958a, 1958b) which, interestingly, contain little material from the UK other than the standard works of Burt and Tredgold. Whereas, in the US, argument had centred on the use of IQs in classifying 'defectives', in the UK the reverse was taking place, namely a debate on the lack of a 'scientific' measure such as IQ for segregating 'defectives' from 'non-defectives'. The various grades of the 1913 Act were still in force, and were still subject to a great deal of variety in interpretation, and very little academic work had been done between the wars on the issue of 'mental deficiency', especially on problems of classification. The 'clinical autonomy' of the psychiatric profession, as it was beginning to be established, meant that each medical superintendent's interpretation of 'mental deficiency' was usually enough to justify continued certification and the looseness of terminology in the Act was sufficient for practically any opinion to be justified by the patient's actual behaviour. The small amount of work that had started on classification *per se* concerned the numbers of institutionalised 'defectives' who had higher than expected IQs. Thus O'Connor and Tizard (1954), who surveyed a sample taken from twelve thousand patients in institutions, found that the average IQ of those classed as 'feeble-minded' was over seventy, which for the tests used represented two standard deviations below the mean. The point, therefore, which other authorities defined as the maximum level for 'deficiency' was merely the average of O'Connor and Tizard's sample. Similarly, Hilliard and Mundy (1954), in a survey of admissions to the Fountain hospital, found many of the 'feeble-minded' had intelligence in the 'dull–normal range', i.e. between one and two standard deviations below the mean. Most of the English research of the fifties, however, was devoted to the potential abilities of people with learning disabilities rather than their classification, together with experiments in alternative forms of care (see Chapter 4).

Thus, although pressure was brought to bear for reform of the Mental Deficiency Acts, and a Royal Commission was set up in 1954, its major concern was not with classification (except for the debate over the 'moral defective' category) but with the procedures for provision of care and admission to psychiatric hospitals. It is therefore not surprising that the definitions and classifications used in the resultant Mental Health Act of 1959 were not particularly clear, nor particularly helpful in removing the distinction between people with mental health problems and those with learning disabilities. Since it remained the legal definition of 'mental disorder' for the next twenty or more years, however, it is neccessary at this point in the history of classification to examine the wording of the 1959 Act. Section Four is reproduced in full below.

(1) In this Act 'mental disorder' means mental illness, arrested or incomplete development of mind, psychopathic disorder, and any other disorder or disability of mind; and 'mentally disordered' shall be construed accordingly.

(2) In this Act 'severe subnormality' means a state of arrested or incomplete development of mind which includes subnormality of intelligence and is of such a nature or degree that the patient is incapable of living an independent life or of guarding himself against serious exploitation, or will be so incapable when of an age to do so.

(3) In this Act 'subnormality' means a state of arrested or incomplete development of mind (not amounting to severe subnormality) which includes subnormality of intelligence and is of a nature or degree which requires or is susceptible to medical or other special care or training of the patient.

(4) In this Act 'psychopathic disorder' means a persistent disorder or disability of mind (whether or not including subnormality of intelligence) which results in abnormally aggressive or seriously irresponsible conduct on the part of the patient, and requires, or is susceptible to, medical treatment.

(5) Nothing in this section shall be construed as implying that a person may be dealt with under this Act as suffering from mental disorder,

or from any form of disorder described in this section, by reason only of promiscuity or other immoral conduct.

(Mental Health Act, 1959)

Once again the definitions are essentially subjective, and related to contemporary norms of behaviour. In fact, the addition of sub-section 5 implicitly recognises the dangers generated by the previous Act, whereby illegitimate pregnancy, or petty theft, could warrant certification as 'moral defectiveness' and compulsory admission to an institution. No definition is given of what constitutes 'subnormality of intelligence' either in terms of points below the mean or in terms of any particular intelligence 'measure'. Fitting an individual into one of the legal classifications thus remained a matter for the personal judgement of consultant psychiatrists.

In a survey following publication of the Act, Castell and Mittler (1965) sought the views of twenty hospitals (although these were not representative of all hospitals since a prerequisite was that they employed a psychologist) on what constituted 'subnormality' and 'severe subnormality' in terms of IQ. The authors then compared the hospital assessments of their patients in terms of whether they were 'subnormal' or 'severely subnormal' with test performance on the Wechsler Adult Intelligence Scale (Wechsler, 1955). This test has a standard deviation of fifteen points, and a consensus of psychologists in the study put the upper limit for 'subnormality' at between one and two standard deviations below the mean, i.e between seventy and eighty-five. The upper limit for 'severe subnormality' was said to be three standard deviations below the mean, i.e. an IQ of fifty-five. Testing on the group classified as 'subnormal' revealed a mean of 71.4, with 26.3 per cent scoring over eighty and 6.8 per cent over ninety. For the 'severely subnormal' group the mean IQ was 60.4, with 48.8 per cent scoring over sixty. The authors concluded that the levels of intelligence associated in the minds of psychologists with the two classes of 'subnormality' in the 1959 Act did not compare with the measured levels of intelligence of those actually classified under one heading or the other. Their findings suggest, of course, that the re-classification of patients admitted under the old Act merely split the hospital population into two and called the 'better' half 'subnormal' and the 'worse' half 'severely subnormal'.

The lack of any serious attempt to obtain IQ scores for institutionalised patients revealed by Morris (1969) was criticised by Townsend in his introduction to her book: 'Ignorance and inertia in obtaining scientific information about ability seem to be poor foundations for a service which owes its legal justification to a definition of subnormality which includes subnormality of intelligence.'

The government White Paper 'Better Services for the Mentally Handicapped' (DHSS, 1971, hereinafter referred to as the 1971 White Paper) used the term 'mentally handicapped' which it claimed covered the conditions legally described by 'subnormality' and 'severe subnormality'. This particular term grew in parallel with the development of a greater variety of services and the greater involvement of non-medical staff in the care of people with learning disabilities. Though they started as the 'Society for Backward Children' and also toyed with the American and WHO term 'mental retardation', the National Society for Mentally Handicapped Children undoubtedly spread the term 'mental handicap' into common usage. Their influence on the 1971 White Paper on this issue seems to be indicated by the statement in that document which explains the use of the term mental handicap 'in preference to any of the alternative terms because this helps to emphasise that our attitude should be the same as to other types of handicap', an opinion widely propounded by the National Society. Beyond this opinion about 'attitude' the White Paper does not provide any view on, or attempt at, classification, and thus common usage was again at odds with legal and academic terminology.

In America, following the debate over classification by IQ alone, the American Association of Mental Deficiency set up a study group to produce a standardised definition and classification of people with learning disabilities. Following the work of Doll, other authors put forward their classifications to include the concept of 'social competence' or 'adaptive behaviour' as it was beginning to be called. Di Michael proposed four classifications, similar to the earlier grades used in America, but including a descriptive grouping according to employability. These were:

(1)   Mentally Defective or idiot (IQ up to 25) – persons incapable of taking care of themselves, who require institutionalisation;
(2)   Borderline Defective or imbecile (IQ 25–49) – persons who may be able to care for themselves. A very few at the upper range capable of simple work in a sheltered workshop or outside;
(3)   Mentally Retarded or moron (IQ 50–74) – persons who are able to take care of themselves. Many can do unskilled work, rarely semi-skilled;
(4)   Functionally mentally retarded or borderline subnormal (IQ 75–85) – persons who can care for themselves. Most can do unskilled work, some semi-skilled, very few skilled.

(Di Michael, 1949)

Notice here, however, that IQ levels still define the groups and their behavioural descriptions are fairly vague. Sloan and Birch (1955) went further, and stated that an IQ level was not sufficient. Drawing on Di Michael's classification, they noted four 'levels of Mental Retardation', the latter term coming into use to imply 'retardation of growth' in the mind rather than a 'defect' of the mind. Unlike Di Michael, Sloan and Birch's four levels are not given general names such as idiot, moron, etc., but merely called 'Levels I to IV'. They are also taken to apply to 'adults' which implies those over 21 years old.

Level I – some motor and speech development, but incapable of self-maintenance. Needs complete care and supervision;

Level II – can contribute partially to self-support under complete supervision. Can develop self-protection skills to a minimum useful level in a controlled environment;

Level III – capable of self-maintenance in unskilled or semi-skilled occupations. Needs supervision and guidance when under mild social or economic stress;

Level IV – capable of social and vocational adequacy with proper education and training. Frequently needs supervision and guidance under serious social or economic stress.

(Sloan and Birch, 1955)

Eventually, the AAMD group produced a 'manual for classification' (Heber, 1959), which initially came down heavily in favour of the IQ definition of 'mental retardation'. This defined 'levels of retardation' by the 'level of deviation in measured intelligence' but was quickly amended to take account of the growth of the 'adaptive behaviour' school so that in a revision published two years later (Heber, 1961), 'mental retardation' is defined as 'subaverage general intellectual functioning which originates during the developmental period *and is associated with impairment in adaptive behaviour*' (author's emphasis). The urge to classify remained, however, and the revision continued its search for 'scientific' definition by giving levels, not only of IQ but of 'adaptive behaviour'. The units of 'adaptive behaviour', however, were not specified for each level, although Heber refers to the Vineland Scale (Doll, 1953) as being the only 'scientific measure' available, and thus presumably was thinking in terms of Doll's 'Social Quotient'. For descriptive purposes, however, he was forced to revert to the four levels of Sloan and Birch, which correspond with the four 'levels of deviation in adaptive behaviour'.

Criticism of the IQ classification continued, including the publication of further findings in the follow-up studies of Baller, Charles and Miller. Miller (1965), reporting on the later attainments of people classified in 1935 as 'defective' and observed earlier by Charles concludes that most of this group were really 'dull normal' or 'borderline' with the only major differences from a control group being in the mortality rate, which was much higher for the 'defectives' and presumably relates to the higher representation in this group of those with specific syndromes then associated with a high mortality rate, such as Down's syndrome. Baller, Charles and Miller (1967) in a third paper on the 1935 subjects, again found a higher death rate amongst those classed as deficient, but confirmed the findings regarding the ability and attainments of the 'defectives'. In addition, re-testing for IQ, using the Weschler Adult Intelligence Scale, the authors found significantly higher levels than those reported from the Stanford–Binet tests. Generally, however, as Tizard (1965) pointed out, these follow-up studies merely served to correct early mistakes in the classification of people with learning disabilities rather than proving necessarily that they were capable of independent living.

The need for a 'scientific' measure of 'adaptive behaviour' to complement the already deeply imbued professional commitment to IQ testing in America and, increasingly, in the UK, was the next area of academic debate. This was despite certain voices, notably Cantor (1961) who argued against the need for 'entitising' people. Eventually, various scales for assessment of adaptive behaviour were produced, notably those of Nihara and his colleagues (1969) and some received strong professional support. The basic descriptive classification remained, however, and an essentially similar system was adopted by the World Health Organization in its division of 'mental retardation' into 'mild', moderate', 'severe' and 'profound'.

In the seventies, particularly in America but also in the UK, the development of the ideas around 'normalisation' (see Wolfensberger, 1972), part of which, in its early formulation, emphasised the effect of 'labelling', meant that debates in some quarters took place over the language being used to describe people. Whilst this produced a variety of general alternatives to 'mental handicap', such as 'developmental disability', 'developmental handicap' and, from the education field, 'special needs' these did not satisfy the continuing urge of professionals to classify and categorise. In the US therefore, the term 'mental retardation', divided into the WHO categories described above, remained in common usage. In the UK developments were more prosaic. The use of 'mental handicap' became commonplace, borrowing the 'severe' and 'mild' labels from the old 'subnormality' division. In legal terms, the 1983 Mental Health Act, instead of removing mental handicap from its provisions, and thus clearly defining the difference between it and mental illness, provided various definitions of mental disorder. Section 1(2) of the Act is as follows:

> 'mental disorder' means mental illness, arrested or incomplete development of mind, psychopathic disorder and any other disorder or disability of mind and 'mentally disordered' shall be construed accordingly;
> 'severe mental impairment' means a state of arrested or incomplete development of mind which includes severe impairment of intelligence and social functioning and is associated with abnormally aggressive or seriously irresponsible conduct on the part of the person concerned and 'severely mentally impaired' shall be construed accordingly.

This was sufficiently confusing as to be largely ignored by people working in the field, who either kept the simple division of 'mild' and 'severe' mental handicap, or, particularly in the case of the Health Service and other planners, began to use a classification devised by the National Development Team (NDT). The NDT, as will be described later, was set up by the Secretary of State for Health and Social Security, Barbara Castle, in 1974 and was involved in a series of investigations of services, mainly hospitals. They then adopted a set of definitions from the Wessex Case Register (Kushlick and Blunden, 1974), to produce the following categories. (The categories have no labels other than Groups I–IV.)

Table 1.1 National Development Team classification

Group I:	Criteria:	Competent in all areas of self-help, ambulant, continent, no behaviour problems, not disruptive in any way.
	Opinion:	Could be discharged home or to hostel immediately without any special facilities necessary for management, apart from those normally provided in a local authority hostel. Some may be appropriately placed in group homes.
Group II:	Criteria:	Continent, ambulant, almost completely self-sufficient with mild problems of behaviour which could be corrected with a short period of treatment and self-help training. A number could be considered for self-care training units.
	Opinion:	Should be suitable for discharge home or to a hostel after a period of pre-discharge training.
Group III:	Criteria:	Continent with lapses at night. Some are mildly overactive with occasional mild behaviour problems. All are said to be easily managed and would benefit from specific training. If discharged to a hostel, staff ratios would need to be higher than for those in Groups I and II.
	Opinion:	Considered suitable for care in the community after intensive training and with greater supervision than is usually required by those in Groups I and II.
Group IV:	Criteria:	Severe double incontinence, multiple physical handicaps, severe epilepsy, extreme hyperkinetic behaviour, aggression to self and others.
	Opinion:	The majority require some form of residential care with a higher staff ratio than is required by those in Groups I, II and III.

Source: National Development Team, 1978

Despite their lack of labels, the use of 'NDT Group x' as a categorisation assumed some currency for a period, especially in discussions of who should, or should not, be in hospital. As with so many categorisations in this chapter, the NDT combines a judgement on the *effect* of handicap with a particular model of service. This, too, led to the continued use of terms such as 'hospital dependency' being used to describe people, and the difficulties of classification continued into the eighties. 'Mental handicap', divided into 'severe' and 'mild' was used in most publications in that decade, including those based on research across the literature (e.g. Office of Health Economics, 1986). With the growth of teaching of normalisation, however, and more particularly in the ideas and practice of citizen advocacy (O'Brien and Wolfensberger, 1988) and self-advocacy (Brechin and Walmsley, 1989) their effects on terminology were as marked, perhaps more so, as their effects on services, which will be described in Chapter 4. Though both of these sets of ideas were developed in the US, originally by Wolfensberger and his colleagues, the impact on classification was perhaps more immediately felt in the UK, with 'mental retardation' still being more commonly used in America than 'developmental disability'. In fact there now seems to be such a plethora of alternatives in that country, trying to avoid offence, that total confusion and a good deal of mutual recrimination as regards 'politically correct' language are rife (see, for example, Davis, 1992).

In the UK, whilst disagreement still exists, those who have made efforts to listen to people with learning disabilities themselves have tended to use the term 'learning difficulties'. MENCAP, in a 're-launch' process, used the term 'learning disability' in general descriptions and in their 'manifesto' (MENCAP, 1993), though for 'commercial reasons' the abbreviation MENCAP was not changed. Nor, in fact, has the society's official title of the Royal Society for Mentally Handicapped Children and Adults. Similar bet-hedging seems apparent in recent government circulars (e.g. LAC(92)15 from the Department of Health) where the term learning disabilities (mental handicap) is used. According to the Centre for Research and Information into Mental Disability (CRIMD) (1992), on the other hand, the term learning disability was 'introduced by the Department of Health in 1991 to replace "mental handicap"'. They go on to use the definitions developed by the World Health Organization in order to 'clarify' the 'confusion of terminology'. This gives them the following three definitions, which they then amplify.

> *Impairment* is defined as 'any loss or abnormality of psychological, physiological, or anatomical structure or function.
> *Disability* is defined as 'any restriction or lack (resulting from an impairment) of an ability to perform an activity in the manner or within the range considered normal for a human being'. The degree to which a person is actually disabled by an impairment depends on the effect of any treatment for the disease or the availability of prostheses and aids to daily living to correct the impairment.
> *Handicap* is 'a disadvantage for a given individual, resulting from an impairment or disability, that limits or prevents the fulfilment of a role (depending on age, sex and social or cultural factors) for that individual'. The degree to which a person is handicapped depends on the availability of services which compensate for the impairment or disability.
>
> (CRIMD, 1992)

The use by CRIMD of the additions beginning 'the degree to which . . .' in the last two categories returns us, of course, to the core argument of a social, rather than scientific, definition. That a person's 'handicap' is by this definition wedded to the availability of services would amuse some people, and anger others. It certainly reveals where the power still lies.

As for current practice, most organisations providing services in the UK use either 'learning difficulties' or 'learning disability'. The debates seem to be becoming more shrill, perhaps reflecting the 'political correctness' arguments from the US, and its accompanying backlash. To those who seek understanding, rather than confrontation, the usefulness of a general definition appears to have diminished. Even fifteen years ago the Jay Committee, wrestling with their attempt to provide a radical solution to the conservative lump that was the service system of their day (see Chapter 4) found tensions between a categorisation of sub-groups, which would enable services to be targeted, and an individualised service, which was then so vague in eligibility that organisations could escape their responsibilities by denying that people had 'special' needs. As services have fragmented in the eighties, at least in terms of a coherent set of ideas informing their provision, so the application of a global characterisation to a finite set of services has declined in usefulness. Those who agree with Ryan that 'the assertion of difference between people is seldom neutral' and that in the case of people with learning disabilities the differences 'have mostly been seen negatively' (Ryan and Thomas, 1987), have tended to shy away from, even oppose, definitions. Those involved in planning and providing services, especially since the NHS and Community Care Act of 1990, do not have this luxury. They still have to deal with the basic dilemma Yespen identified, as long ago as 1941. Quoted by Cantor (1961) in his discussion of the issues involved in terminology, Yespen concludes that after analysing 'one hundred or more criteria and descriptions making up the definitions which have appeared in the literature . . . none actually defines mental deficiency. All are descriptive of the results of mental deficiency.' Over fifty years later one cannot but reflect that current definitions, classifications, and the ferocious arguments they engender, still lead to the same conclusion.

REFERENCES

Acts of Parliament

De Praerogativa Regis, 1325, 17 Edward II
Poor Law Amendment Act, 1834, 4 and 5 Will IV, C.76
Lunatic Asylums Act, 1853, London, HMSO.
Idiots Act, 1886, London, HMSO.
Lunacy Act, 1890, London, HMSO.
Mental Deficiency Act, 1913, London, HMSO.
Mental Deficiency Act, 1927, London, HMSO.
Mental Health Act, 1959, London, HMSO.
Mental Health Act, 1983, London, HMSO.
NHS and Community Care Act, 1990, London, HMSO.

General references

American Association for the Study of the Feebleminded (1921) *Statistical Manual for the Use of Institutions for the Feebleminded*, New York, AASF.
Baller W.R., Charles D.C. and Miller E.L. (1967) Mid-life attainment of the mentally retarded – a longditudinal study, *Gen.Psychol.Mon.*, 75, 235–329.

Brechin A. and Walmsley J. (1989) (eds) *Making Connections: Reflecting on the Lives and Experiences of People with Learning Difficulties*, Milton Keynes, The Open University.

Burt C. (1937) *The Backward Child*, 24th edition, London, Univ. London Press.

Butler F. (1951) Sterilization in the U.S., *Am.J.Ment.Def.*, 56 (2), 360–3.

Cantor G. (1955) On the incurability of mental deficiency, *Am.J.Ment.Def.*, 60, (2), 362–5.

Cantor G. (1961) Some issues involved in Category VIII of the AAMD terminology and classification manual, *Am.J.Ment.Def.*, 65 (5), 561–5.

Castell J.H.F. and Mittler P.J. (1965) Intelligence of patients in subnormality hospitals: a survey of admissions in 1961, *Brit.J.Psychiat.*, 111, 219–25.

Centre for Research and Information into Mental Disability (1992) *Healthcare for People with a Learning Disability*, A Discussion Document, Department of Psychiatry, University of Birmingham.

Charles D.C. (1953) Ability and accomplishment of persons earlier judged mentally deficient, *Gen.Psychol.Mon.*, 47, 3–71.

Davis H. (1992) Living with labels, *Citizen Advocacy Forum*, 2 (4), 10–12.

Department of Health (1992) *Social Care for Adults with Learning Disabilities (Mental Handicap)*, LAC(92)15., London HMSO.

Department of Health and Social Security (1971) *Better Services for the Mentally Handicapped*, Command 4683, London, HMSO.

Dexter L.A. (1958) A social theory of mental deficiency, *Am.J.Ment.Def.*, 62, (5), 920–8.

Di Michael S.G. (1949) Employment of the Mentally Retarded, *J. Rehabilitation*, 2, 19–43.

Doll E.A. (1941) The essentials of an inclusive concept of mental deficiency, *Am.J.Ment.Def.*, 46, 214.

Doll E.A. (1948) What is a Moron? *J.Abn.Soc.Psychol.*, 43, 495–501.

Doll E.A. (1953) *A Manual for the Vineland Social Maturity Scale. The Measurement of Social Competence*, Minneapolis: Education Test Bureau.

Doll E.A. (1964) *The Vineland Scale of Social Maturity*, Minneapolis: American Guidance Service.

Heber R. (1959) *A Manual on Terminology and Classification in Mental Retardation*, Pineville: AAMD.

Heber R. (1961) Modifications in the manual on terminology and classification in Mental Retardation, *Am.J.Ment.Def.*, 65 (4), 499–500.

Hilliard L.T. and Mundy L. (1954) Diagnostic problems in the feebleminded, *Lancet*, 2, 644–6.

Jastak J. (1949) A rigorous criterion of feeblemindedness, *J.Abn.Soc.Psychol.*, 44, 367–78.

Kingsley L.V. and Hyde R.W. (1945) The health and occupational adequacy of the mentally deficient, *J.Abn.Soc.Psychol.*, 40, 37–46.

Kushlick A. and Blunden R. (1974) The epidemiology of mental subnormality, in Clarke A.M. and Clarke A.D.B. (eds), *Mental Deficiency – The Changing Outlook*, 3rd edition, London, Methuen.

Lewis E.O. (1929) Report on an investigation into the incidence of mental deficiency in six areas, 1925–1927, in *Report of the Mental Deficiency Committee*, Part IV, London, HMSO.

Locke J. (1689) *An Essay Concerning Human Understanding*.

Matthews F.B. (1954) *Mental Health Services*, London, Shaw.

Mencap (1993) *Manifesto for Change*, London, Royal Society for Mentally Handicapped Children and Adults.

Mental Deficiency Committee (1929) *The Wood Report*, London, HMSO.

Miller E.L. (1965) Ability and social adjustment at midlife of persons earlier adjudged mentally deficient, *Gen.Psychol.Mon.*, 72, 139–98.

Morris P. (1969) *Put Away: A Sociological Study of Institutions for the Mentally Retarded*, London, Routledge and Kegan Paul.

National Development Team for the Mentally Handicapped (1978) *First Report 1976–1977*, London, HMSO.

Nihara K., Foster R., Shellhaus M. and Leland H. (1969) *Adaptive Behavior Scale*, 1st edition, Washington D.C., AAMD.

O'Brien J. and Wolfensberger W. (1988) *CAPE: Standards for Citizen Advocacy Program Evaluation*, Syracuse N.Y., Person to Person Citizen Advocacy Association.

O'Connor N. and Tizard J. (1954) A survey of patients in twelve mental deficiency institutions, *Brit. Med. J.*, i, 16–20.

Office of Health Economics (1986) *Mental Handicap – Partnership in the Community*, London, HMSO.

Pearson K. (1914) *On the graduated character of mental defect and on the need for standardising judgements as to the grade of social inefficiency which shall involve segregation*, Questions of the Day and of the Fray, no. VIII, Mendelism and the Problems of Mental Defect, Dept. Applied Statistics: UCL.

Pearson K. and Jaederholm G.A. (1914) *On the continuity of mental defect*, Questions of the Day and of the Fray, no. VIII, Mendelism and the Problems of Mental Defect, Dept. Applied Statistics: UCL.

Ryan J. and Thomas F. (1987) *The Politics of Mental Handicap*, 2nd edition, London, Free Association Books.

Sarason S.B. (1953) *Psychological Problems in Mental Deficiency*, New York, Harper Bros.

Sarason S.B. and Gladwin T. (1958a) Psychological and cultural problems in mental subnormality, a review of research, *Gen.Psychol. Mon.*, 57, 3–289.

Sarason S.B. and Gladwin T. (1958b) Psychological and cultural problems in mental subnormality, a review of research, *Am.J.Ment.Def.*, 62 (6), 1115–307.

Sloan W. and Birch J. (1955) A rationale for degrees of retardation, *Am.J.Ment.Def.*, 60, (2), 258–64.

Tizard J. (1965) Introduction, in Clarke A.M. and Clarke A.D.B. (eds) *Mental Deficiency – The Changing Outlook*, 2nd edition, London, Methuen.

Tredgold A.F. (1909) The feebleminded – a social danger, *Eugenics Rev*, 1, 97 104.

Tredgold A.F. (1952) *A Textbook on Mental Deficiency (Amentia)*, 8th edition, London, Balliere, Tindall and Cox.

Wechsler D. (1944) *The Measurement of Adult Intelligence*, Baltimore, University Park Press.

Wechsler D. (1955) *Wechsler Pre-School and Primary Scale of Intelligence*, New York, Psychological Corporation.

Wolfensberger W. (1972) *The Principle of Normalisation in Human Services*, Toronto, National Institute for Mental Retardation.

Wolfensberger W. (1974) *The Origins of our Institutional Models*, Toronto, National Institute for Mental Retardation.

2 Causes of learning disabilities

David Race

With such historical differences between workers in the field of learning disabilities regarding classification, it is virtually inevitable that there should be disagreement regarding causation. Where no clear understanding exists of what constitutes a 'person with learning disabilities', it is difficult for a properly developed science of causation to be formed. Some would argue that since learning disabilities are socially, rather than biologically, defined, no objective science is possible in any case. To their view is added, from within the 'scientific' world, developments in understanding and methodology in the biological sciences, and genetics in particular, which have shown earlier pronouncements of 'scientific fact' in their true speculative light.

A considerable amount of work has been undertaken, however, on the aetiology of learning disabilities. Researchers have tended to concentrate on three main areas of causation, sometimes in isolation, sometimes examining interactions. These three areas are, first, inherited disorders; secondly, disorders due to pre- or post-natal injury or disease to the nervous system; and thirdly, environmental factors acting on the learning processes and conditioning of the individual. The first may be called genetic factors, the second and third environmental, and the great debate over the years has been the relative contribution of these two sets of factors to the development of the human organism. This has, of course, gone beyond the narrow confines of learning disabilities and still remains the subject for heated argument. As this is written a fierce debate is being carried out at all levels of the media as to the causes of delinquency in children – a more academic, but no less bitter, controversy on a related issue was the decline, fall, and attempted rehabilitation of Cyril Burt, following accusations of inconsistencies in certain publications, and counter charges of left-wing witch hunts. Both have roots in the inheritance/environment argument, in which this chapter, having as its aim an overview of the state of knowledge of the causes of learning disabilities, will try, without a great deal of hope of success, to avoid becoming embroiled.

The Eugenics Society has already been mentioned, and it is certain that ill-founded opinions on the degree of inheritance of learning disabilities led to concern, in powerful circles, about 'national degeneracy' and pressure for segregation of the 'unfit' from society to prevent their propagation. Tredgold, even in the later editions of his classic *Textbook* (1952), persists with his view that the majority of 'mental deficiency' is inherited. He defines inherited 'deficiency' as 'primary amentia' and considers that such cases constitute approximately 80 per cent of all cases. The remainder he terms 'secondary amentia'. Quoting figures to support his own from a number of sources and countries the only major disagreement he finds comes from Penrose (1933) who gives a figure of 29 per cent for 'primary amentia'. Penrose considered that most of the cases he investigated were due to the interaction of inheritance and environment. Later, in his classic study of 'defectives' in the Colchester Institution, Penrose (1938) continued with this view, pointing out that, although an association existed, which was greater than that for the rest of the population, between the frequency of 'defect' among the parents and siblings of his patients, those families shared a large number of other factors in the biological and social environment as well as genetic background, and thus any correlation did not imply a causal relationship.

The intrusion of the 'scientific' IQ measurement into the study of the mind had, earlier, brought out further hypotheses when it was observed, in Pearson and Jaederholm's paper (1914) and then many more, that the distribution of IQ scores did not follow the classic Gaussian curve but was skewed to the left. It was observed that most of the 'higher-grade defectives' fell at the lower end of the normal distribution of IQ scores, and the asymmetrical portion contained most of those described as 'low-grade'. Lewis (1933) suggested that the lower end represented the 'pathological' cases of deficiency whilst the 'high-grade defectives' constituted a 'subcultural' group who simply have a 'lower measure of intelligence', i.e. they are at the bottom end of the 'normal biological distribution' found in physiological attributes such as height, weight, etc. This view was supported in a slightly different form by Roberts (1952) who returned to Pearson and Jaederholm's original data to make the hypothesis of two kinds of 'defect'; the lower end of the distribution of 'general intelligence' and the abnormal 'low-grade' group who are 'a highly diverse collection of entities' from, he says, a great variety of causes. Berg (1962) also suggested that the main cause of 'deficiency' in the 'feeble-minded' group is 'normal' biological variation, although he conceded that social adversity played a contributory role.

Apart from the fundamental question of why intelligence should be normally distributed anyway, which tends to throw doubt on the logic behind this division, the series of investigations by Berg and Kirman (Berg, 1963; Berg and Kirman, 1959a; 1959b), did much to cast doubt upon the usefulness of this division in aetiological terms. First of all, Berg and Kirman's division of patients whose IQs put them into the 'high-grade', i.e. subcultural group and 'low-grade', that is pathological, group found considerable overlap in terms of identifiable pathological conditions in some of the 'high-grade' group. Then the study of Berg (1963), in analysing some 800 'severely subnormal' patients admitted to the Fountain Hospital, could identify specific aetiological factors of distinct syndromes in only one-third of the cases. For more able patients, therefore, the uncertainty must increase (see also Davis, 1961; Stott, 1961).

In general the continued lack of agreement on classification for people with learning disabilities, combined with the 'nature versus nurture' argument, meant that most people concerned with aetiology turned away from general statements covering large groups and concentrated on the precise role of heredity in specific syndromes or the existence of specific environmental contributions to handicap. Advances in genetics have made the identification of specific syndromes e.g. Down's, at the prenatal stage possible, though identification and abortion, rather than attempts at prevention prior to conception, have dominated the output of such efforts.

A considerable number of syndromes have been identified which arise from a determined genetic effect, but all occur rarely, other than Down's syndrome, which accounts for some 30 per cent of all severe learning disabilities in children of school age (Office of Health Economics (OHE), 1986). No attempt will be made here to consider all of these special syndromes, for which Hilliard and Kirman (1965), Penrose (1963), Dutton (1975) or Clarke (1986) are suitable references. The action of genetic factors can, however, be summarised under four main headings, which cover most of the known syndromes, although excluding certain conditions, such as spina bifida and anencephaly which have a more complex causality, including some genetic defects. The four groups are (after OHE, 1973):

(1) *Dominant conditions*, due to genes whose effects manifest themselves in the heterozygote – very rarely occurring, examples are the group known as the phakomatoses.

(2) *Recessive conditions*, due to genes which have effect only in the homozygote – the largest group of single major gene defects, they have an incidence of approximately 1 in 50,000 of the population (Holmes *et al.*, 1972). Examples are phenylketonuria, maple syrup urine disease and galactosaemia.

(3) *Sex-linked inheritance*, carried by females who do not manifest the traits but whose male children stand a one in two chance of being affected – examples are glucose-6-dehydrogenose deficiency and sex linked hydrocephalus.

(4) *Conditions resulting from chromosome abnormalities*, either defect of number of chromosomes or loss or rearrangement of chromosomal material – Down's Syndrome is the most widely occurring condition. This is usually due to the presence of an extra chromosome identical to the members of the normal pair 21. There are also cases of Down's Syndrome (some 5 per cent) where translocation, an extra 21 chromosome attached to another chromosome, is the cause. The other main chromosomal cause of learning difficulties is Klinefelter's Syndrome, although not all who suffer from this syndrome have learning dif-

ficulties and recent attention has been given to an X-linked disorder known as 'Fragile X syndrome'.

(OHE, 1986)

Environmental factors are not usually associated with particular syndromes. Adverse environmental conditions have, however, been found to exist in greater frequency for parents and families of children with learning disabilities than those without. Such factors may be divided into two groups. First, those conditions surrounding the birth of a child and secondly, the social and economic conditions of the family in general.

A number of clearly recognisable causes of handicap have been identified as occurring during, and immediately after, pregnancy. Birch and colleagues (1970) found strong associations between the physical stature of mothers, particularly height, and the conditions of children at birth. Dietary excess or deficiency, specifically leading to imbalances of vitamin A, but also imbalance of other vitamins, have been associated with foetal abnormalities (Penrose, 1972; Heaton Ward 1975). Evans (1973) is quoted by Clarke and Clarke (1975) as showing that 'within very deprived families, children receiving diet supplementation for the first two years of life have almost a 12 point IQ advantage in middle childhood over their siblings'. They do not indicate whether the extra diet was accompanied by a general improvement in the social conditions of the family, which may also be having an effect. To return to the more objectively established clinical causes of handicap occurring during pregnancy, Crome (1965) lists irradiation, misuse of drugs, intrauterine infection (including the effects of maternal rubella) and endocrine causes as established reasons for a number of handicapping conditions. Berg (1965) adds maternal age and birth order as being relevant in the chance of the pregnancy resulting in an abnormal birth, and Clarke (1986, op. cit.) includes anoxia of the foetus during pregnancy.

Complications during birth have added to the confusion and debate over learning disabilities. For some, the blanket term 'birth injury' sufficed as a reason for a multitude of subsequent handicaps (Schwartz, 1961) whilst others denied its significance as a major factor (Campbell *et al.*, 1950; Drillien, 1963). As usual the answer seems to lie somewhere between the two extremes and further evidence is difficult to produce because of the difficulty of diagnosis immediately after birth. Birch and colleagues (1970, op. cit.) estimated that 'clinically recognisable obstetric factors' were responsible for subnormality in just over 10 per cent of their sample. Clarke (1986, op. cit.) uses a figure of 1 per cent for 'birth injury' causes.

Other studies have related low birth weight to later learning disabilities (Illsley and Mitchell, 1984), though these are confused as to whether the low weight *per se* produces the condition or the resultant susceptibility to perinatal problems. The same would apply to the relationship between prematurity and later learning disabilities, Dutton (1975, op. cit.)

Post-natal causes are rather more clearly recorded, with meningitis being one of the most common in Berg's (1962) study of admissions. Interestingly, as Berg points out, improvements in treatment have meant that, as more are cured, some people who would have died of tuberculosis or meningitis now survive, but in a 'handicapped' state. In general, improvements in immediate post-natal care have reduced the risk of infection to newborn children, and thus learning disabilities resulting from such conditions as infantile gastro-enteritis (Schlesinger and Welch, 1952), whooping cough (Berg, 1963, op.cit.) and severe jaundice (Crome, 1955) are also less common. On the other hand, vaccination-induced conditions have occurred, and raised some public anxiety, particularly with regard to whooping cough vaccine.

Going beyond the 'biological environmental' factors in the aetiology of learning disabilities to the 'cultural and material' factors (to use the terms of the Office of Health Economics (1973, op.cit.) leads back to the 'nature versus nurture' debate at its height. Claims for *either* heredity or environment have now been established as meaningless, since, as Crome puts it 'dynamic interaction between the individual or its precursor cells with the environment is the very essence of life'. In addition, the argument has been broadened to consider not just interactions, but correlations arising from a genotype choosing its environment because of an ability to do so or because a set of genotypes happen to be in a particular environment. A number of studies have been mounted, however, to establish the environmental 'causes' of learning difficulties, and have demonstrated in general the unsurprising fact that more amenable surroundings produce a greater response from the individual in terms of intellectual performance and that social and economic disadvantage is certainly associated with a degree of learning disability. This 'disad-vantage' has included, in some writers' estimation, the effects of the supposed caring environment itself (Goffman, 1961; Wolfensberger, 1974) and this will be considered shortly, but on the basic issue of social and economic factors, several writers can be mentioned. A lot of the work in the fifties which developed the body of opinion for more 'community care' was concerned with the effects of more stimulating environments on people with learning disabilities. Clarke and Clarke (1954, 1959) and Clarke and col-leagues (1958) all report evidence to show that improvements in IQ levels of the 'feeble-minded' occur if better conditions and a more stimulating environment are produced. Bourne (1955), after dividing his sample of admissions to hospital with IQ below 50 into 'organic' and 'residual' causes, found a much greater incidence of adverse home background in the 'non-organic' group. Woodward (1960) found that disturbed 'social response' in children varied according to early family experiences. Cashdan and Jeffree (1966, 1971) confirmed the effects of this lack of parental stimulation on the retardation of intelligence. On a more general level, Jackson (1968, 1974) found a considerable association between the incidence of learning dis-abilities and various social malaise indicators, findings borne out in the Report of the Committee on Child Health Services (Court Report), 1976.

As mentioned earlier, caring environments themselves have been criticised as providing poor surroundings for those diagnosed as 'mentally handicapped', and thus contributing to the handicap. Woodward (1963) again showed the effect of early home experiences on social response of patients with learning disabilities, but also discovered that poor social response was related to the number of previous admissions undertaken by such patients and hypothesised that the hospital itself was having an effect. Lyle (1959, 1960a, 1960b), in a series of papers, first established the superiority of non-hospitalised 'imbecile' children in verbal ability when matched with those from a hospital, and then reported on the development of children in the 'Brooklands' experimental unit, also discussed in Tizard (1964). This unit attempted to provide a more stimulating environment for previously hospitalised children by setting up a small residential unit, with special staffing facilities. Both writers reported a greater verbal development by the children in the unit than with hospitalised controls. Following up this study, Lyle (1964) observed that the pre-hospital environment did have an effect on later development but that improvements could be made in all hospital patients with a more stimulating environment. Other studies, for example Mundy (1957), confirmed the undesirable comparison between hospital and other environments but most, implicitly or explicitly, make the intellectual jump from the observed improvement with more stimulating conditions to an assumption that a 'bad', i.e, non-stimulating, environment produces or contributes to the original learning disability. There is a danger here of confusing the argument for an environmental contribution to learning disability with a polemic against various institutional regimes and one must not get carried away by certain obvious mistakes, for example, in admission policy. However as Frankenstein (1965) argues, the evidence for the contribution of social and economic environmental factors is overwhelming. What is difficult, however, as Masland (1962) points out, is the evaluation of the effects of these factors.

Inevitably, such detailed studies as those mentioned hitherto will lead to greater understanding about the aetiology of learning disability. The direction of research, however, has proved more controversial as methods of identification are becoming regarded as methods of prevention, i.e. early identification in the embryo resulting in abortion. Embryological research, one main source of such efforts, is itself still subject to a moral debate with the Warnock Committee (Report of Inquiry into Human Fertilisation and Embryology, 1984) suggesting guidelines which were morally neutral and which found their expression in the Human Fertilisation (Embryology) Act of 1990. Genetic counselling is also subject to strictures from those who look to the inter-war 'euthanasia' programme in Germany and can see parallels in the 'scientific' elimination of undesirable genes at the foetal stage (Wolfensberger, 1987). These issues are not for this book, except to repeat the point that identification is not the same thing as causation, and that still, for the vast majority of those described as having learning disabilities, no known cause can be identified. In addition, for a book on services, Clarke's (1986, op. cit.) caveat is appropriate. 'In most cases a knowledge of causation will not help someone in the daily care of a mentally handicapped child or adult. Indeed this clinical emphasis has often been at the root cause of inappropriate patterns of care.' One might add that it is becoming the root cause of inappropriate attitudes to, and threats to, the lives of people with learning disabilities (Williams, 1992).

REFERENCES

Acts of Parliament

Human Fertilisation and Embryology Act (1990) London, HMSO.

General references

Berg J.M. (1962) Meningitis as a cause of severe mental defect, *Proc. Lond. Conf. Scient. Stud. Ment. Defic.*, 1960; 1, 160–4.

Berg J.M. (1963) Causal factors in severe mental retardation, *Proc. 2nd. Int. Congr. Ment. Retard., Vienna*, 1961; 1, 170–3.

Berg J.M. (1965) Aetiological aspects of mental subnormality: pathological factors, in Clarke A.D.B. and Clarke A.M. (eds) *Mental Deficiency – The changing outlook*, 2nd edition, London, Methuen.

Berg J.M. and Kirman B.H. (1959a) Some aetiological problems in mental deficiency, *Brit. Med. J.*, ii, 848–52.

Berg J.M. and Kirman B.H. (1959b) Discussion on the aetiology of mental defect, *Proc.Roy.Soc.Med.*, 52, 787–91.

Birch H.G., Richardson S.A., Baird D., Horobin G. and Illsley R. (1970) *Mental Subnormality in the Community*, Baltimore, Williams and Williams.

Bourne H. (1955) Protophrenia – a study of perverted rearing and mental dwarfism, *Lancet*, 2, 1156–955.

Breg W.R. (1962) Genetic aspects of mental retardation, *Quart.Rev.Pediat.*, 17, 9–23.

Campbell W.A.B., Cheeseman E.A. and Kilpatrick A.W. (1950) The effects of neonatal asphyxia on physical and mental development, *Arch.Dis.Childh.*, 25, 351–9.

Cashdan A. and Jeffree D. (1966) The influence of the home background of S.S.N. children, *Brit.J.Med.Psychol.*, 39, 313–18.

Cashdan A. and Jeffree D. (1971) The home background of the S.S.N. child – a second study, *Brit.J.Med.Psychol.*, 44, 27–33.

Clarke A.D.B. and Clarke A.M. (1954) Cognitive changes in the feebleminded, *Brit.J.Psychol.*, 45, 173–9.

Clarke A.D.B. and Clarke A.M. (1959) Recovery from the effects of deprivation, *Acta Psychologica*, 16, 137–44.

Clarke A.D.B. and Clarke A.M. (1975) *Recent Advances in the Study of Subnormality*, 2nd edition, London, MIND (National Association for Mental Health).

Clarke A.D.B., Clarke A.M. and Reiman S. (1958) Cognitive changes in the feebleminded – three further studies, *Brit.J.Psychol.*, 49, 144–57.

Clarke D. (1986) *Mentally Handicapped People: Living and Learning*, London, Balliere Tindall.

Crome L. (1955) Morphological nervous changes in survivors of severe jaundice in the newborn, *J.Neurol.Neurosurg.Psychiat.*, 18, 17–23.

Crome L. (1965) Causes of mental defect, in Hilliard L.T. and Kirman B.H. (eds) *Mental Deficiency*, London, Churchill.

Davis D.R. (1961) A disorder theory of mental retardation, *Brit.J.Ment.Subn.*, 7, 13–21.

Drillien C.M. (1963) Obstetric hazard, mental retardation and behaviour disturbances in primary school, *Developm.Med.Child.Neurol.*, 5, 3–13.

Dutton G. (1975) *Mental Handicap*, London, Butterworths.

Evans D.C. (1973) Malnutrition and intellectual development: the effects of early dietary supplementation, unpublished PhD thesis, University of Cape Town.

Frankenstein C. (1965) Environmental varieties of mental retardation – causes and patterns, *Acta Psychologica*, 24, 283–313.

Goffman E. (1961) *Asylums: Essays on the social situation of mental patients and other inmates*, Garden City, N.Y., Doubleday.

Heaton-Ward W.A. (1975) *Mental Subnormality*, 4th edition, Bristol, John Wright.

Hilliard L.T. and Kirman B.H. (eds) (1965), *Mental Deficiency*, London, Churchill.

Holmes L.B., Moser H.W., Halldorsen S., Mack C., Pant S. and Matzilevich B. (1972), *Mental Retardation – An atlas of diseases with associated physical abnormalities*, New York, Macmillan.

Illsley R. and Mitchell R.J. (eds) (1984) *Low Birth Weight*, London, John Wiley and Sons.

Jackson R. (1968) Urban distribution of educable mental handicap, *J.Ment.Def.Res.*, 12, 312–16.

Jackson R. (1974) The ecology of educable mental handicap, *Brit.J.Ment.Subn.*, 20, Pt.1, 18–22.

Lewis E.O. (1933) Types of mental deficiency and their social significance, *J.Ment.Sci.*, 79, 298–304.

Lyle J.G. (1959) The effect of an institution environment upon the verbal development of imbecile children – I. Verbal intelligence, *J.Ment.Def.Res.*, 3, 122–8.

Lyle J.G. (1960a) The effect of an institution environment upon the verbal development of imbecile children – II. Speech and language, *J.Ment.Def.Res.*, 4, 1–13.

Lyle J.G. (1960b) The effect of an institution environment upon the verbal development of imbecile children – III. The Brooklands residential family unit, *J.Ment.Def.Res.*, 4, 14–23.

Lyle J.G. (1964) Environmentally produced retardation – institution and pre-institution influences, *J.Abn.Soc.Psychol.*, 69, 329–32.

Masland R.L. (1962) Current knowledge regarding the pre-natal environmental factors in mental deficiency, Dagenham, May and Baker Ltd.

Mundy L. (1957) Environmental influence on intellectual function as measured by intelligence tests, *Brit.J.Med.Psychol.*, 30, 194–201.

Office of Health Economics (1973) *Mental Handicap*, London, OHE.

Office of Health Economics (1986) *Mental Handicap – Partnership in the community*, London, HMSO.

Pearson K. and Jaederholm G.A. (1914) *On the Continuity of Mental Defect*, Questions of the Day and of the Fray No. VIII, Mendelism and the Problem of Mental Defect, Dept. Applied Statistics, University College London.

Penrose L.S. (1933) *Mental Defect*, London, Sidgwick and Jackson.

Penrose L.S. (1938) *A Clinical and Genetic Study of 1,280 Cases of Mental Defect*, London, HMSO.

Penrose L.S. (1963) *The Biology of Mental Defect*, 3rd edition, London, Sidgwick and Jackson.

Penrose L.S. (1972) *The Biology of Mental Defect*, 4th edition, London, Sidgwick and Jackson.

Report of the Committee on Child Health Services (1976) *Fit for the Future (The Court Report)*, Command 6684, London, HMSO.

Report of Inquiry into Human Fertilisation and Embryology (1984) *The Warnock Inquiry*, Command 9314, London, HMSO.

Roberts, J.A.F. (1952) The genetics of mental deficiency, *Eugenics Review*, 44, 71–9.

Schlesinger B. and Welch R.G. (1952) Infantile gastroenteritis as a cause of mental deficiency, *Gt.Ormond St.J.*, 3–4, 14.

Schwartz P. (1961) *Birth Injuries of the Newborn – Morphology, pathogenesis, clinical pathology and prevention*, The Swiss Institute, Basel.

Stott D.H. (1961) A re-appraisal of Lewis's classification of mental defect, *Brit. J. Ment. Subn.*, 7, 23–31.

Tizard J. (1964) *Community Services for the Mentally Handicapped*, London, Oxford University Press.

Tredgold A.F. (1952) *A Textbook on Mental Deficiency (Amentia)*, 8th edition, London, Balliere Tindall and Cox.

Williams P. (1992) Ethical issues in prevention and treatment, *Proceedings of the Annual Conference of the British Institute of Mental Handicap*, September 1992.

Wolfensberger, W. (1974) *The Origins of our Institutional Models*, Toronto, National Institute for Mental Retardation.

Wolfensberger, W. (1987) *The New Genocide of Handicapped and Afflicted People*, Syracuse, N.Y., Training Institute.

Woodward M. (1960) Early experiences and later social responses of SSN children, *Brit.J.Med.Psychol.*, 33, 174–84.

Woodward M. (1963) Early experiences and behaviour disorders in severely subnormal children, *Brit.J.Soc.Clin.Psychol.*, 2, 174–84.

3 Epidemiology of learning disabilities

David Race

As with causation, the problems concerning classification, described in Chapter 1, have affected another fundamental question regarding people with learning disabilities; namely, 'how many are there?' Ever since E.O. Lewis attempted to answer this question for the Mental Deficiency Committee in the twenties, a whole series of surveys have revealed different figures for the numbers of people with learning disabilities existing in a given population.

Since this book is primarily about services for people, rather than numbers, no detailed analysis will be made of those surveys to try and discover which is 'right' – a highly dubious undertaking in any case. What this chapter will try to do is, first, look at the problem of attempting to assess the prevalence of people with learning disabilities. Second, by reviewing some of the major surveys it will try to give the reader a sense of the 'size of the issue', but without any claims to exhaustive coverage.

We have seen the somewhat chequered career of attempts at classification, and this is undoubtedly the greatest factor contributing to the confusion over prevalence rates. Of eleven surveys reported by Kushlick and Blunden (1974), six have definite IQ criteria, but different for each survey, and the other five simply have the criteria of being 'known to the various services agencies'. Conley (1973) lists nine American studies, of which seven use IQ criteria, again all different, and the other two use a combination of IQ and social competence criteria. E.O. Lewis's original survey, the starting point for most studies of epidemiology, attempted, as he puts it, to classify 'mental defectives . . . in accordance with the grades defined in the Mental Deficiency Act of 1913, bearing in mind also in the case of the feeble-minded child, the definition of the "mentally defective child" in the Education Act' (Lewis, 1929). In other words an opinion had to be sought, in this case from 'many persons in responsible administrative, industrial and social positions' as to who fitted the definitions of the Act, rather than any attempt to make a personal assessment of what actually constituted 'mental deficiency' and then go out and measure its prevalence.

This leads on to the second major problem of prevalence surveys – the means used to count the numbers. Conley (1973, op.cit.) divides his list into two types: 'agency surveys' and 'household surveys'. In 'agency surveys', as the name implies, clients of various agencies are either reported to those conducting the survey, who then carry out some test using their own criteria, or the agencies themselves provide an assessment of their clients. In 'household surveys' attempts are made to discover, usually by some form of sampling, the presence of people with learning disabilities in a given population. It comes as no surprise that the prevalence reported in 'agency surveys' is normally lower than that reported in 'household surveys'. The latter provide an approximation to what Tizard (1964) calls the 'true' prevalence rate, i.e. the numbers actually conforming to the particular definition used in the survey. This, as Tizard goes on to point out, is not the same thing as an 'administrative' prevalence rate, which he defines as 'the numbers for whom services would be required in a community which made provision for all who needed them', since some of the 'true' population might not need any services. The 'agency surveys' described by Conley provide a third type of prevalence since, in part at least, they reflect the adequacy of services provided by agencies and the agencies' abilities, or even desire or lack of it, to identify people with learning disabilities.

For the purpose of observing changes in the 'size of the issue' therefore, one should, theoretically at least, attempt to discover 'true' prevalence, and note changes over time. In practice this has not generally been a feasible proposition except in cases, such as Down's syndrome, where the definition is clear. Otherwise the definitional differences make any comparison over time fairly meaningless. In this regard Clarke and Clarke (1975) had reasonable grounds for stating that the 'incidence' of certain types of 'mental handicap', i.e. the number of *new* cases arriving in a given number of births, was declining, whereas the 'prevalence', i.e. the *total* number of cases at a given point in time in proportion to the total population, was increasing. This is, however, complicated in more recent times by the question, academically interesting if morally fraught, of whether aborted children with some identified 'abnormality' are counted in the 'incidence' figures; they certainly would not appear in the 'prevalence'. In the main, however, such questions are of considerably less use to practitioners than the second major use of surveys, which is in the planning of services. Those who have attempted such planning have, in the main, endeavoured to assess Tizard's 'administrative' prevalence but, as noted earlier, have had to rely heavily on agencies' knowledge of individuals in their geographical area. Planning has been further hampered by the way in which the link is made between how many of a certain type of person with learning disabilities exist in a given area, and the 'appropriate' sort of provision which can be planned on those figures. This leads to the debate on the provision of services, the history of which will be described in the next chapter, and so no further detail will be discussed here, except to stress the caution with which surveys who quoted 'x per hundred thousand population' as being in 'need' of some sort of provision should be treated. What such statements are really saying is 'there are x per hundred thousand people of this sort, and we think that this sort of person needs a certain type of provision'. Such a sequential argument should not be taken for granted.

Planning of services does have to take place, however, particularly since the NHS and Community Care Act of 1990, and adequate planning needs some sort of information on the numbers of people with learning disabilities in a given area, together with the likely demands, in terms of severity and variety of learning disabilities that such numbers are likely to make on the service system. (Interestingly, little authoritative guidance is given on this specific aspect in the plethora of circulars sent to local and health authorities regarding implementation of the 1990 Act.) Probably the most useful, and certainly the most used, sources of such data have been 'registers', specifically set up as an aid in planning services. To fulfil the second purpose of this chapter, therefore, that is to provide the reader with an 'order of magnitude' of the numbers involved, we will consider the results of some of these surveys. As Kushlick and Blunden (1974, op.cit.) point out, surveys have a fair measure of agreement on what was defined as 'severe subnormality' or 'severe retardation', commonly supported by an IQ level of less than fifty. Here, the agreed rate is between 350 and 400 per hundred thousand population aged between 15 and 19. This is the age at which the greatest number of adults become known to the services, i.e. at the point of leaving school. Subsequent surveys not included in the Kushlick and Blunden analysis (for example, Mackay, 1971; Wing and Fryers, 1975; and Martindale, 1976) tend to support their figures for the 'severely subnormal' group although it should be noted that no more recent surveys than 1976 seemed to have been published by the time of the Office of Health Economics' review ten years later (OHE, 1986).

Before the age of 15 the prevalence rate of people described as having a 'severe mental handicap' (per hundred thousand *total* population) tended to be similar to the above (see Martindale, 1975, for example). With the advent of the 1981 Education Act, the need for the ascertainment of numbers for 'statementing' purposes as well as for planning produced local variations in these figures. Earlier examples of integration (i.e. before the 1981 Act) had meant that children benefiting from the use of ordinary schools were not included in the 'agency' surveys, since they were not at special schools. The need for statements then added to the confusion by providing local counts of all children defined as having 'special needs', only some of whom had learning disabilities (Meacher, 1976; Martindale, 1976, op.cit.)

To provide a more probably 'true' prevalence rate for both children and adults with severe learning disabilities we therefore return to the surveys of the seventies, and to the 1971 White Paper figures of 69.2 and 167.84 per hundred thousand *total* population which derived from some of those surveys. For people with 'mild' learning disabilities, more doubt exists as to precise numbers. This is most clearly illustrated by the 1971 White Paper which, whilst prepared to use the survey results of Wessex, Newcastle and Camberwell, in its 'official' prevalence rates of 'severe subnormality', only produces rates of 'mild subnormality' for those in hospital or other residential care, commenting that: 'Those living at home are not all known to the authorities . . .; the numbers recorded in the surveys varied widely and do not form a useful basis for estimating service needs'. In this sub-category of learning disabilities, of course, the problem of definition is at its greatest. Simply using those in attendance at special schools to estimate future numbers of 'mildly handicapped' adults is scarcely a sufficient criterion, as many of these pupils go on to lead perfectly normal lives without requiring the help of the services, as evidenced indirectly by the many follow-up studies quoted earlier, and directly by the dramatic fall in numbers on various case registers after the immediate post-school period (Kushlick and Blunden, 1974, op.cit.)

In addition, of course, the effects of the 1981 Act on the numbers in special schools and the counting process has been such that little benefit to planning can now be obtained, given the wide variation in implementation of the Act across the country (Swann, 1986).

In order to establish any numbers at all for people with mild learning disabilities, therefore, the tendency has been to observe the total number of people known to the services as 'mentally handicapped' and to subtract those with severe learning disabilities from this figure, without using any set definition of learning disabilities. In the first edition of this book (Malin *et al.*, 1980) those surveys or registers which applied this pragmatic method were used, as being likely to be as accurate as any using a more theoretical approach based on, say IQ levels. Further, the fact that such surveys or registers were an integral part of the service delivery, such as those in Sweden, or the register set up as part of the Sheffield Development Project, and were routinely maintained, led the authors of that book to rely more heavily on their accuracy than the 'one-off' surveys. The Sheffield register (Martindale, 1975; 1976, op.cit.) was probably the best maintained count of the numbers of mentally handicapped people in an English urban area, and this provided a gross figure of 490 per 100,000 total population (this included all those at ESN(M) schools as defined by the 1970 Education (Handicapped Children) Act). In Sweden, where registers are part of the routine, and have thus been going for some time, a range of numbers was found, from 320 per 100,000 in the industrial county of Stockholm, to 710 per 100,000 in the extreme northern rural county of Vasternorrland (Grunewald, 1974). At 490 per 100,000, the Sheffield figure was higher than most of the industrialised counties of Sweden, and the Swedish national average of 430 per 1,000. However, the figure for adults from Sheffield, at about 360 per 1,000 is much closer to the Swedish figures for urban areas. The contrast between rural and industrial areas is, of course, much greater in Sweden than in the UK, in terms of both the proximity of large towns and the population density and thus, if the prevalence of learning disabilities does tend to rise with an increase in rurality, the differences between areas in the UK should be much less. This is borne out by the data from Wessex, which covered both urban and rural areas, and revealed that prevalence rates between the two did not differ greatly (Kushlick and Blunden, 1974, op.cit.). Taking account of the Sheffield data, therefore, and remembering that this included 'ESN(M)' school pupils, most of whom would not now be classed as having learning disabilities, the total number of people for whom some special provision might have to be made which was given in that book is reproduced as Table 3.1.

Table 3.1 General estimates of numbers of 'mentally handicapped' people requiring services in a total population of 100,000 (rounded figures)

	Children	*Adults*	*Total*
Severe	69	168	237
Mild	149	104	253
Total	218	272	490

Source: Malin *et al.* (1980, op. cit.)

The 1980 review of progress on the 1971 White Paper (DHSS, 1980) attempted to provide a more 'administrative' definition using the case registers from that White Paper and the more contemporary ones of Sheffield and Lambeth. Their definitions are worth reproducing, since they are probably the last attempt to assess the size of the issue for planning purposes. They approached the case registers, and requested figures which were to:

Include: the following Mentally Handicapped People as needing special services. All those now receiving full time residential care, ESN(S) schooling, day care, or if they are receiving none of these services, having some problems with ambulance, continence or behaviour and not able to feed, wash and dress themselves, [or designated severely subnormal].
Exclude: the following Mentally Handicapped People as not in need of special services. *Children* in ESN(M) schools not covered by the above. *Adults* not covered by the above who are ambulant, continent, have no behavioural problems and can feed, wash and dress themselves. In general these clients have had no contact with the special services for many years except possibly for an occasional visit from the social worker.

(DHSS, 1980, op.cit.)

The DHSS go on to state that this may be an 'over-estimate', though their range from 290 per 100,000 to 340 per 100,000 population is lower than the figure of 490 given by Malin and colleagues (1980). This is largely accounted for by the exclusion, from DHSS figures, of those at ESN(M) schools and those aged 0–4, but still highlights the continuing difficulties of epidemiology in this area.

Let us therefore repeat the purpose of this chapter; it is to enable the reader to have some awareness of the *approximate* scale of the issue of learning disabilities. For those who wish to pursue the detail of epidemiological surveys, Kushlick and Blunden (1974, op.cit.) and Conley (1973, op.cit.) are suitable starting points, though a more interesting question might be to examine why such surveys have not been well maintained. Advice to Local Authorities in 1992, Department of Health (1992), giving a vague range of 120,000 to 160,000 adults with 'learning disabilities' (and thus still accepting the 1980 DHSS figures) lends further weight to the thought that surveys of need, if not matched by resources, can become an embarrassment.

Let us also, before the chapter closes, repeat the warning made earlier regarding the use of such figures. Without some resolution of the debate on appropriate forms of service for people with learning disabilities it is, in our view, a highly dangerous activity to state that such figures therefore show that certain percentages of people 'are, or are not, in need of continuous medical and nursing care' (as, for example, in McKeown and Leck, 1967; Quinn *et al.*, 1974; Kushlick, 1969; Browne *et al.*, 1971; Williams, 1971; National Development Team for the Mentally Handicapped, 1978; Clarke, 1986, op. cit.). Nor should such activities involve predicting, from birth and mortality rate, the numbers who will require care from *existing facilities* in the future (as, for example in Primrose, 1966; Heaton-Ward, 1968; Richards, 1969; Richards and Sylvester, 1969; Royal College of Psychiatry (RCP), 1976). Still less should planning decisions about the needs of individuals be based on generalised statements about which group of people society will tolerate (Primrose, 1971; Browne *et al.*, 1971, op.cit.; RCP, 1976, op.cit.). Effective planning can only come when policy issues are resolved, and as we shall see in the next chapter, policy on provision for people with learning difficulties is still very much a matter for debate.

REFERENCES

Acts of Parliament

Education (Handicapped Children) Act 1970, London, HMSO.

General References

Browne R.A., Gunzburg H.C., Johnston Hannau L.G.W., Maccoll K., Oliver B. and Thomas A. (1971) The needs of patients in subnormality hospitals if discharged to community care, *Brit.J.Ment.Subn.*, 17, 1–18.

Clarke A.D.B. and Clarke A.M. (1975) *Recent Advances in the Study of Subnormality*, 2nd edition, London, MIND.

Clarke D. (1986) *Mentally Handicapped People: Living and Learning*, London, Bailliere Tindall.

Conley R. (1973) *The Economics of Mental Retardation*, Baltimore, Johns Hopkins University Press.

Department of Health (1992) LAC 92 (15), *Social Care for Adults with Learning Disabilities (Mental Handicap)*, London, HMSO.

Department of Health and Social Security (1980) *Mental Handicap: Progress, Problems and Priorities*, London, HMSO.

Grunewald K. (1974) *The Mentally Retarded in Sweden*, Stockholm, The Swedish Institute.

Heaton-Ward W.A. (1968) The life expectation of mentally subnormal patients in hospital, *Brit.J.Psychiat.*, 114, 1591–2.

Kushlick A. (1969) Care of the mentally subnormal, *Lancet*, 2, 1196–7.

Kushlick A. and Blunden R. (1974) The epidemiology of mental subnormality, in Clarke A.M. and Clarke A.D.B. *Mental Deficiency – The Changing Outlook*, 3rd edition, London, Methuen.

Lewis E.O. (1929) Report on an investigation into the incidence of mental deficiency in six areas, 1925–1927, in *Report of the Mental Deficiency Committee, Part IV*, London, HMSO.

Mackay D.N. (1971) Mental subnormality in Northern Ireland, *J. Ment. Def. Res.* 15, 12–19.

McKeown T. and Leck I. (1967) Institutional care of the mentally subnormal, *Brit.Med.J.* 3, 573–6.

Malin N., Race D. and Jones G. (1980) *Services for the Mentally Handicapped in Britain*, London, Croom Helm.

Martindale A. (1975) *Services in Sheffield for the Mentally Handicapped*, Report No. 1, Sheffield case register, Sheffield Area Health Authority.

Martindale A. (1976) A case register as an information system in a development project for the mentally handicapped, *Brit.J.Ment.Subn.*, 20 (2), 70–6.

Meacher M. (1976) Living in harmony, *Community Care*, January 1976, 10–11.

National Development Team for the Mentally Handicapped (1978) *First Report 1976–77*, London, HMSO.

Office of Health Economics (1986) *Mental Handicap - Partnership in the Community*, London, HMSO.

Primrose D.A.A. (1966) Natural history of mental deficiency in a hospital group and in the community it serves, *J.Ment.Def.Res*, 10, 159–89.

Primrose D.A.A. (1971) A survey of 502 consecutive admissions to subnormality hospital from 1st January 1968 to 31st December 1970, *Brit.J.Ment.Subn.*, 17, 25–8.

Quinn M., Martindale A. and Hunter E. (1974) Community accommodation for the mentally handicapped, *Brit.J.Ment.Subn*, 20, Part 2, 86–9.

Richards B.W. (1969) Age trends in mental deficiency institutions, *J.Ment.Def.Res.*, 13, 171–83.

Richards B.W. and Sylvester P.E. (1969) Mortality trends in mental deficiency institutions, *J.Ment.Def.Res*, 13, 276–92.

Royal College of Psychiatry (RCP) Mental Deficiency Section (1976) Memorandum on the present and future development and organisation of mental handicap services, *Brit.J.Psychiat*, News and notes, August 1976.

Swann W. (1986) *Special Needs in Education*, Milton Keynes, Open University Press.

Tizard J. (1964) *Community Services for the Mentally Handicapped*, London, Oxford University Press.

Williams C. (1971) A study of the patients in a group of mental subnormality hospitals, *Brit.J.Ment.Subn*, 17, Part 1.

Wing L. and Fryers B. (1975) *Psychiatric Services in Camberwell and Salford, 1964–1973*, Salford, Salford Area Health Authority.

4   Historical development of service provision

David Race

People with learning disabilities are typically marked out from the rest of their immediate society by an inability to cope satisfactorily in that society. Awareness of problems they may have, and the steps taken to remedy them, inevitably reflect the standards of behaviour demanded by the peer group and the wider society, and the tolerance of deviation from those standards. It is not surprising, therefore, that in many countries outside what is called the 'developed' world, the issue of learning disabilities is little studied, still less provided for, since the level of poverty of the bulk of the population, combined with the less complex technical demands of a non-industrial state, means that people with learning disabilities are less susceptible to being labelled 'abnormal'.

As well as the lack of technological development, with its concomitant demands on the coping power of the individual, rural and tribal societies have, as a generality, tended to display a greater acceptance of responsibility for their few severely handicapped members. Similarly, in the United Kingdom prior to the industrial revolution, the 'problem' of learning disabilities did not exist to such an extent. Most villages were able to cope with the 'idiots' in their midst, sometimes at the expense of ridicule and exploitation, sometimes with an almost reverent regard for their simplicity.

With the industrial revolution, however, came large towns, the crowding together of workers dependent on the local factory, mill or pit for their livelihood, and the measurement of people by their ability to cope with the new technological and commercial processes. In addition, there came an increase in education, and in the need for the more abstract skills of reading and writing to be mastered if any sort of social status was to be achieved.

The person with learning disabilities thus began to stand out as being educationally and practically of low competence, but not, in the greater part of the nineteenth century, a specific threat to society, or a specifically undesirable person. Certainly many people with various handicaps were incarcerated in workhouses, along with all the unemployed or unemployable poor of most parishes, but there also prevailed a mood of optimism in academic circles concerning the educability of those classified as 'idiots' or 'imbeciles'. The first impetus came from the continent, with Itard's much publicised training of *The Wild Boy of Aveyron* (1801). This was a youth found running on all fours in the wood whom Itard managed to imbue with a few basic skills by arousing interest and attention in the boy and then teaching by imitation. Itard's pupil Seguin took his theories further and proposed the hypothesis that 'idiots and imbeciles' had the use of their intellectual faculties but lacked the power to apply them because of a lack of resistance to competing stimuli.

Itard's, and then Seguin's, fundamental technique was to attract and keep their subject's attention prior to education and therefore the pioneering institutions of such people as Guggenbuhl in Switzerland and Reed in England were designed as places where the people with learning disabilities could be kept in conditions amenable to their 'training and education'. The fact that the asylums also separated people from their community was really secondary in the minds of the early workers. Their basic premise was that, given suitable attention and training, 'idiots' or 'imbeciles' were capable of learning simple tasks, sufficient to enable them to survive in certain parts of society. The prospects for development of this training and education therefore seemed bright, despite the fact that the confused terminology of the Lunatic Asylums Act of 1853 and the Idiots Act of 1886 meant that many authorities fulfilled their duties under the latter Act to provide 'care, education and training' in special asylums by putting all their mentally disordered people in the same place.

The bright prospects of a developing service for people with learning disabilities were, however, dimmed at the turn of the century, by a complete change of outlook on the part of leaders of opinion in the scientific and medical world. The change was, in essence, from optimism about the potential for education to a belief that such education was not possible except in a limited way and that 'the handicapped' would always be a drain on society. To this pessimism was added the fear that the 'drain' would increase, because of the supposed excessive reproduction of people with learning disabilities. Tizard (1958) is of the view that the two major events which caused this change of opinion and 'set back the service by fifty years' were the beginnings of the science of genetics and the development, by Binet in Paris, of a standardised instrument to 'measure intelligence' (see Chapter 1). This idea of an inherited intellectual ability, which is unaltered by training or education, was not new at the turn of the century, but it was in the minority until the detailed work of Binet, attacking the 'empiricism' of his pre-decessors and calling for a 'scientific' approach to education, persuaded many of the invariance of basic 'intelligence'. Since he also provided them with a 'scientific' test with which to measure this inherent ability, it is not surprising that Binet's name is still associated with the 'innate intelligence' school, and with the opinion that certain people are 'ineducable', which held sway in this country for the first half of this century. In fact, as O'Connor (1965) points out, Binet himself published the view that 'defectives' could and should be taught to read, although this would take longer to achieve than for a normal person, for the sheer practical usefulness this would give them.

Nevertheless, the opinion germinated by Binet at the turn of the century took hold of medical opinion and was fostered by the 'eugenic' ideas then beginning to circulate. Undoubtedly the leader of opinion in this field was Tredgold, who published the first edition of his *Textbook of Mental Deficiency* in 1908, and was a member of the Royal Commission that reported in that year. Many studies appeared at this time which appeared to provide sound evidence of the 'inheritance of mental defect' together with the observation of a relatively high birth rate among the poor and handicapped sections of the population. This led to the view given by Tredgold, in his famous paper in the *Eugenics Review* (1909) that segregation to prevent propagation was the only way to protect society. He says:

> 1. In the first place the chief evil we have to prevent is undoubtedly that of propagation. 2. Next, society must be protected against such of these persons as either have definite criminal tendencies, or are of so facile a disposition that they readily commit crimes at the instigation of others. 3. Lastly, even where these poor creatures are relatively harmless, we have to protect society from the burden due to their non-productiveness.
>
> (Tredgold, 1909)

In this view people with learning disabilities were at worst a danger, at best a burden, to society. Tredgold's view on the means to alleviate this problem then follow.

> I have come to the conclusion that, in the case of the majority of the feeble-minded, there is one measure, and one measure only, which will fulfil all these *desiderata* and which is at the same time practically possible, namely the establishment of suitable farm and industrial colonies . . . Society would thus be saved a portion, at least, of the cost of their maintenance, and more important, it would be secure from their depredation and danger of their propagation.
>
> (Tredgold, 1909)

There is no doubt that this view was highly influential in the formation of the ensuing Mental Deficiency Act, despite certain vigorous objections in Parliament. These objections had arisen at the appearance in 1912 of a Mental Deficiency Bill, with very solid eugenic views, including a clause prohibiting the marriage of any person held to be 'mentally defective'. Although opposition caused this Bill to be withdrawn that year, a new Bill, leading to the Act of 1913, was, in many respects, harsher than the original. The clause prohibiting marriage had disappeared, but instead great stress was laid on the proposed facilities for keeping people in institutions once they had been admitted. At this time, following the Local Government Act of 1886, all asylums were controlled by county councils, and their Boards of Control were given powers under the new Act to prevent discharge of anyone they thought unfit to leave. This power of detention was the more contested when it was seen how, and which individuals were made 'subject to be dealt with'.

Section 2 of the 1913 Act provided that a person who was 'a defective' might be dealt with by being sent to an institution for defectives or placed under guardianship:

(a) at the instance of his parent or guardian;
(b) if in addition to being a defective he was a person:
(i) who was found neglected, abandoned, or without visible means of support, or cruelly treated or . . . in need of care or training which could not be provided in his home; or
(ii) who was found guilty of any criminal offence, or who was ordered to be sent to an approval school;
(iii) who was undergoing imprisonment, or was in an approved school; or
(iv) who was an habitual drunkard; or
(v) who had been found incapable of receiving education at school, or that by reason of a disability of mind might require supervision after leaving school.

If a parent or guardian was attempting to place their child in an institution, they required two medical certificates from qualified medical practitioners, one of whom was approved for the purpose by the local health authority or the Minister of Health. The other reasons for 'a defective' being sent to an institution (i.e. (b) above) could be cited by a number of people, for example, relatives, friends or a local authority officer, in a petition to a 'judicial authority' again accompanied by two medical certificates. An order for admission lasted for one year. After that time the Board of Control was provided with reports on the person by the 'visitors' of the institution and by the medical officer of the institution, stating whether they should continue to be detained. If they were, the order was continued for a further year, and then for five-year periods. The Board of Control retained the ultimate power to decide whether a person should be discharged.

Although the caveat 'in addition to being a defective' is used above, and in the definition of a 'moral defective' used in the Act, it is certain that, following the initial inertia brought about by the First World War, many people who had merely exhibited the behaviour described in Section 2(b), without necessarily having learning disabilities, were committed to institutions. 'Certification' had a permanence about it, probably enhanced by the prevailing views of invariance of intellectual abilities and certainly compounded by the essentially subjective nature of the definitions of the Act. The motivation behind the Act was segregation of undesirable social 'inefficients' and, to a large extent, this was achieved. The Act applied to both children and adults, and part of the new power to be exercised by the local authority was to ascertain the numbers of children who were incapable, by reason of 'mental defect', of benefiting from the instruction in special schools or classes which had been set up in a small way under the Elementary Education (Defective and Epileptic Children) Act of 1899. From an early age, therefore, people with learning disabilities could be certified as incapable of benefiting from any education, likely to be a burden on society, both in terms of draining its resources and lowering its stock, and thus subject to permanent detention in an institution. This is the extreme, of course, but it should also be remembered that the Mental Deficiency Act remained essentially the same until 1959, and there are many people, even 35 years later, in institutions who were committed under this Act (including, in a notable case, relatives of the Royal Family). For a graphic personal account, see Barron (1989).

After the First World War and for the ensuing twenty years, more and more people became 'subject to be dealt with' under the Mental Deficiency Acts. Tredgold (1952) gives figures for those under the various forms of care provided by the Acts (Table 4.1) and these show that between the wars the number 'requiring care' rose more than sevenfold. The pressure this put on the institutional services meant that, for primarily economic reasons, the size of institutions grew, until as O'Connor (1965, op.cit.) notes, 'the tendency to build large institutions for about 2,000 patients in isolated country areas was a definite policy'.

Table 4.1 Total number of 'defectives' under the care and control of the Mental Deficiency Acts

Year	Total no. (rounded)
1920	12,000
1926	37,000
1939	90,000
1950	100,000

Source: Tredgold, A.F., *A Textbook on Mental Deficiency* (1952)

O'Connor might have added that economy also brought about the conversion of large numbers of workhouses and lunatic asylums into the category of 'suitable' institutions. The essence of this policy, however, was, as Tredgold had demanded, for the large and isolated 'colony' to be set up. The Report of the Mental Deficiency Committee (the Wood Report, 1929) sums up the position with frightening clarity.

The modern institution is generally a large one, preferably built on a colony plan, takes defectives of all grades of defect and all ages. All, of course, are properly classified according to their mental capacity and age. The Local Mental Deficiency Authority has to provide for all grades of defect, all types of care and all ages, and an institution that cannot, or will not, take this case for one reason and that case for another is of no use to the Authority. An institution which takes all types of ages is economical because the high-grade patients do the work and make everything necessary, not only for themselves, but also for the lower grade. In an institution taking only lower grades, the whole of the work has to be done by paid staff; in one taking only high grades the output of work is greater than is required for the institution itself and there is difficulty in disposing of it. In the all-grade institution, on the other hand, the high-grade patients are the skilled workmen of the colony, those who do all the higher processes of manufacture, those on whom there is a considerable measure of responsibility; the medium-grade patients are the labourers, who do the more simple routine work in the training shops and about the institution; the best of the lower-grade patients fetch and carry or do the very simple work.

(Wood Report, 1929)

The inter-war years were not, of course, noted for great developments in enlightened attitudes to the unfortunate members of society. Economic pressures brought a much more demanding dichotomy between the 'deserving' and 'undeserving' poor, and the hard times can be said to have had their effect on thinking in the field of learning disabilities. The eugenics movement continued to be active, especially in academic and medical circles, and its more extreme end found a ready outlet in Germany, and a ready vehicle for a policy of euthanasia in the Nazi party. The work of Binding and Hoche, published in 1920, was one of many academic papers advocating the disposal of those 'unfit' who were a burden on society. With the coming to power of Hitler and his party, the way was cleared for an active *'euthanasie'* policy that was to prove the prototype for the holocaust (Wolfensberger, 1987).

In the United Kingdom the combination of the prevailing view of permanent inadequacy with, it must be remembered, a service which depended on maintenance of numbers for continued financial support, left little changed by the end of the Second World War. The works of Burt and Penrose were the only noticeable English contributions to the literature in the twenties and thirties and these were mainly devoted to the study of the aetiology and classification of 'mental deficiency' rather than desirable forms of care for the existing population.

After the Second World War, however, research findings began to have some influence on opinion regarding the potential for employment of people with learning disabilities. It is interesting to note that most of these studies originated from outside the contemporary bodies who were directly responsible for the institutions in which most people were housed. Within the direct caring professions, however, the pessimistic pre-war views were maintained. This is important when consideration is given to the fact that many of those undergoing training in the late forties and fifties are now in positions of considerable responsibility within the system of care provision for people with learning disabilities (see Heaton-Ward (1989) for a graphic illustration of this point). In 1948 implementation of the National Health Service Act of 1946 passed control of certified institutions from local councils to the Minister of Health and, through him, to the Regional Hospital Boards set up by that Act. 'Colonies' became 'hospitals' overnight and trainee nurses, administrators and doctors in the new health service would consider in their studies the accumulated wisdom of 40 years of segregation. Tredgold seems to take most of the brickbats for the views of his day, but this is not surprising when statements such as those found as late as the eighth (1952) edition of his *Textbook* are considered in terms of their effect on the development of attitudes of some current senior staff dealing with people with learning disabilities. Thus, on euthanasia of 'the 80,000 or more idiots or imbeciles in the country' he writes,

> These are not only incapable of being employed to any economic advantage, but their care and support, whether in their own home or in institutions, absorb a large amount of the time, energy and money of the normal population which could be utilised to better purposes. Moreover, many of these defectives are utterly helpless, repulsive in appearance and revolting in manners. Their existence is a perpetual source of sorrow and unhappiness to their parents, and those who live at home have a most disturbing influence upon other children and family life. With the present shortage of institutional accommodation there are hundreds of mothers who are literally worn out in caring for these persons at home. In my opinion it would be an economical and humane procedure were their existence to be painlessly terminated.
>
> (Tredgold, 1952)

Even on a less contentious matter than preservation of the 'fitter' stock, one of the issues on which the world had just gone to war (though, interestingly, no punishment for the German euthanasia programme seems to have been handed out at Nuremberg), students in the forties and fifties would read on the matter of employability that 'we may at once dismiss idiots and imbeciles, for although the latter may be occupied in certain routine tasks, their financial value is practically nil' (Tredgold, 1952, op.cit.). In education, too, the 1944 Education Act, set up with some considerable influence from Burt, had continued to define a class of children as 'incapable of receiving education at school' and these were to be excluded from the 'universal' education system set up by that Act.

Within the ranks of those involved with direct caring for people with learning disabilities, therefore, the pessimism of the inter-war years remained. From others, mainly psychologists in England, came findings which suggested that improvements were possible at all levels of 'defect'. These, combined with direct observation and several inquiries into the state of mental hospitals in the fifties, led to a change of view in some quarters to something approaching optimism for patients' capabilities and criticisms of the perceived inadequacies of the existing provision for them. It also of course, provided a vehicle for the fledgling psychology profession to flex their muscles against the power of the medical and psychiatric establishment.

The Second World War had provided, in the form of those rejected for military service on 'mental deficiency' grounds, an easily available sample of 'defectives' for study. In America, a number of 'follow-up' studies had already been started before the war, observing the successes and failures in society of those judged 'mentally deficient' at school. Kingsley and Hyde (1945) studied 600 people rejected by the military for reasons of mental deficiency. They found that a majority, more than the authors expected, were both socially and economically self-supporting. Charles (1953) in his careful study following Baller's (1936) group of persons adjudged mentally deficient traced 151 of the original 206. Among his findings on this group he discovered that 80 per cent were married, with less children per family than the national average, few of whom were themselves 'retarded'. Eighty-three per cent of the follow-up samples were considered to be self-supporting and Charles concludes that the prognoses for these people had been unduly pessimistic. Similar results were produced by Hartzler (1951) who found that 73 per cent of girls discharged from a state institution were wholly or partially successful in adjustment to life in the community. All of the above authors stressed the importance of emotional factors in the ability to adjust, a conclusion confirmed by Hiatt (1951) in his report on successful placements of 'defectives'. Garrison (1951) found that improvements in social skills and attitudes could be achieved by a programme of training, and once again, achievement was not related to IQ level.

In England, the work of Tizard, O'Connor and the Clarkes dominated a number of studies concerning the potential of 'mental defectives', and the higher than expected IQ levels to be found among inmates of mental hospitals. O'Connor and Tizard (1954) surveyed a 2 per cent sample of patients in twelve mental deficiency institutions. The average IQ of the 'feeble-minded' group (remembering the classification of the 1913 Act) was over 70, and 50 per cent of the sample were reported as not requiring special nursing or supervisory care. This survey followed the authors' earlier criticisms of existing training methods in hospitals as being irrelevant to outside employment, and as seriously underestimating the potential of the trainees for working in the community (Tizard and O'Connor, 1952). The criticisms were supported by more concrete evidence from Hilliard (1954) who observed 175 female 'defectives' in a ten-year experiment to find them work in the community and give them generally greater freedom than was available in the institution. Hilliard concludes from this study that certification was a waste of potential. The same author found, in another study of admissions to a large hospital, that higher than expected IQ levels existed amongst the patients (Hilliard and Mundy, 1954). He again concluded that hospitals were not the right place for many of these people and called for more accurate diagnoses and more effective rehabilitation.

The Clarkes, after challenging the supposition of permanent defect as measured by an IQ test (Clarke and Clarke, 1953, 1954) set up a series of experiments with various colleagues, to examine the learning potential of the 'ineducable imbeciles and idiots'. In an early paper, Clarke and Hermelin (1955) quote the views of Tredgold and others on the lack of potential for industrial work possessed by 'imbeciles' and then report experimental work showing them capable of various assembly and other industrial tasks after training. The Social Psychiatry Research Unit set up in two mental deficiency hospitals, started to organise sub-contracted industrial work for the patients and various experimental results were obtained on the employment potential of people with learning disabilities. General aspects are discussed by O'Connor and Tizard (1956) but specific studies showed that there was definite potential for learning industrial tasks, not related to IQ, and improved by incentives (Claridge and O'Connor, 1957; O'Connor and Claridge, 1958; Gordon, *et al.*, 1954, 1955). Separate work by Walton and Begg (1958) confirmed the effect of incentives on performance and noted the sometimes forgotten fact that first performances of a task were not always the best. In America, along with further follow-up studies of successful rehabilitation (Harold, 1955; Fry, 1956; Krishef and Hall, 1955), the effects were always being studied. Gottsegen (1957) used the Vineland Society Maturity Scale to plan an educational programme and found improvements in 'social age' after training had been given. Smith (1957) reported on the introduction of sheltered employment in an institution and Cromwell and Moss (1959) note the effect of incentives on improving performance.

With the backing of their own studies, researchers were not only demonstrating the potential ability of people with learning disabilities, but were beginning to criticise, either implicitly or explicitly, the facilities for care in existence during the fifties. More studies by Clarke and others began to associate the environmental background, which included the institutions, with IQ and other measurements of ability, and found associations between stimulating environments and performance (Clarke *et al.*, 1958; Clarke and Clarke, 1959). The psychologists' ideal environment at that time was described by Gunzburg (1957) who saw the hospital primarily as a rehabilitation centre, preparing people with handicaps for community living.

The change of mood amongst research workers was, therefore, well established in the fifties, to one of confidence in the abilities of people with learning disabilities to respond to training and fulfil useful tasks in industrial employment. This did not, however, transmit itself to most of those directly involved with caring for people with learning disabilities, or for those with power over admission and discharge from hospital. It is significant that the major causes of the Royal Commission on the Law Relating to Mental Illness and Mental Deficiency and subsequent legislation were the more negative ones of bad conditions in hospitals, more particularly for people with mental health problems, and allegedly wrongful detention of certain people. The bad conditions were reported in terms of general inhumanity to the inmates, rather than a lack of opportunity for rehabilitation. The National Council for Civil Liberties (1951) published details of several cases of alleged wrongful detention under the 1913 Act which, together with the activities of the newly formed National Association for Parents of Backward Children (now MENCAP, the Royal Society for Mentally Handicapped Children and Adults), brought public attention to the way the Mental Deficiency Acts were operating and to the sort of institutions in which people were being detained. A report of the King Edward's Hospital Fund in 1955 summarised the position:

> In general it may be said that the average age of the mental hospitals is well over 50 years and that the majority date from the time when the mentally ill (*sic*) were looked on primarily as potential dangers to the community . . . some of these nineteenth and early-twentieth century build-ings and airing grounds suggest than 'prison' would be a truer designation even than 'asylum'. Second to the protection of the community came the custodial care of the inmates. These were herded in enormous wards, of a size not found in any other type of hospital, with cells for the solitary confinement of the more disturbed patients. Sometimes dormitories were provided for the patients from two or three wards and contained perhaps 160 beds or more in close-packed rows. Patients were not expected to have any possessions, and no lockers were provided. In some hospitals, the patients' clothes were still rolled and tied to their beds at night, since no storage space is provided for them. Washing, bathing and toilet facilities were primitive and inadequate, even by the standards of the last century, and, in some cases, have remained so until the present day. Overcrowding occurs to a degree unknown in other hospitals.
>
> (King Edward's Hospital Fund, 1955)

The extremely poor physical conditions and the permanent detention of patients was, therefore, the main motivation behind the pressures for change given in the evidence to the Royal Commission. This was not confined to the United Kingdom, and, at the same time as the Royal Commission was sitting, the World Health Organization published a report by its Joint Expert Committee (1954) giving guiding principles on mental deficiency legislation. These can be summarised as follows:

(1) The main function of legislation should be protective – children must be protected against cruelty, adolescents against exploitation, families against the pressure of a handicapped child and the community against antisocial actions.

(2) Over-protection should be avoided, and the law reviewed regularly in this connection.

(3) Legislation for children with learning difficulties should, as far as possible, be made within the framework of legislation protecting all children.

(4) In the same way duties enforced on local authorities should be for the care of all children.

(5) Total responsibility, amounting to legal guardianship, may be necessary in some cases.

(6) Legislation should ensure that adequate supervision of institutions is provided.

(7) Legislation regarding admission and detention should be carefully considered to avoid, on the one hand, total loss of control of parental rights where this is unnecessary, and, on the other, exploitation by unscrupulous or incompetent parents.

(8) Legal compulsory detention should only be adopted as a last resort.

(9) A distinction should be drawn up between, and different provision provided for, 'the mentally ill and mentally handicapped'.

(World Health Organization, 1954)

Notice that even this 'ideal' state of legislation contains no recommendations as to the type of care to be provided for the 'protection' of people with learning disabilities nor any duty to ensure adequate education or employment for them. Its main concern, like the Royal Commission, was with the compulsory detention of patients and the responsibilities of the administering authorities. Thus, though the report of the Commission spends some time on the ideal of a move towards 'community care', the major conclusions, and the major effect of the 1959 Mental Health Act, was to abolish, except in certain defined circumstances, the *compulsory* detention of the newly, and as has been noted, confusingly, created categories of 'mentally disordered' persons. 'Informal admission' and the removal of 'certification' were the two key measures in what became known as the 'open door' policy, and much of the Act is taken up with procedures for compulsory admission, courts of protection and review tribunals, etc. In terms of provision, no specific methods of care are proposed, the only clue to action being in paragraph 6 of the Act, wherein local health authorities are required to exercise an existing duty of Section 28 of the National Health Service Act 1946 for 'disordered persons' in the following way:

(a) the provision, equipment and maintenance of residential accommodation and the care of persons for the time being resident in accommodation so provided;

(b) the provision of centres or other facilities for training or occupation, and the equipment and maintenance of such centres;

(c) the appointment of officers to act as mental welfare officers under the following provision of this Act;

(d) the exercise by the local health authority of their functions under the following provisions of this Act in respect of persons placed under guardianship thereunder . . . and

(e) the provision of any ancillary or supplementary service for, or for the benefit of any such persons as are referred to in subsection (1) of this Act.

It is worth noting that although this provision was imposed as a duty on the local health authorities, in practice the care of those in need of accommodation remained in the hands of the Ministry of Health through the hospital service as administered by Regional Hospital Boards and their appointed Hospital Management Committees. This was because local interpretation of the duty to provide 'residential accommodation' and 'training or occupation' was, in some cases, restricted merely to the appointment of mental welfare officers to deal with admissions to, and discharges from, the local mental hospital. These, incidentally, were now 'undesignated', i.e. they could admit all forms of 'mentally disordered' persons, both those with mental health problems and those with learning disabilities. Other authorities did make more of an attempt to meet their prescribed duties under the Act, but were, of course, suffering from the lack of a base of capital provision on which to build. Thus, with the 'residential' side taken care of by hospitals, those authorities doing anything at all after the 1959 Act tended to concentrate on setting up training centres, both 'Junior' for 'ineducable' children and 'Adult' for all those over the school-leaving age (then 15). For many reasons, therefore, the 1959 Mental Health Act was unpopular with a significant group of those concerned with people with learning disabilities, the major reason being that it effectively maintained the status quo of the large hospital as the alternative in terms of residence to keeping the person at home. The stigma of 'certification' had been removed, some of the fears of 'unlawful' detention had been removed, but the institutions remained. As in the fifties, the major disagreements came from outside the direct caring services. The 'psychologists' group' continued to publish their results on progress of handicapped people in acquiring skills, given adequate training and stimulating environment (Clarke and Blakemore, 1961; Gunzburg, 1961; Claridge, 1961). From within the services, which mainly meant the psychiatric consultants, sentiments were much more mixed. Some of this group were opposed to any infringement of the right of the clinician to the ultimate decision over the provision of service, and viewed with alarm the planned number of 'hostels' being allowed into the ten-year plan for England and Wales (Ministry of Health, 1962). 'Hostels' were, in any case, not yet in an established form, and the only definition in operation by the end of the fifties was essentially that of 'residential accommodation in small units'. However, by comparison with hospitals of 500 beds and more, quite a large number may be considered 'small'. Generally, however, hostel size became determined by a mixture of cost-conscious efforts at economies of scale, published material on the likely numbers requiring care in a local authority setting, and reproduction of an established pattern of size or provision for other long-stay groups, e.g. children in care.

Jones *et al.* (1979) note a political move at this time, in a 'somewhat intemperate speech', by Enoch Powell, the Minister of Health, announcing in 1961 'the run down of the mental hospital'. Though Jones calls this a 'real shift of emphasis' it should be remembered that the speech concerned a number of groups, not just people with learning disabilities. Equally, the publication of the so-called Blue Book 'Health and Welfare: the Development of Community Care' in 1963 saw very general advice to Local Authorities, and had no earmarked funding – as an interesting foretaste of events twenty years later it is worth noting the opposition to Enoch Powell's speech from Professor Richard Titmuss, on the ground that the 'primary motive was economic'. In reality, effects were felt much more quickly in the areas of mental health and services to elderly people. In terms of people with learning disabilities, other events were to push the debate forward.

A major influence on the future design of hostel provision was the experimental unit set up at Slough by the National Society of Mentally Handicapped Children (Baranjay, 1971). Although the 'Slough experiment' had a much wider intention than mere residential care, being combined with an on-site training centre and run as an experiment in 'social training' for maximum functioning in the community, there is no doubt that the residential facilities at Slough had a considerable influence on the size of hostels over the next decade. This is not to give the impression of a spate of new buildings in the sixties. As mentioned earlier, many authorities, faced with the choice between training centres for the many or hostels for the few, chose to invest in the former, and by the time of publication of the White Paper in 1971 the government admitted that 'residential accommodation is still far short of what is needed'. Thus, in the sixties, most people with learning disabilities in need of residential accommodation continued to be housed in hospital. To use one particular set of figures for the moment, from the 1971 White Paper, 52,100 in-patient beds were provided in 1969 for adults in NHS hospitals and 4,850 places in 'community' residential care. The latter figure included various forms of accommodation, and is not totally made up of new buildings. Given this sort of difference in quantity of provision, it is not surprising that much influence on the development of services in the sixties continued to be exercised by the medical profession, maintaining the 'medical model' of care for people with learning disabilities as the service for the majority with a selected few subject to the new provision of 'community care' in hostels and local authority training centres.

This was despite more studies being published on the success of rehabilitation experiments and the continuing debate on the appropriateness of an institutional environment to provide the sort of training necessary for such rehabilitation. It should be remembered, of course, that the studies already noted had shown that many people certified under the 1913 Act as 'moral defectives' or 'feeble-minded' had much higher IQ levels and greater chances of success in the community than those in the field expected and thus experiments in the sixties, particularly on rehabilitation, may have been biased by the contemporary hospital population.

As well as these specific studies however, several authors used their findings to join the debate on a general level. As usual, there is a variation from very little hospital care being proposed to very little community care, and this seems to depend on the authors' proximity to the hospital service. Near one end of the spectrum, Tizard (1964) made out the case for 'an approach to the problem of organising residential care for the mentally subnormal which is based upon small residential units, closely associated with the day care services of a particular area'. This would cover all grades of 'defect' and replace the hospital-oriented approach, with nursing care only being provided for chair and bed-fast patients. Using Kushlick's (1961) data, Tizard estimated that this latter group could be housed in a 20–40-bedded hospital annexe of a normal hospital. Dutton (1963) adopted a more conservative approach and proposed three different streams, to be given a programme of training. Only the top stream, however, were thought by the author to be capable of returning to the community, and he does not give any estimates of numbers in each stream. A similar approach was adopted by Galloway and Garratt (1964) in their division of the 'mentally handicapped' into three 'care types' with associated provision. The first group, defined as the 'nursing care' group, should, as the name implies, stay in hospital. The second group is defined as those in need of 'control', i.e. those with dangerous or criminal propensities. For this group the authors recommend special secure units. For the third group, those simply in need of 'training', small (20–25 adults) units in the community are recommended. Once again the precise numbers in each group are not well defined. The authors also recommend that the planning units for such care should be the local health authority rather than the Regional Hospital Boards, a fairly radical suggestion for the field of learning disabilities, but one which was gaining momentum in the debate, if not the practice, of care provision. To some, the fact that the debate was taking place implied a change of practice. Pilkington (1964a) summarises the changing role of the hospital, and advocates a joint approach, i.e. hospital and community services, to the problem, reviewing the literature on rehabilitation. However, the implications of his subsequent paper (1964b) in terms of the progress made towards a community care service are rather optimistic when faced with the reality of the day.

In fact very few alternatives to hospital care existed, and the rehabilitation debate turned to the more detailed subject of the appropriate orientation of training rather than the general discussion of whether the right sort of basic residential provision was being planned. It is true that the early work of Tizard's group and the Clarkes had let to a fashion for 'industrially-oriented' workshops in hospitals, and there was now a need for some debate on the appropriateness of this type of training for effective rehabilitation. Thus Speyer (1964) as well as arguing for more training in general, also pointed out the need for comprehensive training, in social as well as industrial skills, for rehabilitation to be successful. Schiphorst (1964) took up the same theme in his argument against the industrial bias of workshops, and, of course, the basis of the Slough experiment (Baranjay, 1971 op.cit.) was to provide a 'comprehensive social and industrial training centre for community care of the mentally handicapped'. The major contributor to the 'social training' movement was Gunzburg. Early versions of his 'Progress Assessment Charts' appeared in the sixties (Gunzburg, 1960; Matthew, 1964), and by the time his detailed work on the subject appeared (Gunzburg, 1968), the charts were in widespread use. In the context of the development of services for people with learning disabilities the significance of the charts is in their general view of social skills being fundamental to rehabilitation.

Gunzburg was concerned with isolation of people with learning disabilities through their lack of socially acceptable abilities. He tended to concentrate on training these skills as an end in itself without initially worrying too much about the precise location, size and organisational pattern of the training and care provision. Various supporting studies emphasised the need for social training, including work training (Price, 1967; Williams, 1967; Moorman 1967), but, like the early works of Gunzburg, they did not consider any precise specification of the type of provision. Later in the sixties and on into the seventies, Gunzburg, with his wife, did become involved with the architecture of environments for the handicapped (A.L. Gunzburg, 1967; Gunzburg and Gunzburg, 1973) but these works still avoid the argument about responsibility for care, and the continuing use of the 'medical model'.

In practical terms, therefore, though the experimenters of the fifties had demonstrated the ability of people with learning disabilities to learn social and industrial skills given adequate training and a stimulating environment, the sixties were noticeable more for a debate on the *desirability* of rehabilitation, a joint approach to care, and the appropriate training to be carried out, than for any real changes in the pattern of direct care provision. This was especially true, as noted earlier, in the case of residential provision, where the large subnormality hospital continued to have a dominant influence on the type of care provided. It is therefore not surprising that studies should continue to be published reaffirming the criticisms of existing institutions and making pleas for more stimulating environments (for example, Tizard, 1966; Cortazzi, 1969; Morris, 1969), and that the finding of Morris's large-scale study of hospitals should have received such attention. In this study the author reported on a sociological survey of 35 subnormality hospitals in England and Wales which had as its object 'to discover what is actually happening in a given situation as well as what it said to be happening, or what is thought ought to be happening'.

Her findings were highly critical of the provision for people with learning disabilities in subnormality hospitals and though she notes the state of transition of service for such people in terms of 'concepts of care', her overriding conclusion, in agreement with the view expressed above, is that 'if the philosophy of treatment is changing, our findings clearly indicate that this is not paralleled by similar changes in the provision available for subnormal patients'.

Remembering the King Edward's Hospital Fund Survey (1955) quoted earlier, hospital provision over the decade between this and Morris's survey (1969) does not appear to have changed greatly. Morris's findings may be summarised as follows, quoting her own words where appropriate.

1 *Physical condition*
'Generally speaking, however, it would be true to say that a high proportion of patients live in buildings which are dilapidated and decrepit, two-thirds of which were put up before 1900 . . . Inside these barrack-like edifices, over one-third of the patients sleep in dormitories of 60 or more, often with only a few inches between the beds and with no room for any other furniture. Patients are not encouraged to have personal possessions; there is nowhere to keep or display them. Physically the day rooms are in rather better condition, but most are too large to be "homely" and do not have sufficient arm-chairs or settees to enable all patients to sit comfortably at the same time. Provisions in sanitary annexes are often extremely rudimentary, being deficient in lavatories and baths, as well as totally lacking in opportunities for privacy.'

2 *Nursing needs of patients*
Morris estimates that over 80 per cent of patients are ambulant and 'apart from epilepsy, the amount of serious physical or mental illness amongst them appears to be small'.

3 *Assessment of patients*
Although acknowledging the deficiencies of IQ tests, Morris points out that such tests are little used in hospitals and that 'furthermore, no alternative methods of assessing capacity are applied in these hospitals'.

4 *Objectives of treatment*
Morris found little agreement amongst the staff of the hospitals regarding treatment objectives. The author's findings indicate that 'for the vast majority of patients, the objective consequences of hospitalisation are those of containment and the relief of familial incapacity to provide care'.

5 *Staff resources*
Because of a shortage of nurses, on average one nurse on duty to 16 patients, 'there is a tendency for the resources of nursing staff to be directed towards those in greatest physical need'. As well as a shortage of basic nursing staff, Morris also found an acute shortage of specialist staff for training and education.

6 *Communications between staff*
When concluding that only a small number of patients benefit from specialist help, Morris does not put all the blame on a lack of resources, but points to the 'construction of channels of communication' within the hospital. 'There appears to be virtually no cross-fertilisation of ideas between medical, nursing and specialist staff.'

7 *The isolation of subnormality hospitals*
Noting the physical location of most hospitals, 'far from the nearest town or village' Morris points to the effect this has on visits from friends and relatives, and to the lack of any identity with a local community felt by the patients. In addition, she notes that the physical barrier is increased by staff

attitudes to outsiders who 'be they relatives, friends, voluntary organisations or interested individuals, are not really welcomed as visitors and there is little opportunity for them to offer personal service to the hospital'. It comes as no surprise when it is further learnt that whilst most patients have living relatives, more than one-third of them had not been visited or gone home during the twelve months preceding the research visit.

Morris's study has been summarised at length, not only because of its important place in the development of attitudes to care for people with learning disabilities, but also because it describes very fully the situation that existed for some 90 per cent of those in residential care in 1969 despite almost two decades of research findings indicating alternatives to hospital provision.

Although Morris's report cast grave doubt on the hospital (at least as then organised) as the appropriate environment for people with learning disabilities, it was again more basic failings of particular hospital regimes which drew public attention to the hospital issue. In fact, Morris's book appeared shortly after one of a number of inquiries into psychiatric hospitals which were to appear over the ensuing years (this particular inquiry, into allegations of cruelty and neglect, was published as the Howe Report, 1969) and for a short time the matter was given the full glare of national publicity. This had little immediate effect in practice, however, though it did win the support of an able and forthright minister, Richard Crossman, to the cause of improving conditions in hospitals. As he reveals in his diaries though (Crossman, 1977), even ministerial support does not always bring about great changes when faced with a solidly established service. Incidentally, the diaries also reveal the reluctance of officials in the Department of Health to publish the Howe Report, and the fact that they, as a Department, had been aware of conditions at the hospital concerned for some time before the inquiry was instigated.

Crossman's main contribution was, first, to give some impetus to improvements in the physical conditions of hospitals and secondly, again after much resistance from the Department, to set up a Hospital Advisory Service, reporting directly to the Minister. Both of these efforts, however, took place during the last years of a Labour government, and were only put into effect in the main, after Crossman had left the DHSS following the Conservative victory in 1970. For those more directly concerned with people with learning disabilities, the debate returned to the level of published argument. The spectrum ranged, as before, from those who argued for complete community care, except for a small number in need of direct nursing in general hospitals, to those who sought to maintain the control of and responsibility for 'the mentally handicapped' in the hands of the clinical consultant.

On a more practical level, significant work on the practice of care for children with learning disabilities had been carried out by a group from the Institute of Education in London (King and Raynes, 1968; Raynes and King, 1968; King et al., 1971; Tizard, 1968). Their findings, more objectively presented than those of Morris (1969), nevertheless contained the same indictment of the hospital system.

They identified four 'interrelated characteristics' of the hospital pattern of care, following Goffman (1961).

1 *Rigidity* – this was the most often presented feature, where the routine of the hospital was such that the same practices were carried out at the same time on the same days, regardless of the changing nature of the patient population.

2 *Block Treatment* – in alliance with the rigidity of the routine, children in hospital were managed as a group, rather than as individuals 'before, during and after routine activities'. This inevitably meant each patient waiting for his or her 'turn' at being bathed, toiletted and so on, often sitting around for several hours in the meantime.

3 *Depersonalisation* – very little evidence was found of any personal clothing or possessions, still less any opportunities for privacy or expressions of individuality.

4 *Social Distance between Staff and Children* – the interaction between staff and patients was limited to basic functional necessities, with very few attempts at personal relationships.

The authors found that this pattern of care contrasted sharply with the approach of the local authority hostels for children: 'The hostel pattern of care typically involved these characteristics to a much lesser degree or else they were absent altogether.' Voluntary homes had a greater variation, some falling near the hospital in terms of care and some near the hostel.

This research is undoubtedly important, like that of Morris, and more so in that it openly proposed an alternative to the criticised hospital system. It thus lent weight to those on the 'community' side of the general argument over care which continued as Hospital Boards began to come under heavy attack for depriving subnormality hospitals of the facilities to carry out any effective rehabilitation (Kushlick, 1969; Bavin, 1970), and for failing to accept their responsibilities as a training environment (Gunzburg, 1970). A principle, originally imported from Scandinavia, known as 'normalisation' (Nirje, 1969), became the catchphrase of a number of those seeking change in the system of care. Once again the group consisted mainly of people outside the medical care staff of hospitals, although a few psychiatrists such as Kirman (1970) supported the idea of community provision. The more common view of psychiatrists at the time is put by Shapiro (1970) who sharply criticises the 'radicals' in the field of mental deficiency and argues for the maintenance of 'mental deficiency' as a clinical speciality only to be practised by those with the appropriate training.

Events seemed, however, at the end of the sixties to be moving towards the 'radical' solution, at least in theory. The report of the Seebohm Committee (Home Office *et al.*, 1968) and the subsequent legislation setting up Social Services Departments provided that 'social care', i.e. community care, should be the responsibility of these new bodies. The Seebohm Report also proposed the abolition of the idea of ineducability, and the takeover of the existing 'Junior Training Centres' by the education service. This was implemented in the Education (Handicapped Children) Act of 1970 which gave local education authorities the responsibility for educating all children, regardless of handicap. Thus local authority services, except education, became the responsibility of the new Social Services Departments, and they were to take over those few hostels and adult training centres that were in existence in the early seventies. However, as the Seebohm Report noted: 'Published plans suggest that for years ahead many parts of the country will not have resources to provide adequate community care services' and the mere continuation of the existing level of provision did not satisfy the critics of the hospital-based system. The pressure of these arguments together with the support of Crossman must have been felt in the senior levels of the Department of Health, since the White Paper *Better Services for the Mentally Handicapped*, published in 1971, gave much credit to the principle of rehabilitation in the community, and noted the 'deficiencies' of the current system (DHSS, 1971). Having done this however, and reviewed the arguments and findings considered above, its conclusions were considered by some to be half-hearted and lacking any real sense of motivation towards effective change (Campaign for Mentally Handicapped (CMH), 1971; 1972). Whilst advocating a reduction in hospital beds for adults from some 90 per cent of residential provision to just over 40 per cent, the White Paper did not really explain why this remaining 40 per cent were needed, and whilst advocating an enormous expansion of local authority services, it gave no firm guidelines on the problems of transferring patients from hospitals to the community provision. Beyond this, of course, it was an advisory document which had no force of legislation behind it, and thus individual local authorities and individual hospitals were left to follow its recommendations more or less strictly.

Reactions from both sides of the fence were therefore hostile. The 'radicals' criticised the White Paper for not going far enough and having no force behind it, for example, Elliott (1972), whilst the psychiatrists' group criticised the fact that their responsibilities were being diminished in response to 'unqualified' pressure, for example the Royal Medico-Psychological Association (RMPA) (1971). The major criticism that this author would make of the White Paper is its naive assumption that the sort of joint planning and organisation necessary for its 'comprehensive' service would be possible with the continued existence of three entirely separate bodies, that is to say, Hospital Boards, education departments and social services departments, with separate finances and separate political control. This problem, as we shall see, has bedevilled the service ever since, even defying the centralising forces of the eighties' Thatcher government. In practice, following the 1971 White Paper, there was a steady but significant growth in local authority services for people with learning disabilities, and a small diminution of the hospital population. Summary figures from a consultative document published in 1976 show the number of residential care places in England in local authority private and voluntary homes rising from 5,900 in 1969 to 9,500 in 1974 and the hospital population falling from 60,000 in 1969 to 55,000 in 1974 (DHSS, 1976). Since the final targets of the White Paper were 33,700 community places and 33,000 hospital places by 1991, considerably faster rates of growth and reduction would be necessary over the ensuing period. This was unlikely, given the economic climate of the time and the continuing debate over responsibility for care and appropriateness of particular types of care. There was a strong body of opinion, led by such as Elliott (1972 op.cit., 1975), Pilkington (1974) and Day (1974) for a unified service to supersede the roles currently undertaken by the social, education and health services. Others, such as Gunzburg (1973) did not go so far as proposing a new service, but stressed the importance of the 'multi-disciplinary team' approach. The problem with this latter approach, as with other attempts at co-operation later, was the divisions caused by the relative status of the team members (Kushlick *et al.*, 1976). Shapiro (1974) maintained that the psychiatrist was the natural leader of such a team, a view not shared by opponents of the 'medical model' of care such as Shearer (1972). Given the relative status, then as now, of clinicians and such people as social workers or residential care staff in the minds of the public at large, it is scarcely surprising that strongly held attitudes were still taken on both sides. Some aspects of the issue were much less debated, however, and the combination of the Education (Handicapped Children) Act and the White Paper had its more immediate effect in setting up models of daytime activity which were unchallenged for a decade. These were the two-tier special school system and the large, 80–150-place adult training centre. As the majority recipients of capital finance in the early seventies these two forms of daytime provision, along with adult hostels, established a powerful place within the service system.

On the basic hospital/community debate, however, Barbara Castle, taking over the job of Secretary of State at the DHSS in 1974, and with ideas of carrying on some of the work of Richard Crossman, also appeared to become disillusioned with progress. Responding to pressure from researchers and others to make a policy statement on the issue, she noted disappointment with the lack of 'change of attitudes' among professionals in the service. She also went further than any other politician in committing herself away from the medical model of care.

On a more practical front, in the same speech to the National Society for Mentally Handicapped Children in February 1975, Mrs Castle announced a number of policy initiatives. First, the setting up of a 'National Development Group (NDG) for the mentally handicapped' under the chairmanship of Professor Peter Mittler to 'play an active part in the development of policy at the DHSS', (Cunningham, 1975). Together with this Development Group, which would generally act at the central level of the DHSS, was a National Development Team (NDT), whose job it would be to go round to local authorities and health areas, advising on the implementation of DHSS policies. This was to replace, in the field of learning disabilities, the activities of Crossman's Hospital Advisory Service, which though it had been extremely critical of facilities of hospitals, had had very little effect on the service in practice. In any case it had been dormant for over a year, following the re-organisation of the NHS in April 1974 and subsequent administrative burdens. Precise details of the Development Team were not given in Mrs Castle's statement, and it was not fully formed until 1976, following consultation with local bodies on its constitution. It was headed by a consultant psychiatrist, Dr. G. Simon.

Two further initiatives were announced by Mrs Castle in 1975: the setting up of a Committee of Inquiry into Mental Handicap Nursing and Care, under Mrs Peggy Jay, one of the initial members of the National Development Group, and a 'reorganisation of the medical role in mental handicap'. The Jay Committee eventually reported in 1979, and their recommendations are considered in more detail later in this chapter. As for the 'review' of the role of the medical specialist in mental handicap, certain administrative changes were made such as appointing consultants to Area Health Authorities rather than special hospitals, but other than that the consultants' positions were unchanged. So was, importantly, their power over admissions and discharges for NHS facilities.

Given the stringent financial constraints on public sector spending in the years between 1975 and 1979, it is difficult to assess the initial impact of the NDG and NDT on services for people with learning disabilities. Certainly the NDG was active in publication, producing pamphlets on a number of topics, beginning in July 1976 with the document *Mental Handicap – Planning Together* (NDG, 1976). Subsequent topics on which the NDG issued its views included children with learning difficulties, school leavers, short-term residential care and day services (NDG, 1977a; 1977b; 1977c; 1977d). Pamphlet 5, on day services, was the most widely used document and, given the furore it raised by its advocacy of a move towards Social Education Centres, its most controversial. Elsewhere, with more powerful interests within the services still at odds, the politics of the situation in the mid-seventies made it perhaps inevitable that a group set up to 'balance' views of the medical, nursing and other professionals should have produced compromises. In particular, though its final two reports (NDG, 1978; 1980) produced far more in terms of direct recommendations about standards, they did so within the context of the status quo of services, i.e. on the assumption that residential care would largely be provided in hospitals and hostels, schooling in special schools and daytime activity for adults in adult training centres. The balance of power within the DHSS, and thus in advice to ministers and policy makers, is also suggested by the fact that the NDG was wound up in the early eighties, whereas the NDT, headed until 1986 by a psychiatrist, continues.

Further evidence of what Ryan and Thomas (1980) accurately described as 'The Politics of Mental Handicap' are shown by two other major developments which began in the middle to late seventies, one firmly fixed in the system of services, the other decidedly not so, though it has considerable influence on any body attempting to analyse that system. The first was the emergence of what became known as 'joint financing' and, accompanying this, the setting up of joint planning teams at local level. Set up initially to try and bridge the financial gap between what was paid through the NHS for people in hospital and what was needed to provide a service in the community, joint finance was originally paid on the basis of a tapering amount over seven years. The tapering period grew to thirteen years in certain circumstances, as did the purpose to which joint financing could be put. These purposes moved from the relatively simple concept of *moving* people out of hospital, to include a great variety of schemes justified on the basis that they *kept* people out of hospital. The two major drawbacks to joint financing were, firstly, that the total amount of money available only represented a fraction of any authority's spending on people with learning disabilities (though an eventual commitment to paying even this amount in full still kept many social services departments at bay). The second, and more important drawback to joint financing and joint planning repeats the author's criticisms of the White Paper given earlier, namely that such planning should be expected to be undertaken by at least three entirely different bodies (education was allowed to be included in the early eighties), with different political control and different systems of financing. As a number of studies have demonstrated (Glennerster *et al.*, 1983; Audit Commission, 1986), you can lead joint planners to the table but you cannot necessarily make them plan. Despite ever more desperate attempts by the DHSS to use financial mechanisms to carry out a policy of 'community care', therefore (DHSS, 1983a; 1984), the difficulties over finance combined with the fact that the debate over hospital and community care had never been really settled meant that the reduction in the population of people in hospital did not meet the targets of the White Paper, and that though elaborate plans to close hospitals were published in the eighties very few were actually closed (Wertheimer, 1986). The exception to this conclusion concerns children in hospital, the numbers of whom reduced to about 1,000 in the mid eighties (Office of Health Economics (OHE), 1986) as opposed to White Paper targets of 6,000. There are now virtually no children with learning disabilities in long-stay hospitals. Despite some help from a special initiative in the early eighties (known as the pound for pound scheme, DHSS, 1983b) the main reason for this reduction would appear to be a combination of fairly rigorous non-admission policies and children in hospital reaching the age of 16, when they ceased to become children for DHSS statistical purposes.

The second significant development beginning in the seventies was, as indicated earlier, much smaller in origin, and came from groups not in policy making positions in the system of services. This was the impact of the developing concept of normalisation. As coined in Scandinavia in the sixties, we have seen that this had already had an impact on the group critical of the medical model of care. As developed by Wolfensberger in his seminal work (Wolfensberger, 1972) and as taken up by a number of individuals in the seventies, the concept had much wider implications. Whereas the Scandinavian definition sought to provide for people with handicaps the same 'rights and obligations' and the same 'pattern of activities' as so-called 'normal' members of society, this still allowed for such activities to take place in segregated institutions, with little contact between handicapped people and others (Grunewald, 1974). Wolfensberger's analysis, to which he then gave substance in the evaluation instrument called PASS (Programme Analysis of Service Systems) (Wolfensberger and Glenn, 1975), went beyond this, and began to concentrate on the way in which society, and services, casts people with handicaps into certain roles and reinforces those roles by the way in which service activities are carried out and the environment in which they are carried out.

This analysis formed the backbone of campaigning by various groups in the late seventies, notably CMH (O'Brien and Tyne, 1981), and had its most direct effect in the principles of the 'Model of Care' proposed in the Jay Committee Report of March 1979. As noted earlier, this Committee had been set up in 1975, with terms of reference implied by its title 'The Committee of Enquiry into Mental Handicap Nursing and Care'. It was also asked to address recommendations of an earlier committee, the Briggs Committee (DHSS *et al.*, 1972) that a separate profession be set up for the care of people with learning disabilities. The Jay Committee chose to interpret its brief, or at least state that it would not carry out its brief without recourse to doing so, by proposing a 'model of care' based on the following broad principles:

a) Mentally handicapped people have a right to enjoy normal patterns of life within the community.
b) Mentally handicapped people have a right to be treated as individuals.
c) Mentally handicapped people will require additional help from the communities in which they live and from professional services if they are to develop to their maximum potential as individuals.

(Jay Committee Report, 1979, p. 35)

The influence of normalisation is clear, and more so in the 'Service Principles' which followed:

a) Mentally handicapped people should use normal services wherever possible.
b) Existing networks of community support should be strengthened by professional services rather than supplanted by them.
c) 'Specialised' services or organisations for mentally handicapped people should be provided only to the extent that they demonstrably meet or are likely to meet additional needs that cannot be met by the general services.
d) If we are to meet the many and diverse needs of mentally handicapped

people we need maximum coordination of services both within and between agencies and at all levels. The concept of a life plan seems essential if coordination and continuity of care is to be achieved.

e) Finally, if we are to establish and maintain high quality services for a group of people who cannot easily articulate and press their just claims, we need someone to intercede on behalf of mentally handicapped people in obtaining services.

(Jay Committee Report, 1979, pp. 36–7)

These principles probably represent the most public acceptance of a change in attitude within the broad 'field' of learning disabilities, and together with 'An Ordinary Life', a proposal for a comprehensive model of residential care based on ordinary housing, which appeared a year later (King's Fund, 1980) the most public challenge to the still medically dominated service. Even here, however, notes of dissent from members of the Committee, especially the minority report by D.O. Williams, Chairman of the Staff Side of the Whitley Council for the Health Services, demonstrated the tremendous professional interests at stake. In between those two publications however, the ascent to power of Mrs Thatcher and a 'radical' Conservative government introduced a whole new dimension to the notion of 'services', for all sorts of people. The fact that services for people with learning disabilities would have been at a turning point with the Jay Committee Report (1979) was rather irrelevant to the much greater upheavals and, as Ryan notes, by 1981 'The Jay report . . . a ground breaking inquiry . . . had been quietly buried and with it the heated controversy and commitment to extra expenditure that the government was too anxious to avoid' (Ryan and Thomas, 1987). Instead, a White Paper in 1981, whilst it 're-emphasises' the government's commitment to community care only mandated a hospital closure programme, and that in very vague terms (DHSS, 1981). Alternatives to both hospital and the predominant local authority form of residential care, the hostel, were not seriously put forward.

As for normalisation, in both the US and UK, the ideals rapidly became 'adopted and adapted' by various parts of the existing service system, to the extent that the word, and the concept, has become seriously misapplied and misunderstood. This is not the place for a debate on how widespread such misunderstanding has become (see Wolfensberger (1980) for the US experience and Brown and Smith (1992) for a much wider discussion though, interestingly, one which does not have a direct contribution from Wolfensberger).

Despite its entry into service language, therefore, the development of normalisation ideas did not, over the country as a whole, have a major impact on the pattern of services, with the exception of residential care, and even there the degree of that impact is arguable. To take two examples; despite the Warnock Committee Report in 1979 (Department of Education and Science, 1979), and the subsequent Education Act of 1981 (not implemented until

1983) the degree of integration into ordinary schools of children with learning disabilities is still extremely limited, though as elsewhere, a vast literature exists on the subject. Similarly, despite efforts at repeating the push to change of the document 'An Ordinary Life' in the field of daytime provision, economic circumstances and the entrenched capital investment in adult training centres have meant that 'An Ordinary Working Life' (King's Fund Centre, 1984) has largely been written off, and a much vaguer sense of the purpose of day services prevails (Department of Health, 1992b).

Even in the residential field, where the ideas of normalisation were said to have taken the greatest hold (and created their own backlash in the formation of RESCARE, a pressure group committed to the halting of hospital closure and the setting up of 'village communities' on hospital campuses (Segal, 1989), real developments in services are limited. Subsequent chapters go into much greater detail but the only result of any scale in the last decade in implementing services based on normalisation has been the growth of a number of projects based on staffed ordinary houses. Even here, such projects are still often described as 'experimental' and, in keeping with the times, have been subject to much more rigorous examinations of 'cost-effectiveness' than was ever the case with hostels in the seventies. At the same time, the eighties have seen a vast expansion of private residential provision, growth of places in which has exceeded the growth of places provided by local authorities and whose model of care seems more based on the economies of an 8–12 bedded home than on its impact on those who are there. The Residential Homes Act (1984), originally brought in as a safeguard to the growing number of private old people's homes, has had little but nuisance value to private accommodation for people with learning disabilities, except those places attempting to prevent the continuing devaluation of residents by the conditions of their physical environment (Race, 1987).

Following the large capital expansion of the seventies, therefore, attempts to resolve the hospital/community debate in the eighties by a simple transfer of people signally failed (Audit Commission, 1986, op. cit.) to the extent that the alternative administrative arrangements of the 1990 NHS and Community Care Act became necessary. The impact of the principle of normalisation has been considerable in terms of debate, less so in terms of the pattern of services, though a number of individual actions have emerged (Ward, 1988; Williams and Race, 1988). More fundamentally, with reference back to Titmuss's criticisms of Enoch Powell cited earlier (see Jones *et al.*, 1979), services for people with learning difficulties appear to have again become swept along with the economic tide that has altered the position for other care groups. In the sixties, it was predominately services for people with mental health problems, with services for elderly people and those with learning disabilities swept along. Today, the social security bill for elderly people in residential and nursing homes, especially the ever growing private and voluntary ones, appears to be the driving force behind legislative and policy changes. As in 1963, specific alternatives to the hospital are not prescribed by the legislation, and policy advice in 1992 appears to throw the whole argument wide open. Local authorities are advised to 'recognise these entirely legitimate concerns' ascribed to 'parents and carers', though the history of this chapter would not suggest that the professions were altogether disinterested, that 'the essential needs of disabled people' including access to specialist health care, will be met on a lifelong basis (DoH, 1992, op. cit.). That this advice still comes from the Department of Health is also interesting. The frisson of privatisation of the eighties, added to the economic and ideological imperatives which drove two separate generations of Conservative governments to cut public spending, would suggest a pattern of service development much more akin to that in the United States, where the massive deinstitutionalisation of the seventies, combined with the existing market economy in welfare, has produced a vast range of provision, some very much at the radical edge of services in this country, some light years behind or representing a major backlash towards closed communities (Smith and Kendrick, 1986).

There is one final aspect to this historical review, however, and it concerns something slightly out of current definitions of 'services' which nevertheless seems highly significant in relation to the rest of the book. This aspect concerns the much greater public debate on issues to do with learning disabilities which appears to have occurred in the last five or ten years. Some of this is connected with the efforts of pressure groups on both sides of the community care debate, whose activities have given a much greater public profile to the issue. Beyond this, however, two related aspects have brought people with learning disabilities into the public gaze. The first has been the increasing debate around all the aspects of 'quality of life' as it has emerged on the general issues of embryology and genetic engineering and on special cases to do with, for example, the sterilisation of people with learning disabilities, the abortion of children diagnosed before birth as having learning disabilities, the growing evidence of children with learning disabilities 'not treated' for conditions which routinely have been dealt with in other children (Williams, 1992).

The second has been the growth, limited in practice but vast in literature (see, for example, Brechin and Walmsley, 1989) and enshrined in law in the Disabled Persons (Services, Consultation and Representation) Act 1986, of advocacy for people with handicaps. Advocacy, if the literature is to be believed, represents, at least in its self-advocacy form, the major development affecting services for people with learning disabilities. Influential texts such as *Making Connections* (Brechin and Walmsley, 1989, op. cit.) are at last giving space to the relation of life experiences by people with learning disabilities, hitherto only notable for their rarity, e.g. Deacon (1976). Reference is made in most Community Care plans to the 'views of service users' and even advice from the Department of Health (1992, op.cit.) included reference to 'views of the person with learning disabilities'. Much work has been done in this area, and much heated debate over the relative merits of 'citizen advocacy' where a person without learning disabilities makes a commitment to advocate for the interests of someone with learning disabilities, and 'self-advocacy' where individuals speak for themselves, with or without help to develop skills in doing so. Ironically, as one of the originators of 'citizen advocacy', Wolfensberger has been often a target in this debate, which then impinges on his other ideas, in particular the evolution of Social Role Valorisation (SRV). This, Wolfensberger's preferred terminology for what he has evolved from normalisation, it is said is an imposition of a world view on people with learning disabilities which, detractors also imply, is a criticism of citizen advocacy. Like the debate around SRV, unfortunately, the impact on those at the front line of services, both users and providers, is often the emergence of a degree of cynicism that centres on such arguments being more widespread in current circumstances, than in times when resources are more readily available for direct service provision. In other words they divert the energies of influential people away from the struggle to make such resources adequate.

Advocacy and the 'quality of life' debate raise fundamental questions about the way we regard people with learning disabilities and the nature of commitment to them. Both, ironically, have a number of interesting throwbacks to the issues which began this chapter. However, whereas in the early twentieth century the debate was conducted between a relatively small number of scientists, academics and politicians, a case in 1987 concerning the sterilisation of a young woman with learning disabilities was debated widely in the media and a case (January 1993) of whether or not to cease the artificial feeding of a young man who had been damaged in the Hillsborough disaster of 1989 provoked similar debate and even direct action.

On the sterilisation case, attitudes were alarmingly similar to those displayed in the heyday of Tredgold, the eugenics movement, and the creation of 'colonies' with the addition in the eighties of a vast variety of competing 'experts' on everything from the economics of the quality of life to the trauma of giving birth if you have learning disabilities. An astonishing compendium of all views covered in this historical review were propounded in the course of this one case, including many that had seemed to be buried some time earlier (e.g. the notion of 'mental age'). In the Hillsborough case more profound and to some, alarming decisions about life and death were taken in an ever more utilitarian and individualistic fashion (compare, for example, the view of Phillips (1993) on this case with the general views of Wolfensberger (1987)). The point for those working in services is that such cases gradually reveal publicly the values and attitudes that underlie those services.

Such a relevation can, especially in services with an already stated or implicit value base, be profoundly disturbing (see Williams and Race (1988, op.cit.) for an example from a Christian organisation).

Perhaps, as John Arlott pointed out about cricket, services reflect the wider attitudes and policies of the time more readily than those involved intensely with them would care to admit. It is doubtful that without a eugenics movement in wider society, segregation, and the creation of colonies, would have taken the path it did. Without the power of the medical profession and the inclusion of colonies in the NHS after the war, the dominance of the health professional view and interest would not continue to this day. Without a particular interest from a Labour minister, with the revolutionary spirit of the sixties in full swing, the reforms of the 1971 White Paper and the changes in opinion up to the Jay Committee Report (1979) might well have never occurred. Without a government causing a sea change in attitudes to individualism, competition and the notion of public service, the contrasting ideals that underlie social role valorisation might not have been seen in such sharp focus. Ryan (Ryan and Thomas, 1987, op. cit) concludes that this reveals the 'strains' of a society decreasingly having available what were once socially acceptable forms of 'putting away' and that 'public visibility is itself progress'. Without those wider social factors, however, those looking to develop services that value people with learning disabilities might not be fighting a debilitating battle with those looking to represent the 'rights' of such people, while the big battalions of vested interest look on with mild amusement, seeing their opposition destroy itself. It is therefore with sadness, rather than surprise, that the quotation which concludes this chapter is the same as that from the corresponding chapter in the first edition of this book, and seems as relevant seventeen years later. Replying to a rather optimistic statement from the chairman of the National Development Group, Tyne wrote:

> There have been changes. Yet the pattern of services available to a mentally handicapped person and his family is much the same as it always was. Hospitals are still large and distant from the people they service. Local authorities have improved educational provision, but there is still pressure on day places in adult training centres. Residential provision has developed slowly and in a stereotyped way.
>
> (Tyne, 1976)

What is this 'pattern of services' of which Tyne is so critical? Answering that question for the 1990s is what the rest of this book is essentially about.

REFERENCES

Acts of Parliament

Disabled Persons (Services, Consultation and Representation) (1986), London, HMSO.
Education (Handicapped Children) Act (1970), London, HMSO.
Education Act (1981), London, HMSO.
Elementary Education (Defective and Epileptic Children) Act (1899), London, HMSO.
Residential Homes Act, National Health Service and Community Care Act (1990) London, HMSO.

General references

Baller W.R. (1936) A study of the present social status of a group of adults who, when they were in elementary schools, were classified as mentally deficient, *Gen.Psychol.Mon*, 18, 165–244.

Baranjay E.P. (1971) *The Mentally Handicapped Adolescent*, Oxford, Pergamon.

Barron D. (1989) Locked away; life in an institution, in Brechin A. and Walmsley J. (eds) *Making Connections*, Milton Keynes, Open University Press.

Bavin J. (1970) Subnormality in the seventies – priority in resources, *Lancet*, 2, 285–7.

Binding K. and Hoche A. (1920) *The Release of the Destruction of Life Devoid of Value*, Leipzig, F. Meiner.

Brechin A. and Walmsley J. (eds) (1989) *Making Connections – Reflecting on the Lives and Experiences of People with Learning Difficulties*, Milton Keynes, Open University Press.

Brown H. and Smith H. (eds) (1992) *Normalisation, A Reader for the Nineties*, London, Routledge.

Campaign for the Mentally Handicapped (1971) *The White Paper and Future Services for the Mentally Handicapped*, London, CMH.

Campaign for the Mentally Handicapped (1972) *Even Better Services for the Mentally Handicapped*, London, CMH.

Charles D.C. (1953) Ability and accomplishment of persons earlier judged mentally deficient, *Gen.Psychol.Mon*, 47, 3–71.

Claridge G.S. (1961) The Senior Occupation Centre and the practical application of research to the training of the severely subnormal, *Brit.J.Ment.Subn.*, 8, 11–16.

Claridge G.S. and O'Connor N. (1957) The relationships between incentive, personality type and improvement in performance of imbeciles, *J.Ment.Def.Res*, 1, 16–25.

Clarke A.D.B. and Clarke A.M. (1953) How constant is the IQ?, *Lancet*, 2, 877.

—— (1954) Cognitive changes in the feebleminded, *Brit.J.Psychol.*, 45, 173–9.

—— (1959) Recovery from the effects of deprivation, *Acta Psychologica*, 16, 137–44.

Clarke A.D.B., Clarke A.M. and Reiman S. (1958) Cognitive and social changes in the feebleminded – three further studies, *Brit.J.Psychol*, 53, 321–30.

Clarke A.D.B. and Blakemore C.B. (1961) Age and perceptual motor transfer in imbeciles, *Brit.J.Psychol.*, 52, 125–31.

Clarke A.M. and Hermelin B.F. (1955) Adult imbeciles, their abilities and trainability, *Lancet*, ii, 337–9.

Cortazzi D. (1969) The bottom of the barrel, *Brit.J.Ment.Subn.*, 15, Pt. 1.

Cromwell R.L. and Moss J.W. (1959) The influence of reward value on the stated expectancies of mentally retarded patients, *Am.J.Ment.Def.*, 63, No. 4.

Crossman R. (1977) *The Diaries of a Cabinet Minister*, Vol. 3, London, Hamish Hamilton.

Cunningham J. (1975) Barbara and her begging bowl, *New Psychiatry*, March 13, 1975.

Day K. (1974) Follow the Northern Lights, *New Psychiatry*, Nov. 28, 8–11.

Deacon J. (1976) *Tongue Tied*, London, Human Horizons Press.

Department of Education and Science (1979) *Report of the Committee of Enquiry into the Education of Handicapped Children and Young People* (The Warnock Report), London, HMSO.

Department of Health (1992a) *Social Care for Adults with Learning Disabilities (Mental Handicap)*, LAC(92)13, London, HMSO.

Department of Health (1992b) *Social Care for Adults with Learning Disabilities*, LAC(92)15, London, HMSO.

Department of Health and Social Security (1971) *Better Services for the Mentally Handicapped*, Command 4683, London, HMSO.

—— (1976) *Priorities in the Health and Social Services in England – A Consultative Document*, London, HMSO.

—— (1981) *Care in the Community – A Consultative Document on Moving Resources for Care in England*, London, HMSO.

—— (1983a) *Care in the Community*, HC(83)6, London, HMSO.

—— (1983b) *Getting Mentally Handicapped Children out of hospital*, DA(83)13, London, HMSO.

—— (1984) *Health Services Division; Collaboration between the NHS, Local Authorities and Voluntary Organisations*, HC(84)6, London, HMSO.

Department of Health and Social Security, Scottish Home and Health Department and Welsh Office (1972) *Report of the Committee on Nursing (The Briggs Report)*, London, HMSO.

Dutton G. (1963) The mentally subnormal and the hospital, *Brit.J.Ment.Subn.*, 9, Pt. 1.

Elliot J (1972) Eight propositions for mental handicap, *Brit.J.Ment.Subn.*, 18, 24–30.

—— (1975) Segregated ghetto or better services? *Res.Soc.Work*, 15, 4–5.

Fry L.M. (1956) A predictive measure of work success for high-grade mental defectives, *Am.J.Ment.Def.*, 61, No. 2.

Galloway J.F. and Garratt F.N. (1964) Hospitals for the mentally subnormal and the local health authority, *Brit.J.Ment.Subn.*, 10, Pt. 1

Garrison I.K. (1951) The development of social skills and attitudes, *Am.J.Ment.Def.*, 56, No. 2

Glennerster H., Korman N. and Marsden-Wilson F. (1983) *Planning for Priority Groups*, Oxford, Robertson.

Goffman E. (1961) *Asylums – Essays on the Social Situation of Mental Patients and Other Inmates*, Garden City, N.Y., Doubleday.

Gordon S., O'Connor N. and Tizard J. (1954) Some effects of incentives on the performance of imbeciles, *Brit.J.Psychol.*, 45, 225.

—— (1955) Some effects of incentives on the performance of imbeciles on a repetitive task, *Am.J.Ment.Def.*, 60, No. 2.

Gottsegen M.G. (1957) The use of the Vineland Social Maturity Scale in the planning of an educational program for non-institutional low-grade mentally defective children, *Gen.Psychol.Mon.*, 55, 85–140.

Grunewald K. (1974) *The Mentally Retarded in Sweden*, Stockholm, The Swedish Institute.

Gunzburg A.L. (1967) Architecture for social rehabilitation. Montpelier – a turning point, *Brit.J.Ment.Subn.*, 13, 84–7.

Gunzburg H.C. (1957) Therapy and social training for the feebleminded youth, *Brit.J.Med.Psychol.*, 30, 42–8.

—— (1960) *Social Rehabilitation of the Subnormal*, London, Balliere, Tindall and Cox.

—— (1961) The case for comprehensive training, *Brit.J.Ment.Subn.*, 7, 53–61.

—— (1968) *Social Competence and Mental Handicap*, London, Balliere, Tindall and Cassell.

—— (1970) The hospital as a normalizing training environment, *Brit.J.Ment.Subn.*, 16, Pt. 2.

—— (1973) The role of the psychologist in manipulating the institutional environment, in Clarke A.D.B. and Clarke A.M. (eds) *Mental Retardation and Behavioural Research*, IRMR study group No.4, London, Churchill Livingstone.

Gunzburg H.C. and Gunzburg A. (1973) *Mental Handicap and Physical Environment*, London, Balliere Tindall.

Harold E.C. (1955) Employment of patients discharged from the St. Louis State Training School, *Am.J.Ment.Def.*, 60, No. 2.

Hartzler E. (1951) A follow-up study of girls discharged from the Laurelton State Village, *Am.J.Ment.Def.*, 55, 612–18.

Heaton-Ward A. (1989) The wheel always turns full circle: a history of the growth of villages in the U.K., in Segal S. (ed.) *The Place of Special Villages and Communities*, A.B. Academic Publishers.

Hiatt M.S. (1951) Casework services in community placement of defectives, *Am.J.Ment.Def.*, 56, No. 1.

Hilliard L.T. (1954) Resettling mental defectives: psychological and social aspects, *Brit.Med.J*, i, 1372–6.

Hilliard L.T. and Mundy L. (1954) Diagnostic problems in the feebleminded, *Lancet*, 2, 644–6.

Home Office, Department of Education and Science, Ministry of Housing and Local Government, Ministry of Health (1968) *Report of the Committee on Local Authority and Allied Personal Social Services (The Seebohm Report)*, Command 3703, London, HMSO.

Howe Report (1969) *Report of the Committee of Enquiry into Allegations of Ill-treatment of Patients and Other Irregularities at the Ely Hospital, Cardiff*, Command 3795, London, HMSO.

Itard J.M.G. (1801) *The Wild Boy of Aveyron* (trs. Humphrey G.M.), 1932, New York, New York Press.

Jay Committee (1979) *Report of the Committee of Enquiry into Mental Handicap Nursing and Care*, Command 7468, London, HMSO.

Jones K., Brown J. and Bradshaw J. (1979) *Issues in Social Policy*, London, Routledge and Kegan Paul.

King Edward's Hospital Fund for London (1955) *Report on Mental Illness and Mental Deficiency Hospitals*, London, King's Fund.

King R.D. and Raynes N.V. (1968) An operational measure of inmate management in residential institutions, *Soc.Sci.Med.*, 2, 41–53.

King R.D., Raynes N.V. and Tizard J. (1971) *Patterns of Residential Care: Sociological Studies in Institutions for Handicapped Children*, London, Routledge and Kegan Paul.

King's Fund (1980) *An Ordinary Life – Comprehensive Locally-based Services for Mentally Handicapped People*, London, King's Fund Centre.

—— (1984) *An Ordinary Working Life – Vocational Services for People with Mental Handicaps*, King's Fund Project Paper No. 50, London, King's Fund Centre.

Kingsley L.V. and Hyde R.W. (1945) The Health and Occupational Adequacy of the Mentally Deficient, *J.Abn.Soc.Psychol.*, 40, 37–46.

Kirman B.H. (1970) The mentally handicapped individual in society, *Brit. J. Ment. Subn.*, 16, Pt. 1.

Krishef C. and Hall M. (1955) Employment of the mentally retarded in Minnesota, *Am.J.Ment.Def.*, 60, No. 2.

Kushlick A. (1961) *Report on the Mental Health Services of the City of Salford for the Year 1960* (eds M. Susser and A. Kushlick), Lancashire Regional Hospital Board.

—— (1969) Care of the mentally subnormal, *Lancet* 2, 1196–7.

Kushlick A., Felce D., Palmer J. and Smith J. (1976) *Evidence to the Committee of Inquiry into Mental Handicap Nursing and Care from the Health Care Evaluation Research Team*, Winchester, HCERT.

Matthew G.C. (1964) The social competence of the subnormal school leaver, *Brit.J.Ment.Subn.*, 10, 2, 83–8.

Ministry of Health (1962) *A Hospital Plan for England and Wales*, London, HMSO.

Moorman C. (1967) A Social Education Centre, *Brit.J.Ment.Subn.*, 13, 88–92.

Morris (1969) *Put Away: A Sociological Study of Institutions for the Mentally Retarded*, London, Routledge and Kegan Paul.

National Development Group for the Mentally Handicapped (NDG) (1976) *Pamphlet No.1 – Mental Handicap – Planning Together*, London, HMSO.
—— (1977a) *Pamphlet No.2 – Mentally Handicapped Children: A Plan for Action*, London, HMSO.
—— (1977b) *Pamphlet No.3 – Helping Mentally Handicapped School Leavers*, London, HMSO.
—— (1977c) *Pamphlet No.4 – Residential Short-term Care for Mentally Handicapped People: Suggestions for Action*, London, HMSO.
—— (1977d) *Pamphlet No.5 – Day Services for Mentally Handicapped Adults*, London, HMSO.
—— (1978) *Helping Mentally Handicapped People in Hospital: A Report to the Secretary of State for Social Services*, London, HMSO.
—— (1980) *Improving the Quality of Services for Mentally Handicapped People – A Checklist of Standards*, London, HMSO.
Nirje B. (1969) The normalization principle and its human management implications, in Kugel R.B. and Wolfensberger W. (eds) *Changing Patterns in Residential Services for the Mentally Retarded*, Washington D.C., President's Committee on Mental Retardation.
O'Brien, J. and Tyne, A. (1981) *Normalisation: A Foundation for Effective Services*, London, CMH.
O'Connor N. (1965) The successful employment of the mentally handicapped, in Hilliard L.T. and Kirman B.H. (eds) *Mental Deficiency*, London, Churchill.
O'Connor N. and Claridge G.S. (1958) A 'Crespi effect' in male imbeciles, *Brit.J.Psychol.*, 49, 42–8.
O'Connor N. and Tizard J. (1954) A survey of patients in twelve mental deficiency institutions, *Brit.Med.J.*, I, 16–20.
—— (1956) *The Social Problem of Mental Deficiency*, London, Pergamon.
Office of Health Economics (1986) *Mental Handicap – Partnership in the Community*, London, HMSO.
Phillips M (1993) Crossing the Rubicon?, *Guardian*, 12 March 1993.
Pilkington T.L. (1964a) The hospital's role in the care and treatment of the subnormal, *Brit.J.Ment.Subn.*, 10, 113–17.
—— (1964b) Mental subnormality in Great Britain, *Brit.J.Ment.Subn.*, 10, Pt. 2.
—— (1974) Patterns of Care for the Mentally Retarded in the United Kingdom, *Mental Handicap Bulletin* No.14, London, King's Fund Centre.
Price I.J. (1967) The industrial training and social education of subnormal adults, *Brit.J.Ment.Subn.*, 13, Pt. 1.
Race, D.G. (1987) Beyond ordinary housing – practical issues arising from attempts to implement values based services, *Community Living* November, 21.
Raynes N.V. and King R.D. (1968) *The Measurement of Child Management in Institutions for the Retarded*, Proc. Ist. Cong. Int. Assoc. Sci. Study. Ment. Def., Baltimore, University Park Press.
Royal Medico-Psychological Association (1971) RMPA memorandum on future patterns of care of the mentally subnormal, *Brit.J.Psychiat.*, 119.
Ryan J. and Thomas F. (1980) *The Politics of Mental Handicap*, London, Penguin.
—— (1987) *The Politics of Mental Handicap*, revised and extended edition, London, Free Association Press.
Schiphorst B. (1964) Are we facing the challenge?, *Brit.J.Ment.Subn.*, 10, Pt. 2.
Segal S. (ed.) (1989) *The Place of Special Villages and Communities*, Bicester, Oxford, A.B. Academic Publishers.
Shapiro A. (1970) The clinical practice of mental deficiency, *Brit.J.Psychiat.*, 116, 353–68.
—— (1974) Fact and fiction in the care of the mentally handicapped, *Brit.J.Psychiat.*, 125, 286–92.

Shearer A. (1972) *Normalization?* Campaign for the Mentally Handicapped, Discussion Paper 3, London: CMH.

Smith H. and Kendrick M. (1986) *Safeguarding Community Care: The American Experience*, London, King's Fund Centre.

Smith H.W. (1957) A sheltered employment project in an institution for mental defectives, *Am.J.Ment.Def.*, 61, 665–71.

Speyer N. (1964) Social integration of the mentally handicapped adult, *Brit. J. Ment. Subn.*, 10, 35–41.

Tizard J (1958) Introduction, in Clarke A.M. and Clarke A.D.B. (eds) *Mental Deficiency – The Changing Outlook*, 1st edition, London, Methuen.

—— (1964) *Community Services for the Mentally Handicapped*, London, Oxford University Press.

—— (1966) *The Integration of the Handicapped in Society*, 6th Bartholomew Lecture – delivered at the University of Keele, 4 February, 1966, London, Edutext Publications.

—— (1970) The role of social institutions in the causation, prevention and alleviation of mental retardation, in Haywood H.C. (ed.) *Socio-cultural Aspects of Mental Retardation: Proceedings of the Peabody–NIMH Conference*, New York, Appleton Century Crafts.

Tizard J. and O'Connor N. (1952) The occupational adaption of high-grade defectives, *Lancet*, 2, 620–3.

Tredgold A.F. (1909) The feebleminded – a social danger, *Eugenics Rev*, 1, 97–104.

Tredgold A.F. (1952) *A Textbook on Mental Deficiency (Amentia)*, 8th edition, London, Balliere, Tindall and Cox.

Tyne, A. (1976) Handicap: a rejoinder, *New Society*, 8 July.

Walton D. and Begg T.L. (1958) The effect of incentives on the performance of defective imbeciles, *Brit.J.Psychol.*, 49, 49–55.

Ward L. (1988) Developing opportunities for an ordinary community life, in Towell D. (ed.) *An Ordinary Life in Practice*, London, King's Fund Centre.

Wertheimer A (1986) *Hospital Closures in the Eighties*, London, CMH.

Williams P. (1967) Industrial training and remunerative employment of the profoundly retarded, *Brit.J.Ment.Subn.*, 13, Pt. 1.

Williams P. (1992) Ethical issues in prevention and treatment, *Proceedings of the Annual Conference of the British Institute of Mental Handicap*, September 1992.

Williams P. and Race D.G. (1988) *Normalisation and the Children's Society*, London, Community and Mental Handicap Education and Research Association.

Wolfensberger W. (1972) *The Principle of Normalisation in Human Services*, Toronto, National Institute of Mental Retardation.

—— (1980) *Experiences of Thirty Years of Services for Mentally Retarded People*, Address to Annual Meeting, Toronto, National Institute for Mental Retardation.

—— (1987) *The New Genocide of Handicapped and Afflicted People*, Syracuse, N.Y., Training Institute.

Wolfensberger W. and Glenn L. (1975) *Program Analysis of Service Systems*, 3rd edition, Toronto, National Institute for Mental Retardation.

Wood Report (1929) *Report of the Mental Deficiency Committee*, London, HMSO.

World Health Organization (1954) *The Mentally Subnormal Child*, Geneva, WHO.

5 Residential and day services

Paul Williams

INTRODUCTION

The study of residential and day services is fascinating. Practice reflects the best and worst of our behaviour towards each other. The 1980s have seen a continuation of scandals about institutions (Association for the Protection of Patients and Staff, 1982; National Development Team, 1990a; Blom-Cooper, 1992) and also growing documentation of ill-treatment of people in community settings (Hewitt, 1987; Wolfensberger, 1992). Regular magazines in this field, such as *Care Weekly* and *Community Care*, frequently carry accounts of disasters and abuse in community-based services for all client groups.

On the other hand, each day tens of thousands of skilled and committed people deliver much-needed support and service to the most vulnerable people in society. There is increasing appreciation that residential and day services involve the application of a high degree of professional social work, teaching and caring skills (Shaddock, 1988; Wagner, 1988; Ward, 1993).

This chapter provides a review and resource on developments in residential and day services for people with learning disabilities during the 1980s and early 1990s. The process documented is one of continuing consolidation of moves towards community care. In some ways progress has been slow, with acknowledgement of the risks involved; but there have also been many exciting developments. Tyne (1987) quotes Oscar Wilde: 'An idea that isn't dangerous isn't worth calling an idea.' And Ward (1989) quotes Bogdan and Taylor (1987): 'Despite the disappointments, no-one can legitimately claim that the lives of people with developmental disabilities are not better today than when the current wave of reform began in the early 1970s.'

This chapter will discuss some of the critiques, pitfalls, problems and failures of the move towards community care, but in a context of recognition of the great achievements made in both attitudes and practice.

The chapter will concentrate on services for adults, and draws primarily on British literature produced since 1980.

Statistics

The Department of Health (1992) estimates that about 25,000 adults with severe or profound learning disabilities live in hospitals and NHS community units, around 35,000 live in residential accommodation provided by local authorities or the voluntary or private sector, and some 65,000 live at home with family members. The Department's estimate of the position in 1969 (DHSS, 1971) was that there were some 60,000 places in hospitals and NHS facilities, and only around 6,000 in local authority, voluntary or private provision. There has thus been a major, but still substantially incomplete, move from health-oriented and often institutional provision (see Malin *et al.*, 1980) to more community-based provision.

The Social Services Inspectorate (1989) reported that there were around 50,000 places in local authority day services in 1986, an expansion from 23,000 in 1969. About a quarter of those attending lived in various forms of residential care, the rest with their family. There has thus been a considerable increase in day service provision, but there must still be a substantial number of adults living at home and in residential care who are not receiving any day services, even taking into account alternatives such as college, work, and NHS, voluntary or private provision.

Philosophy underlying community care

Apart from the extensive influence of the principles of normalisation or social role valorisation (see Brown and Smith, 1992b), other themes are identifiable in the thinking behind community care developments. One important issue concerns the identity, aspirations and true needs of service users. The nature of disability as social oppression rather than personal tragedy has been explored by a number of writers (Abberley, 1987; Oliver, 1989, 1992). Much more respect has, belatedly, come to be given to people's cultural, ethnic, gender and personal identity (Connelly, 1988; Dominelli, 1988; Noonan-Walsh, 1988; Brown and Smith, 1989, 1990, 1992a; Baxter *et al.*, 1990).

It has also been acknowledged that people aspire to relationships rather than simply physical settings and conditions (Cattermole *et al.*, 1990). Social role valorisation is fundamentally about improving the relationships of people with others in society, to counteract processes of social devaluation. This task is likely to require commitment to the ideal of inclusive communities (Tyne, 1992), flexibility and lateral thinking (Dowson, 1991), and work to develop 'competent communities' (Bulmer, 1987; Heginbotham, 1987; O'Brien and Lyle, 1987).

General moral principles considered to underlie moves to community care include equality (Baker and Gaden, 1992), fairness, stewardship (avoidance of waste of human and material resources) and responsibility (Tyne, 1987). There are also themes of people's vulnerability to abuse and even death (Brown and Craft, 1989; Wolfensberger, 1990; Baron and Haldane, 1992). A further relevant theme has been the exploration of the philosophical notion of 'community,' seen clearest perhaps in the work and writings of Jean Vanier, founder of the L'Arche movement for lifesharing with people with learning disabilities (Vanier, 1979, 1982, 1990; Spink, 1990).

The ideal has become clearer: it is for the equal acceptance and valuing of people in competent, caring, mutually beneficial communities, based on respect for the personal identity and aspirations of people while acknowledging their vulnerability. It is to be achieved through flexible, creative services that support good relationships for people in society.

Community care policy

The influential paper *An Ordinary Life* (King's Fund Centre, 1980) gave impetus to a number of developments. Research projects in Wessex, South Wales, Sheffield, Kent, Northumberland, Bristol and elsewhere began to turn their attention to the evaluation of ordinary housing options. The pioneer NIMROD project was established in Cardiff to demonstrate the feasibility of comprehensive community-based services (Lowe and de Paiva, 1990), and receptiveness to these possibilities among service planners in Wales led to the *All Wales Strategy* (Welsh Office, 1983; Hudson, 1988; McGrath, 1988; McGrath and Grant, 1992) designed to facilitate community care.

The King's Fund Centre, and its sister body the King's Fund College, continued their influential role in producing discussion papers on policy relating to strategic planning (Towell, 1984, 1990; Hunter and Wistow, 1987; Towell and Beardshaw, 1991) and to the practice of community care (Ward, 1982, 1987b; King's Fund Centre, 1984, 1988; Towell, 1988).

The well-established pressure group CMH (now Values Into Action) continued to press for better community services, and its sister body, the Community and Mental Handicap Educational and Research Association, developed systematic training in Britain in the principles of social role valorisation, primarily through the vehicle of the PASS and PASSING evaluation instruments (Wolfensberger and Glenn, 1975; Wolfensberger and Thomas, 1983). Allied to this work were visits to Britain by a number of American thinkers and activists in the development of community care, notably John O'Brien, bringing to attention a range of formative literature (for example, O'Brien, 1987a, 1987b; Schwartz *et al.*, 1987; O'Brien and Lyle, 1991, 1992).

The Social Services Committee of the House of Commons (1985), the Audit Commission (1986, 1989), the Department of Health (1989) and the Social Services Inspectorate (1989) have been among the government-related bodies producing important policy statements. The Griffiths Report (1988) had a major influence on the legislative structure for community care. The Wagner Report (1988) on residential care identified the need for much greater flexibility and choice in residential provision. As part of the Wagner study, commissioned from the National Institute for Social Work by the Secretary of State for Health and Social Services, a comprehensive review of research in residential care for different client groups was commissioned, and includes an excellent chapter on services for people with learning disabilities (Atkinson, 1988b).

Commentary on developments in community care policy during the 1980s can be found in Walker (1982), Jones and Tutt (1983), Towell (1985), Malin (1987), Ward (1987b), Leighton (1988), Sines (1988), Dalley (1989), Booth (1990), National Development Team (1990b, 1990c) and Welch (1991).

In 1992, the Department of Health produced a Local Authority Circular on *Social Care for Adults with Learning Disabilities* giving guidance on policy. It states that 'few, if any, people need to live in hospitals', but 'in the Government's view there is a wide range of acceptable living arrangements, including sharing with non-disabled people, ordinary housing, hostels, homes and residential communities'.

On day services, the circular states that numbers in local authority day services have risen to 56,000, and it includes an annexe on day service provision that envisages a continuing need for day centres alongside use of community education and leisure opportunities and work. An increase in the need for day provision for people with profound or multiple disabilities is predicted.

Critiques of the move to community care

The development of policy has been accompanied by healthy debate on the appropriateness, efficiency and effectiveness of developments. Critiques of specific services are reviewed later in this chapter, but some general criticisms of trends have also emerged.

A fairly common question that is raised is whether there is any such thing as 'community' in the modern world. Issues relating to this concern are discussed from a number of perspectives in Willmott (1986). Political analyses tend to paint a rather gloomy picture of the position of powerless groups; Wolfensberger (1989), for example, claims that an ever-growing pool of dependent people is required to provide 'fodder' for an ever-expanding service providing industry, essential to the functioning of a 'post primary production economy'.

Criticism of the development of community care has included the complaint that it is too slow and piecemeal (Blunden and Smith, 1988; Hudson, 1990; Collins, 1992a), with serious flaws in funding (Ward, 1988; Clayton, 1992). There has been evidence that institutional practices are easily transferred to community facilities (Allen, 1989; Sinson, 1990, 1992b; Brandon, 1992a). Although the manifest function of services may be claimed to be community integration, the latent function may still be social control (Wolfensberger, 1989; Stainton, 1992). Critiques of normalisation have pointed out that some interpretations have not empowered service users and have failed to incorporate equal opportunities and anti-discrimination principles (Day, 1987; Brown and Smith, 1989; Baxter *et al.*, 1990). The position of women, especially mothers, as informal carers has been commented on by a number of authors (for example, Abbott and Sapsford, 1987).

Among the criticisms of the deinstitutionalisation element in community care policy have been that the closure of hospitals has wasted resources (see Sines and Curry, 1987) and that the development of community services for people coming out of institutions contrasts with relative neglect of the needs of people already living in the community (McCarthy, 1987a, 1987b).

Community care in practice

There are many general accounts of successful community services. Long (1988) describes the relocation of people into communities in Sussex; Humphreys (1987) describes developments that led to the complete closure of an institution in Devon; Wertheimer (1988) reports on new services in Somerset. Cottis *et al.* (1989) describe a number of community care projects established by voluntary organisations.

Two collections of accounts of pioneer community-based projects have been assembled by Shearer (1986) and Ward (1982). Other sources include Ayer and Alaszewski (1984), Baldwin *et al.* (1988), Raynes *et al.* (1987) and Heginbotham (1981).

The experiences of the people

There is no more powerful way of describing both the need for and the practice of community care than documenting the experiences of service users themselves. Alongside developments in community care has been the rise of the self-advocacy movement that has given a voice to people with learning disabilities (Crawley, 1988). A number of studies of community services have collected accounts and views of users (Lowe *et al.*, 1987; Sugg, 1987; Cattermole *et al.*, 1989). Methods for doing so effectively have been developed (Crocker, 1989; Simons *et al.*, 1989; Clare, 1990).

There is some evidence that the involvement of service users themselves in decision taking, either about their own needs and future or about the operation of services, is disappointing (Welsh Office and Social Services Inspectorate, 1989). Nevertheless, the potential to contribute, and indeed the right to contribute, can be seen from a number of projects. Potts and Fido (1991) report an 'oral history' project in an institution; 17 people with an average length of stay of 47 years give a unique account of the history of institutional care from their own direct experience. Atkinson and F. Williams (1990) collected together a fascinating anthology of writings, poetry and art by people with learning disabilities, much of it prepared in and facilitated by residential, day and educational services. Whittaker and colleagues (1991) report on an evaluation of community services in the London Borough of Hillingdon, commissioned by the authority from the self-advocacy organisation People First, and carried out by two people with learning disabilities.

Supplementing these projects are accounts of the experiences of individual people. Barron (1989) describes his own experiences in an institution. Thompson and colleagues (1988a) give an account of the lives of two people five years after leaving hospital, stressing the role of day care. Hill-Tout (1988) describes the programme of activities engaged in by one man. Ford (1987) and Fullerton (1987) also each describe the rehabilitation of one person, the latter after 40 years in hospital.

Two of the most powerful and moving sets of accounts of the lives of individuals have come from research projects in Hampshire and Cardiff. Felce and Toogood (1988) describe the individual impact of a community residential service on the lives of nine people, and Humphreys, Evans and Todd (1987) give accounts of individual people served by the NIMROD project.

RESIDENTIAL SERVICES

As has been implied, there is a wide range of residential settings in which people with learning disabilities live, sometimes by choice, sometimes by planning, sometimes by neither. The following sections cover some of the issues that have emerged in relation to different kinds of provision.

Living alone

Two studies of the experiences of people with learning difficulties who live alone (Donegan and Potts, 1988; Flynn, 1989) have shown that many people in this position lead marginalised, lonely and isolated lives, though there are also positive compensatory experiences, particularly of freedom and control. In discussing the size of groupings facilitated by services, Wolfensberger and Thomas (1983) draw attention to the fact that groups can be too small as well as too big to be conducive to personal development and good experiences. In particular, they caution against viewing living alone as necessarily beneficial.

Living with family

As we have seen, a very large number of adults with learning disabilities live at home with their parents or other family members. A number of issues have been identified. The people themselves may not like that arrangement (Lowe *et al.*, 1987). A much higher proportion of non-disabled adults leave the parental home for arrangements of their own in early adulthood than is the case for people with learning disabilities. Thus, parents and other relatives remain the largest group of carers of adults with learning disabilities. Satisfaction with this varies, but in many cases there has had to be a difficult process of adjustment to lifelong responsibility for and commitment to the caring task (Flynn and Saleem, 1986). It is important in understanding the nature and potential of services, particularly short-term care and day provision, to acknowledge their role in supporting the families in which the people with learning disabilities receive their primary care and experience.

A related issue is the need for careful work with families and people with learning disabilities themselves in preparation for any move out of the family home (Richardson and Ritchie, 1986, 1989b; Cattermole *et al.*, 1988).

Family placements

A possible option for some people is placement with a family other than their own (Gathercole, 1981a). Dagnan and Drewett (1988) describe a family placement scheme in County Durham; they report good experiences, but make the point that in their sample most of the carers had professional experience with people with learning disabilities, so generalisation of the results requires caution.

Lifesharing

Living with a family, your own or another, is one form of experience of what has been called 'lifesharing', the equal sharing of accommodation and home and social life between a person with learning disabilities and non-disabled people. Other forms have been described, such as the home in Cardiff that is shared between people with learning disabilities and university students (Pithouse, 1980) and a scheme in North Wales where the local authority recruits and supports non-disabled people to live alongside people with learning disabilities (Harper, 1989). It is worth noting that this form of care comes out best on measures of services' conformity to the principles of social role valorisation (Williams, 1986), though issues of management and supervision of such arrangements need special creativity (Tyne and Williams, 1987).

Short-term care

Before moving on to other forms of residential care, some issues will be mentioned that relate to the use of any form of care for short periods. It has been acknowledged and documented how useful such a service can be to families, to give them and the person they care for a break (Grant and McGrath, 1990; Sholl *et al.*, 1991). (The word 'respite' is probably best avoided since it implies a burden, a perception that many families would not share.) Schemes offering short-term care for adults with learning disabilities have been described by Tyndall (1987) and Mitchell (1990).

A point made powerfully by Maureen Oswin (1984) in her study of short-term care services for children is that care has to be of high quality to give effective support to families. Hubert (1991) found considerable dissatisfaction amongst families of adults receiving short-term care; so much so that many parents had been put off any prospect of care outside their family and expressed a hope that their son or daughter would not outlive them.

Lodgings

This form of provision needs a mention. It involves people living alone or with others under the supervision of someone who acts as landlord or landlady with some caring responsibilities. Some examples are described by Ferrity and colleagues (1986) and an idea of what can be involved for the 'landlady' is given by Eastwood (1987).

Group homes

This term has come to be used to describe situations where a group of people live independently, without staff on the premises but usually with some input of support by a part-time carer or social worker. The model has been described comprehensively by Gathercole (1981b) and Malin (1983), and findings on the quality of experience of people living in such settings have been reported by Phillips *et al.* (1988) and Booth *et al.* (1989).

Staffed houses

A major form that the expansion in community residential provision has taken is that of the staffed house. Indeed, services for people with learning disabilities have led the way in the use of ordinary housing for residential provision, moving away from two ideas that are prevalent in provision for other groups, for example, elderly people: that large groupings are necessary for economic reasons and for provision of needed facilities; and that services should be 'purpose-designed' and specially built. Normalisation has drawn attention to the damage that can be done to people's development and to their social reputation by living in too large groups and in buildings that stick out like a sore thumb (Wolfensberger and Thomas, 1983).

Staffed housing schemes have been extensively studied by a number of research teams, and it has been shown that they can successfully accommodate people with practically any degree of disability, including people with profound or multiple handicaps or severe behaviour difficulties. Thomas (1985) reports increased social contacts for young people who moved from hospital to ordinary houses in Northumberland. Alaszewski and Nio-Ong (1990) describe a Barnardos' project for young people with profound and multiple disabilities in North-West England. Mansell *et al.* (1987) and Felce (1989) describe experience from the development of ordinary housing schemes in the South of England. During the 1980s a number of community care projects based on staffed ordinary housing provision were established under a government-sponsored 'care in the community initiative'. The projects were extensively researched by a team at the University of Kent (Knapp *et al.*, 1992). A highly localised project involving use of staffed housing in Bristol was also the subject of a comprehensive research study (Ward, 1989). Most thoroughly and lengthily researched of all was the Cardiff NIMROD project, a comprehensive service whose residential care component utilised staffed ordinary houses (Lowe and de Paiva, 1990). This project was also independently evaluated with PASS (Williams, 1992 – see below under 'Evaluating Residential and Day Services', p. 94).

All these studies have shown benefits accruing directly from the accommodation of people in small numbers in ordinary community neighbourhoods. Where comparison have been made between residents of houses and those living in more institutional settings (e.g. Rawlings, 1985a, 1985b), better progress and experience has been demonstrated in the houses. Discussion of some of the issues involved can be found in Russell and Ward (1983), Chamberlain (1988) and Williams (1993).

There have been criticisms of small homes, though. Gunzburg and Gunzburg (1992) and Sinson (1990, 1992b) describe how opportunities for development and community participation are often underused, a phenomenon that Sinson calls 'micro-institutionalisation'. The research studies listed above have also generally found that special efforts have to be made to ensure that opportunities are capitalised on, through some structuring and planning of activities (Saxby *et al.*, 1988).

Hostels

Many local authorities have a legacy of provision, established in the 1960s and 1970s, of hostels accommodating 12 to 30 people in one building. It is an ironic fact that in some areas, Health Authority residential provision is in much smaller, more homely settings than social services provision.

The definitive government-sponsored study of hostel provision was the Sheffield Development Project. Research evaluation of this demonstrated many facets of such provision that make it unsuitable. The project generated much useful data on architectural design and the problems of large-group living (Dalgleish, 1983), but the clear conclusion of the study was that the considerable amount of money put into the scheme represented a wasted opportunity if deinstitutionalisation and community integration were the aim (Heron, 1982).

Others have studied the design of hostels, for example, Auburn and Leach (1989) concluded that certain designs facilitate group interaction while others encourage people to retreat to their individual bedrooms. The problems of communal living in hostels have been documented by Locker and colleagues (1983, 1984) and by Booth, W. *et al.* (1990). Brandon and Ridley (1985) interviewed the residents of a hostel about their views.

A finding of Sumpton and colleagues (1987) (see also Raynes, *et al.*, 1987), who followed up a number of children Raynes had studied almost 20 years earlier, was that once a person has experienced hostel care they are likely to have embarked on a long-term 'career' in institutional settings. Harper (1990) has described a concerted attempt by a local authority, Clwyd in North Wales, to replace its hostel provision with ordinary housing.

'Village communities'

There is a pressure group – RESCARE, the National Society for Mentally Handicapped People in Residential Care – that offers a forum for families and professionals who believe that large-scale provision should be retained (Tonkin, 1987; Jackson, 1991). The model of provision that is usually put forward is that of the 'village community', and it is argued that many existing institutions, instead of being closed, could be turned into such communities. A number of well-known village communities have existed for many years in Britain, for example, Ravenswood, run by a Jewish Foundation in Berkshire, the Camphill villages in Yorkshire and Scotland, and the communities established by the Home Farm Trust, CARE (Cottage and Rural Enterprises) and others. L'Arche has a large community in France, though it utilises ordinary dispersed housing for its provision in Britain.

These 'villages' enjoy a good reputation for care. Many of them are based on philosophies that engender special respect for people with learning disabilities, such as the Rudolf Steiner philosophy of 'anthroposophism' that underlies Camphill, or the lifesharing philosophy of Jean Vanier's L'Arche. A recent book (Segal, 1990) argues the case for village communities and describes a wide range of provision considered to come under that heading. In a review of the book, Williams (1991) points out the danger that the benign philosophies underlying this model of provision are often confused with negative perceptions of people as a menace or nuisance in ordinary society. Isolation from society is a major issue for this model, irrespective of how good the care inside can be.

Hospitals

Hospitals are the legacy of some very negative perceptions of people with learning disabilities in the past (Wolfensberger, 1975; Brandon, 1992d). Nevertheless, they have been the repository of professional expertise in the care of people with learning disabilities (Jones and Fowles, 1984; Alaszewski, 1986) and debate still continues about whether there are any people whose special needs require them to live in a hospital environment (Keene and James, 1986; Walker and Naylor, 1990). At present, 25,000 people still do so. The degree of their disabilities compared to those of people in community settings has been reported by a number of studies (Farmer *et al.*, 1990; Jawed *et al.*, 1993; Krishnan *et al.*, 1993; Dickinson and Singh, 1991; Kiernan and Moss, 1990). These studies have found that, although overall the people living in hospitals have more severe disabilities and problems of behaviour, there is a large overlap with people cared for in community settings. There are certainly examples of people with very severe degrees of disability or behaviour problem being cared for successfully in ordinary staffed housing (see, for example, Felce and Toogood, 1988). However, there remains some scepticism amongst hospital staff that *everyone* could be discharged (Summerfield, 1988). The complete closure of a large hospital, Darenth Park in Kent, has been the subject of extensive study (Wing, 1989; Korman and Glennerster, 1990).

Research has generally shown that people with very severe disabilities fare better in community settings than in hospitals (for example, Rawlings, 1985a, 1985b; Beail, 1988), even if sometimes a little disappointingly (Bratt and Johnston, 1987; Allen, 1989). There has also been a continuing series of reports of extremely poor conditions in hospitals (Martin, 1984); such settings seem to have characteristics that can easily foster poor and abusive treatment (Ryan and Thomas, 1987). Staff in hospitals are often well aware of this. The National Development Team as recently as 1990 reported on one hospital:

> We were saddened, and shared the despondency of many of the staff we met, about the neglect in people's lives and about the physical environment, which on many of the wards was as poor as we have seen anywhere on our visits. The question being asked by District and Unit level managers was 'Is the hospital really as bad as we are being told?' Our answer is Yes!
> (National Development Team, 1990a)

There are concerns that the process of relocation of people from hospitals to community provision is slowing down (Collins, 1992b). There have also been criticisms of the way in which it has been done. The National Development Team (1988) criticised one scheme for the wholesale transfer of residents from one large institution to another in order to close one of them. Brandon (1992b) has drawn attention to the relocation of people far away from any community with which they might have links. Halliday and Potts (1987) describe the long delays there often are in getting people out. Francis (1987b) discusses some problems involved in the transfer of staff from hospital to community settings.

A growing body of research shows the benefits to people of discharge from hospital to community (Hemming *et al.*, 1981; Hulbert and Atkinson, 1987; Atkinson, 1988a; Booth, T. *et al.*, 1990; Booth and Phillips, 1991). However, a small number of people are readmitted to hospital following a period in a community setting; the reasons have been studied by Hemming (1982) and Causby and York (1990, 1991).

Special security provision

Some people with learning disabilities have committed serious offences or are considered a danger to themselves or others. There are Regional Secure

Units attached to some hospitals for people with learning disabilities. Stay in these is intended to be limited; longer-term provision is in the form of places at the three Special Hospitals in England – Broadmoor, Rampton and Ashworth – or Carstairs in Scotland. In England, Rampton concentrates on people with learning disabilities, although there is also provision at Ashworth. The special hospitals are managed by a Special Hospitals Service Authority rather than being part of health service provision. In the past, staff, although having official identity and training as nurses, have also belonged to the Prison Officers Association.

A key issue in this type of service is the difficulty of reconciling good care and rehabilitation (see, for example, Bennett, 1989) with a high level of security. A punitive culture can easily develop. Following a television programme about the death of a patient in seclusion at one special hospital, an inquiry called for a complete change of culture towards a more therapeutic regime – a tall order for an establishment of some 700 residents and 1400 staff (Blom-Cooper, 1992).

A related issue is the need for great care in the process of dealing with people with learning disabilities accused of offences. There have been a number of instances of serious miscarriage of justice. Guidance has been given by Hewitt (1989), Thomas (1989), Perske (1991) and Letts (1992).

DAY SERVICES

Day provision plays a large part in the community life of most people with learning disabilities, though as we have noted there are many people who do not receive a day service. The main form of such provision has been the Adult Training Centre, some of which were renamed Social Education Centres after the influential report of the National Development Group (1977) or have more recently adopted the title of Resource Centre. Typically such centres cater for 80 to 100 people. Many were built to a factory-type design and located in industrial areas at a time when they were oriented towards sheltered work rather than the broader educational aims now current.

There have been other developments in day provision, in the areas of leisure and recreation, education in colleges, and work.

The emergence of the 'resource centre'

Jan Carter (1981) in a comprehensive study of day services for all client groups, sponsored by the National Institute for Social Work, discovered a wide variety of aims being pursued: social contact, leisure and recreation, practical help and advice, education and training, assessment and treatment, individual therapy, group therapy, rehabilitation, prevention of admission to residential care, preparation for leaving the family home, relief of families, industrial production, work finding and preparation for work. Many day services for people with learning disabilities are based on the expectation that all these aims will be pursued at once by the same service. Furthermore, the service users will range from people with a mild or borderline degree of learning disability, to people with profound and multiple disabilities or severe behaviour difficulties.

Barnes (1990), utilising an analysis by Dartington and colleagues (1981), collapses the above aims into three models: 'warehousing' or containment-oriented, 'horticultural' or training-oriented, 'enlightened guardian' or advice and activity-oriented. He adds, and argues for, a fourth model – 'disabled action', in which day services offer support and give control to people pursuing their own interests, choices and definitions of need.

The 1980s began with a period of great confusion about the function of day centres for people with learning disabilities as they moved away from a 'containment' model, often masquerading under the guise of sheltered work, to the more educational model proposed by the National Development Group. During the 1980s a number of groups and organisations entered the debate about the aims and future of day services; these included the Independent Development Council for People with Mental Handicap (1985), MENCAP (1985), the National Association of Teachers of the Mentally Handicapped (1985), Bridges (the Association of Professions for People with Mental Handicaps) (Woolrych, 1989) and Values Into Action (Puddicombe, 1991).

Three themes began to emerge that represented a step towards Barnes' 'disabled action' model: the growth of the self-advocacy movement, especially in the form of users' groups in day centres (Crawley, 1988); recognition of the importance of working towards good relations for people in ordinary society as identified by normalisation theory (Couchman *et al.*, 1987); and growing appreciation of the needs of individual people for personal growth, confidence and empowerment (Shaw *et al.*, 1992). These considerations have led to the development of two models of day provision: the 'choice' model (Taylor, 1987; Carter, 1988) and the 'community dispersal' model (Bender, 1986). In the first, a 'menu' of opportunities is provided from which each person can have an individual programme reflecting their choices; modern centres that have adopted this model can have as many as fifty activities available in an extremely complex timetable. The second model involves the dispersal of the service into small local 'enclaves' from which use can be made of a wide range of community facilities.

The Social Services Inspectorate (1989) (see also Gray, 1990) carried out a survey of day centres which illustrated continuing confusion, but pointed to the emergence of a 'resource centre' model. This model is an unclear combination of the 'choice' and 'dispersal' models. Extensive use of generic community facilities and activities is envisaged, but there is nothing to dissuade authorities from building new large segregated centres, which some are doing at a current cost of around £1.5 million a time (Puddicombe, 1991). Many services are of course based in older buildings rendered unsuitable by changing perceptions of the task (Rose and Adamson, 1990).

Colleges

The educational model for day provision is extremely important; the varied facets of it have been reviewed by Sutcliffe (1990). It has become common for people with learning disabilities to attend colleges of further education, especially between the ages of 16 and 19. Sometimes this provision involves good integration with non-disabled students (Willis and Kiernan, 1984; Sutcliffe, 1992). Specific opportunities provided for people in this way can be a liberation for individuals (Cottis, 1989). Sinson (1992a) describes the work of an independent specialist college for adults with learning disabilities.

Some criticisms have been levelled at current practice in college education. Whittaker (1991) points to continued segregation of people within colleges. Brandon (1991) and Steele (1993) question the relevance of college curricula. Lister and Ellis (1992) point out that only 10 per cent of people in supported employment schemes come from education services, and they conclude: 'This suggests that school leavers are oriented towards the more traditional forms of service provision and that Colleges of Further Education do not yet routinely see employment as a logical outcome for the majority of their students.' The Further Education Unit (1992) has issued guidance to try to remedy this situation.

Leisure and recreation

Brief mention can be made of developments in support for leisure and recreation for people with learning disabilities. A strong structure exists to enable people to engage in sporting activities, and British performers have done well in international sporting events. There are also flourishing drama, art and music groups of people with learning disabilities. For accounts of current developments see Garrett (1989), McConkey and McGinley (1991) and Judith Russell's chapter (Chapter 8).

Work

Britain pioneered interest in the work potential of people with severe learning disabilities through the post-war work of Jack Tizard, Neil O'Connor, Alan Clarke and others (see O'Connor and Tizard, 1956). This interest was pursued in the best Adult Training Centres, but was dissipated by the National Development Group's (1977) proposals for a wider educational function for centres. Interest is now, however, being strongly revived.

Lister and Ellis (1992) report that there are currently over 70 supported employment services in Britain, about half operating as independent agencies and the rest under the auspices of day centres. They are mostly small enterprises; 40 per cent support less than ten clients, and less than half have full-time staff. Nevertheless, some 1600 people are being supported in open jobs. Furthermore, Lister and Ellis report that:

70 per cent were within the mild or moderate category of degree of learning disability. However it is extremely encouraging to note that services were catering for 418 people defined as having severe learning disabilities, and 15 people defined as having profound learning disabilities.

(Lister and Ellis, 1992)

Accounts of the development of work-oriented support services are given by Porterfield and Gathercole (1985), Wertheimer (1987, 1992), and Brothers of Charity (1992). Important to this development has been the introduction to Britain of a method of analysing the support needs of people in a work context, known as 'Training in Systematic Instruction' (see Wertheimer, 1992). Szivos (1990) has provided one word of warning: she reports that work does not necessarily increase the self-esteem of people with learning disabilities; there remain needs for support in developing identity, confidence and self-worth.

SOME GENERAL ISSUES IN RESIDENTIAL AND DAY SERVICES

In the final section of this chapter we will briefly review some general issues that relate to the task of both residential and day services: the development of friendships and community networks, provision for people with special needs, the evaluation of services, staff training, and the wider context to the professional task in group care.

Friendships and networks

Central to the community care task is the fostering of friendships and good personal relationships in the community (Atkinson and P. Williams, 1990). General issues in understanding the nature of this task are discussed by Abraham (1989), Evans and Murcott (1990) and Cullen (1991). The experiences of people with learning disabilities of community relationships have been described by Dalgleish and colleagues (1983), Atkinson and Ward (1986, 1987) and Atkinson (1987).

Reactions of neighbours and the public to the establishment of community residential services have been described by Francis (1987a), Groarke (1987), Mills (1988) and Pittock and Potts (1988). Strategies for ensuring good relations have been proposed by Hay (1987), Dudley (1989) and Hogan (1989).

Practical ways of supporting people in gaining friends and community networks are described by Raynes (1986), King's Fund Centre (1988), Perske (1988), Richardson and Ritchie (1989a), Firth and Rapley (1990) and Schneider (1992).

People with special needs

Community services must expect to support people with very severe disabilities (Department of Health and Social Security, 1984); these will include people with a profound degree of learning disability, people with multiple handicaps, and people with severe behaviour difficulties. As we have seen, many people with this degree of disability now live in community residential provision, and many live at home with their families; most day centres also cater for these special needs (Crawford *et al.*, 1984). Brief mention will be made here of some developments in provision for these people.

The needs of people with profound and multiple handicaps are discussed by Hogg and Sebba (1986) and Thompson and colleagues (1988b). Practical approaches to a developmental curriculum for people with these needs have been suggested by Norris (1982, 1988), Sebba (1988) and Longhorn (1988). A development that has been incorporated in a number of day centres is 'Snoezelen'; this involves provision of equipment, often in a special room, to give sensory stimulation to aid development and enjoyment. The possible benefits from such provision are being researched (Haggar and Hutchinson, 1991; Hutchinson, 1991). The idea has come in for criticism on the grounds of its unnatural and potentially segregatory nature (Whittaker, 1992).

The community care needs of people with behaviour difficulties are discussed in Blunden and Allen (1987) and by Maher and Russell (1988). One development has been the introduction of training in Britain in the methods known as 'gentle teaching', which involve the careful development of a trusting relationship with the person with difficult behaviour (McGee *et al.*, 1987; Hobbs, 1993).

Many people with very severe disabilities or with behaviour difficulties are likely to have been prescribed medication. Attention has been drawn by Hubert (1992) to the dissatisfaction of many parents with the use and administration of medication for their sons or daughters.

Evaluating residential and day services

A number of indicators of quality of services have emerged over the last decade (Centre for Policy on Ageing, 1984; Independent Development Council, 1986; Evans *et al.*, 1987; Chamberlain, Samuel and Rogers, 1990a, 1990b; Department of Health and Social Services Inspectorate, 1992a, 1992b). Evaluation in terms of financial costs has also been reported (Davies, 1987).

In view of the place of normalisation in the development of community care and practice, use of the PASS and PASSING evaluation instruments (Wolfensberger and Glenn, 1975; Wolfensberger and Thomas, 1983), which evaluate a service's conformity to normalisation principles, is particularly interesting. The validity and usefulness of PASS and PASSING in Britain have been studied by Pilling and Midgley (1992). The Community and

Mental Handicap Educational and Research Association has carried out a number of commissioned evaluations of services, the results of some of which have been made available (for example, Tyne and Williams, 1987; Williams, 1992).

Figure 5.1 (reproduced from Williams, 1986) shows the score on PASS achieved by 52 residential services, divided into nine categories. As might be predicted, institutional provision comes out very badly; small homes within institution grounds, and village communities, fare little better; ordinary housing and social services hostels approach, but do not reach, the level of minimum acceptability in terms of normalisation. The only kind of provision to exceed minimally acceptable practice is ordinary housing that involves 'lifesharing' with non-disabled people.

In a sample of 13 adult training centres evaluated with PASS (Williams, 1987), performance above the minimum acceptable level was achieved in areas concerned with the physical location of services and access to com-

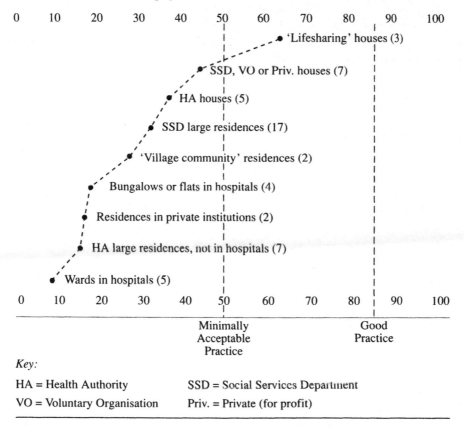

Figure 5.1 Median total scores on PASS of 52 residential services for adults with mental handicaps

Source: Williams (1986)

munity resources, in developmental challenges within the centres, and in some aspects of age-appropriateness. There was very poor performance in areas of imagery, consumer participation, grouping together of large numbers of people with different needs, autonomy and rights, appropriate activities, community integration, efficient use of time, and 'model coherency'. The latter concept involves an expectation that a service will utilise space, time and resources, and will provide programme content and process, that are appropriate to specific needs. For example, work preparation and support will involve places of work, work equipment, staff skilled and experienced in supporting employment, timing and duration that are associated with work, etc. Education will be given in education establishments by teachers, with appropriate lengths of courses with defined aims. The precise opposite of model coherency is the large multi-purpose day centre, where client and staff identity and programme aims, content and duration are ill-defined. It can be noted that this issue is not resolved in the current models of 'choice', 'community dispersal' or 'resource centre'.

Evaluations with PASS can also help to clarify management needs in community services. For example, evaluations of staffed houses have tended to highlight issues of staff role and behaviour in small houses where 'ownership' of the setting should clearly belong to the residents (see Williams, 1992).

Staff training

The management of community services, especially small, dispersed provision, requires special attention to staff support needs (Shaddock, 1988; Harris, 1992) and training is an important part of this. The training needs of staff in the emerging patterns of community-based services have been reviewed by a number of authors (Shearer, 1983; Whiffen, 1984; Hogg and Mittler, 1987; Raynes and Sumpton, 1987a, 1987b; Central Council for Education and Training in Social Work (CCETSW), 1992). The potential impact of staff training on service users and on organisations has been described by Scally and Bayer (1992a, 1992b). Many of the research studies of community services previously mentioned have generated suggestions for and experience of the requirements for staff training, for example, the study of the Wells Road project in Bristol (Ward, 1985, 1987a; Ward and Wilkinson, 1985).

Systematic training in the principles of normalisation and social role valorisation have been available in Britain, through the Community and Mental Handicap Educational and Research Association and others. Organisations providing relevant in-service training courses have included Castle Priory College, the staff training centre of the Spastics Society, and the British Institute of Learning Disabilities (formerly BIMH). Multidisciplinary BA degree courses in learning disabilities have recently been established in

Winchester, Stockport and London, and post-qualification MA courses are provided in Kent, Portsmouth, Birmingham, Hull, York, Keele and Reading.

The main forms of professional qualification have continued to be mental handicap nursing, and qualifications in social work under the auspices of CCETSW. Since the Jay Report (1979), there have been a number of experiments in joint training of nurses and social workers, but none has become established (see Donovan, 1989). Training of specialist mental handicap nurses will continue under the Project 2000 proposals for nurse training, while the Diploma in Social Work (replacing CQSW and CSS) will be the form of professional qualification for residential and day service work. The new structure of NVQ training, involving on the job training and assessment of specific skills, should be helpful to the identification and meeting of staff training needs (Henderson and Crowhurst, 1991).

Publications and aids to staff training have been developed (see, for example, Open University, 1986, 1990; Averill *et al.*, 1989; Brandon and Brandon, 1989; Brandon, 1992c; Brown and Benson, 1992; Alcoe and Parker, 1993).

The general context of group care

There is a wealth of general literature on residential and day service work that has relevance to work with people with learning disabilities. Also, the development of community services for people with learning disabilities has had innovative aspects of importance to the wider field of community care. For both these reasons, it is important for those who work in this specialist field to develop a broad interest and perspective that extends to more general concerns. Some general resources on issues in residential care are Walton and Elliott (1980), Davis (1982), Douglas and Payne (1985), Wagner (1988) and Atherton (1989). Concerns relating to group care in general, including work in day services, are covered, for example, by Brown and Clough (1989) and by Ward (1993). The latter summarises his book by saying:

> Group care is complex and demanding work, requiring understanding, skills and professional teamwork of a high order. This work has positive potential to make a real difference to people's lives, and there is a need for group care workers to sustain this belief and to be supported in it.
>
> (Ward, 1993)

In few other fields is this demonstrated as much as in the community care of people with learning disabilities.

REFERENCES

Abberley, P. (1987) The concept of oppression and the development of a social theory of disability. *Disability, Handicap and Society*, 2, 5–21.

Abbott, P. and Sapsford, R. (1987) *Community Care for Mentally Handicapped Children*. Milton Keynes: Open University Press.

Abraham, C. (1989) Supporting people with a mental handicap in the community: a social psychological perspective. *Disability, Handicap and Society, 4*, 121–30.

Alaszewski, A. (1986) *Institutional Care and the Mentally Handicapped*. London: Croom Helm.

Alaszewski, A. and Nio-Ong, B. (1990) *Normalisation in Practice: Residential Care for Children with a Profound Mental Handicap*. London: Routledge.

Alcoe, J. and Parker, C. (1993) *Training Materials for the Caring Services*. Hove: Pavilion Publishing.

Allen, D. (1989) The effects of deinstitutionalisation on people with mental handicaps: a review. *Mental Handicap Research, 2*, 18–37.

Association for the Protection of Patients and Staff (1982) *Vulnerable People*. London: APPS.

Atherton, J. (1989) *Interpreting Residential Life: Values to Practise*. London: Tavistock.

Atkinson, D. (1987) How easy is it to form friendships after leaving long-stay hospitals? *Social Work Today*, 15 June, 12–13.

Atkinson, D. (1988a) Moving from hospital to the community: factors influencing the lifestyles of people with mental handicap. *Mental Handicap, 16*, 8–10.

Atkinson, D. (1988b) Residential care for children and adults with mental handicap. In: Wagner, G. (ed.) *Residential Care: The Research Reviewed*. London: National Institute for Social Work and HMSO.

Atkinson, D. and Ward, L. (1986) *A Part of the Community: Social Integration and Neighbourhood Networks*. London: Values Into Action.

Atkinson, D. and Ward. L. (1987) Friends and neighbours: relationships and opportunities in the community for people with a mental handicap. In: Malin, N. (ed.) *Re-assessing Community Care*. London: Croom Helm.

Atkinson, D. and Williams, F. (eds) (1990) *Know Me As I Am: An Anthology of Prose, Poetry and Art by People with Learning Difficulties*. London: Hodder and Stoughton.

Atkinson, D. and Williams, P. (1990) *Networks – Workbook 2 of Mental Handicap: Changing Perspectives*. Milton Keynes: The Open University.

Auburn, T. and Leach, S. (1989) An evaluation of the physical environment of two community-based homes for the mentally handicapped. *British Journal of Mental Subnormality, 35*, 83–93.

Audit Commission (1986) *Making a Reality of Community Care*. London: HMSO.

Audit Commission (1989) *Developing Community Care for Adults with a Mental Handicap*. London: HMSO.

Averill, L., Lee, H. and Felce, D. (1989) *A Guide to Training Resources in Mental Handicap*. Kidderminster: BIMH Publications.

Ayer, S. and Alaszewski, A. (1984) *Community Care and the Mentally Handicapped*. London: Croom Helm.

Baker, J. and Gaden, G. (1992) Integration and equality. In: Fairbairn, G. and Fairbairn, S. (eds) *Integrating Special Children: Some Ethical Issues*. Aldershot: Avebury.

Baldwin, S., Parker, G. and Walker, R. (eds) (1988) *Social Security and Community Care*. Aldershot: Avebury.

Barnes, C. (1990) *Cabbage Syndrome: The Social Construction of Dependence*. London: Falmer Press.

Baron, S. and Haldane, J. (eds) (1992) *Community, Normality and Difference: Meeting Special Needs*. Aberdeen: Aberdeen University Press.

Barron, D. (1989) Slings and arrows: what it was like on the receiving end of services. In: Brandon, D. (ed.) *Mutual Respect: Therapeutic Approaches to Working with People who have Learning Difficulties*. New Malden: Hexagon Publishers.

Baxter, C., Poonia, K., Ward, L. and Nadirshaw, Z. (1990) *Double Discrimination: Issues and Services for People with Learning Difficulties from Black and Ethnic Minority Communities.* London: King's Fund Centre.

Beail, N. (1988) A comparative observational study of the care provided in hospital with the care provided at home for profoundly multiply handicapped children. *Behavioural Psychotherapy, 16,* 285–96.

Bender, M. (1986) The inside out day centre. *Community Care,* 23 October, 14–15.

Bennett, B. (1989) *Education in a Special Hospital.* Nottingham: University of Nottingham Department of Adult Education.

Blom-Cooper, L. (1992) *Report of the Committee of Inquiry into Complaints about Ashworth Hospital.* London: HMSO.

Blunden, R. and Allen, D. (eds) (1987) *Facing the Challenge: An Ordinary Life for People with Learning Difficulties and Challenging Behaviour.* London: King's Fund Centre.

Blunden, R. and Smith, H. (1988) Leaving long-stay hospitals: caring in patches. *Community Care Supplement,* 27 October, i–ii.

Bogdan, R. and Taylor, S. (1987) Conclusion: the next wave. In: Taylor, S., Biklen, D. and Knoll, J. (eds) *Community Integration for People with Severe Disabilities.* London, Ontario: Teachers College Press.

Booth, T. (ed.) (1990) *Better Lives: Changing Services for People with Learning Difficulties.* Sheffield: Joint Unit for Social Services Research, University of Sheffield.

Booth, T. and Phillips, D. (1991) From hospital to a home in the community. *British Journal of Mental Subnormality, 37,* 73–9.

Booth, T., Phillips, D., Barritt, A., Melotte, C., Matthews, J. and Pritlove, J. (1989) Home from home: a survey of independent living schemes for people with a mental handicap. *Mental Handicap Research, 2,* 152–66.

Booth, T., Simons, K. and Booth, W. (1990) *Outward Bound: Relocation and Community Care for People with Learning Difficulties.* London: Open University Press.

Booth, W., Booth, T. and Simons, K. (1990) Return journey: the relocation of adults from long-stay hospital into hostel accommodation. *British Journal of Mental Subnormality, 36,* 87–97.

Brandon, D. (1991) Colleges favourites to win the new Nobel prizes. *Community Living, 4* (3), 8.

Brandon, D. (1992a) How we create new institutions from the ashes of the old. *Community Living, 6* (2), 10.

Brandon, D. (1992b) Must moving out mean moving on? *Community Living, 5* (4), 18.

Brandon, D. (1992c) *Staff Practice Handbook.* Salford: Centre for Health Studies, University College Salford.

Brandon, D. (1992d) *Strange Places.* Salford: Centre for Health Studies, University College Salford.

Brandon, D. and Brandon, A. (1989) *Putting People First: A Handbook on the Practical Application of Ordinary Living Principles.* New Malden: Hexagon Publishers.

Brandon, D. and Ridley, J. (1985) *Beginning to Listen: A Study of the Views of Residents Living in a Hostel for Mentally Handicapped People.* London: Values Into Action.

Bratt, A. and Johnston, R. (1987) Changes in lifestyle for young adults with profound disabilities following discharge from hospital care into a second generation housing project. *Mental Handicap Research, 1,* 49–74.

Brothers of Charity (1992) *Innovations in Employment Training and Work for People with Learning Difficulties.* Chorley: Lisieux Hall Publications.

Brown, A. and Clough, R. (eds) (1989) *Groups and Groupings: Life and Work in Day and Residential Centres*. London: Tavistock/Routledge.

Brown, H. and Benson, S. (1992) *A Practical Guide to Working with People with Learning Difficulties*. London: Care Concern.

Brown, H. and Craft, A. (eds) (1989) *Thinking the Unthinkable: Papers on Sexual Abuse and People with Learning Difficulties*. London: Family Planning Association.

Brown, H. and Smith, H. (1989) Whose ordinary life is it anyway? *Disability, Handicap and Society, 4*, 105–19.

Brown, H. and Smith, H. (1990) Whose ordinary life is it anyway? *Journal of Practical Approaches to Developmental Handicap, 14* (2), 17–24.

Brown, H. and Smith, H. (1992a) Assertion not assimilation: a feminist perspective on the normalisation principle. In: Brown, H. and Smith, H. (eds) *Normalisation: A Reader for the Nineties*. London: Tavistock/Routledge.

Brown, H. and Smith, H. (eds) (1992b) *Normalisation: A Reader for the Nineties*. London: Tavistock/Routledge.

Bulmer, M. (1987) *The Social Basis of Community Care*. London: Allen and Unwin.

Carter, J. (1981) *Day Services for Adults: Somewhere To Go*. London: George Allen and Unwin.

Carter, J. (1988) *Creative Day Care for Mentally Handicapped People*. Oxford: Blackwell.

Cattermole, M., Jahoda, A. and Markova, I. (1988) Leaving home: the experience of people with a mental handicap. *Journal of Mental Deficiency Research, 32*, 46–57.

Cattermole, M., Jahoda, A. and Markova, I. (1989) We want a real say. *Nursing Times*, 11 January, 65–7.

Cattermole, M., Jahoda, A. and Markova, I. (1990) Quality of life for people with learning difficulties moving to community homes. *Disability, Handicap and Society, 5*, 137–52.

Causby, V. and York, R. (1990) Social support and the success of deinstitutionalisation. *Journal of Applied Social Sciences, 14*, 197–219.

Causby, V. and York, R. (1991) Predictors of success in community placement of persons with mental retardation. *British Journal of Mental Subnormality, 37*, 25–34.

Central Council for Education and Training in Social Work (1992) *Learning Together: Shaping New Services for People with Learning Disabilities*. London: CCETSW.

Centre for Policy on Ageing (1984) *Home Life: A Code of Practice for Residential Care*. London: Centre on Policy for Ageing.

Chamberlain, P. (1988) Moving into ordinary houses supported by staff. In: Horobin, G. and May, D. (eds) *Living with Mental Handicap: Transitions in the Lives of People with Mental Handicaps*. London: Jessica Kingsley Publishers.

Chamberlain, P., Samuel, R. and Rogers, C. (1990a) A measure of community services. *Nursing Times*, 5 September, 36–9.

Chamberlain, P., Samuel, R. and Rogers, C. (1990b) What cost quality of life? *Nursing Times*, 12 September, 51–3.

Clare, M. (1990) *Developing Self-Advocacy Skills with People with Disabilities and Learning Difficulties*. London: Further Education Unit.

Clayton, N. (1992) Cracks in the community. *Community Care*, 2 April, 12–13.

Collins, J. (1992a) Changing places. *Community Care*, 11 June, 22–3.

Collins, J. (1992b) *When the Eagles Fly*. London: Values Into Action.

Connelly, N. (1988) *Care in the Multi-Racial Community*. London: Policy Studies Institute.

Cottis, S. (1989) Art work, art share: community care in action. *Journal of Social Work Practice, 4*, 54–61.

Cottis, T., Cervenka, H. and Shelton, P. (1989) Ships in a harbour are safe, but that's not what ships are built for: care in the community. *Journal of Social Work Practice*, 4, 88–99.

Couchman, W., Gray, B. and Kenny, B. (1987) Three steps to normalisation. *Senior Nurse*, 6, 11–12.

Crawford, N., Taylor, P. and Thobroe, E. (1984) Special care in 19 adult training centres. *Mental Handicap*, 12, 54–6.

Crawley, B. (1988) *The Growing Voice: A Survey of Self-Advocacy Groups in Adult Training Centres and Hospitals in Great Britain.* London: Values Into Action.

Crocker, T. (1989) Assessing consumer satisfaction with mental handicap services: a comparison between different approaches. *British Journal of Mental Subnormality*, 35, 94–100.

Cullen, C. (1991) Experimentation and planning in community care. *Disability, Handicap and Society*, 6, 115–28.

Dagnan, D. and Drewett, R. (1988) Community based care for people with a mental handicap: a family placement scheme in County Durham. *British Journal of Social Work*, 18, 543–75.

Dalgleish, M. (1983) Environmental constraints on residential services for mentally handicapped people: some findings from the Sheffield Development Project. *Mental Handicap*, 11, 102–5.

Dalgleish, M., Barnes, S. and Matthews, R. (1983) External contacts of residents in hospitals and hostels for mentally handicapped adults. *Community Medicine*, 5, 227–34.

Dalley, G. (1989) Community care: the ideal and the reality. In: Brechin, A. and Walmsley, J. (eds) *Making Connections: Reflecting on the Lives and Experiences of People with Learning Difficulties.* London: Hodder and Stoughton.

Dartington, T., Miller, E. and Gwynne, G. (1981) *A Life Together.* London: Tavistock.

Davies, L. (1987) Ordinary life – does it cost more? *Health Service Journal*, 97, 221–3.

Davis, L. (1982) *Residential Care: A Community Resource.* London: Heinemann.

Day, P. (1987) Mind the gap: normalisation theory and practice. *Practice*, 1, 105–15.

Department of Health (1989) *Caring for People: Community Care in the Next Decade and Beyond.* London: HMSO.

Department of Health (1992) *Social Care for Adults with Learning Disabilities (Mental Handicap): Local Authority Circular.* London: Department of Health.

Department of Health and Social Security (1971) *Better Services for the Mentally Handicapped.* London: HMSO.

Department of Health and Social Security (1984) *Helping Mentally Handicapped People with Special Problems.* London: HMSO.

Department of Health and Social Services Inspectorate (1992a) *Caring for Quality: Day Services.* London: HMSO.

Department of Health and Social Services Inspectorate (1992b) *Guidance on Standards for the Residential Care Needs of People with Learning Disabilities/ Mental Handicap.* London: HMSO.

Dickinson, M. and Singh, I. (1991) Mental handicap and the new long stay. *Psychiatric Bulletin of the Royal College of Psychiatrists*, 15, 334–6.

Donegan, C. and Potts, M. (1988) People with mental handicap living alone in the community: a pilot study of their quality of life. *British Journal of Mental Subnormality*, 34, 10–22.

Donovan, H. (1989) The revolution is over. *Nursing Times*, 11 January, 67–9.

Dominelli, L. (1988) *Anti-Racist Social Work.* Basingstoke: Macmillan.

Douglas, R. and Payne, C. (1985) *Developing Residential Practice: A Sourcebook of References and Resources for Staff Development.* London: National Institute for Social Work.

Dowson, S. (1991) *Moving to the Dance: Service Culture and Community Care.* London: Values Into Action.

Dudley, J. (1989) The role of residential programme staff in facilitating positive relations with the neighbourhood: what should it be? *Administration in Social Work, 13*, 95–111.

Eastwood, L. (1987) A group home/landlady scheme. In: Malin, N. (ed.) *Re-assessing Community Care*. London: Croom Helm.

Evans, G. and Murcott, A. (1990) Community care: relationships and control. *Disability, Handicap and Society, 5*, 123–35.

Evans, G., Todd, S., Blunden, R., Porterfield, J. and Ager, A. (1987) Evaluating the impact of a move to ordinary housing. *British Journal of Mental Subnormality, 33*, 10–18.

Farmer, R., Holroyd, S. and Rhode, J. (1990) Differences in disability between people with mental handicaps who were resettled in the community and those who remained in hospital. *British Medical Journal, 301*, 646–7.

Felce, D. (1989) *The Andover Project: Staffed Housing for Adults with Severe or Profound Mental Handicaps*. Kidderminster: BIMH Publications.

Felce, D. and Toogood, S. (1988) *Close to Home: A Local Housing Service and its Impact on the Lives of Nine Adults with Severe and Profound Mental Handicap*. Kidderminster: BIMH Publications.

Ferrity, B., Ford, D. and Bratt, A. (1986) The private sector: just landladies or carers? *Mental Handicap, 14*, 166–9.

Firth, H. and Rapley, M. (1990) *From Acquaintance to Friendship: Issues for People with Learning Disabilities*. Kidderminster: BIMH Publications.

Flynn, M. (1989) *Independent Living for Adults with Mental Handicap: A Place of My Own*. London: Cassell.

Flynn, M. and Saleem, J. (1986) Adults who are mentally handicapped and living with their parents: satisfaction and perceptions regarding their lives and circumstances. *Journal of Mental Deficiency Research, 30*, 379–87.

Ford, S. (1987) Into the outside. *Nursing Times*, 20 May, 40–2.

Francis, W. (1987a) Ignorance of the right kind? *Community Care*, 21 May, 18–19.

Francis, W. (1987b) Setting the wheels in motion. *Community Care*, 27 August, 24–5.

Fullerton, M. (1987) Out in the world. *New Society*, 24 July, 20–1.

Further Education Unit (1992) *Developing Competence: Guidelines on Implementing Provision Leading to Employment-led Qualifications for Learners with Disabilities and Learning Difficulties*. London: Further Education Unit.

Garrett, B. (1989) *Not Just Play: The Evaluation of PLAYTRAC*. London: Save the Children Fund.

Gathercole, C. (1981a) *Family Placements*. Kidderminster: BIMH.

Gathercole, C. (1981b) *Group Homes – Staffed and Unstaffed*. Kidderminster: BIMH.

Grant, G. and McGrath, M. (1990) Need for respite care services for care givers of persons with mental retardation. *American Journal of Mental Retardation, 94*, 638–48.

Gray, G. (1990) Notes on the Social Services Inspectorate report on the inspection of day services for people with a mental handicap. *Newsletter of the Association of Professions for Mentally Handicapped People*, Spring, 4–9.

Griffiths, R. (1988) *Community Care: Agenda for Action*. London: HMSO.

Groarke, A. (1987) Community living for persons with mental handicap: a survey of public attitudes. *Journal of Practical Approaches to Developmental Handicap, 11* (1), 20–5.

Gunzburg, H. and Gunzburg, A. (1992) Normal home environments: indifferent or stimulating? In: Gunzburg, H. (ed.) *Despite Mental Handicap: Learning to Cope with Adult Daily Life*. Stratford-upon-Avon: British Society for Developmental Disabilities.

Haggar, L. and Hutchinson, R. (1991) Snoezelen: an approach to the provision of a leisure resource for people with profound and multiple handicaps. *Mental Handicap, 19*, 51–5.

Halliday, S. and Potts, M. (1987) Moving into the community: views from the staff involved on the causes and effects of delays in one move. *British Journal of Mental Subnormality, 33*, 31–42.

Harper, G. (1989) Life-sharing. *Community Living, 2* (4), 6–7.

Harper, G. (1990) A better life on the outside. *Community Living, 3* (4), 14–16.

Harris, P. (1992) Support, respect and value: the keys to high staff morale. *Community Living, 6* (2), 12–13.

Hay, D. (1987) Planning blight? *Nursing Times*, 1 July, 47–9.

Heginbotham, C. (1981) *Housing Projects for Mentally Handicapped People.* London: Centre on Environment for the Handicapped.

Heginbotham, C. (1987) Putting trust back in the community. *Social Work Today*, 26 January, 19–21.

Hemming, H. (1982) Mentally handicapped adults returned to large institutions after transfers to new small units. *British Journal of Mental Subnormality, 28*, 13–28.

Hemming, H., Lavender, T. and Pill, R. (1981) Quality of life of mentally retarded adults transferred from large institutions to new small units. *American Journal of Mental Deficiency, 86*, 157–69.

Henderson, R. and Crowhurst, G. (1991) On-the-job training for residential staff. *Mental Handicap, 19*, 155–7.

Heron, A. (1982) *Better Services for the Mentally Handicapped? Lessons from the Sheffield Evaluation Studies.* London: King's Fund Centre.

Hewitt, S. (1987) The abuse of deinstitutionalised persons with mental handicaps. *Disability, Handicap and Society, 2*, 127–35.

Hewitt, S. (1989) *Interviewing Persons with Mental Handicaps and the Codes of Practice.* Bath: S. Hewitt.

Hill-Tout, J. (1988) Personal services. *Community Care*, 4 February, 22–4.

Hobbs, D. (1993) *Learning Together: Gentle Teaching Training Package.* New Malden: Hexagon Publishing.

Hogan, R. (1989) Managing local government opposition to community-based residential facilities for the mentally disabled. *Community Mental Health Journal, 25*, 33–41.

Hogg, J. and Mittler, P. (eds) (1987) *Staff Training in Mental Handicap.* Beckenham: Croom Helm.

Hogg, J. and Sebba, J. (1986) *Profound Retardation and Multiple Impairment. Vol.1: Development and Learning.* London: Croom Helm.

Hubert, J. (1991) *Home-Bound: Crisis in the Care of Young People with Severe Learning Difficulties – A Story of Twenty Families.* London: King's Fund Centre.

Hubert, J. (1992) *Too Many Drugs, Too Little Care.* London: Values Into Action.

Hudson, B. (1988) Tried and tested in Wales. *Health Service Journal, 98*, 596–7.

Hudson, B. (1990) Looking for a way out. *Health Service Journal, 100*, 1354–5.

Hulbert, C. and Atkinson, D. (1987) On the way out and after. *British Journal of Mental Subnormality, 33*, 109–17.

Humphreys, E. (1987) A sharing experience. *Social Services Insight*, 28 August, 11–13.

Humphreys, S., Evans, G. and Todd, S. (eds) (1987) *Lifelines.* London: King Edward's Hospital Fund.

Hunter, D. and Wistow, G. (1987) *Community Care in Britain: Variations on a Theme.* London: King Edward's Hospital Fund.

Hutchinson, R. (ed.) (1991) *The Whittington Hall Snoezelen Project.* Chesterfield: North Derbyshire Health Authority.

Independent Development Council for People with Mental Handicap (1985) *Living*

Like Other People: Next Steps in Day Services for People with Mental Handicap. London: IDC.

Independent Development Council for People with Mental Handicap (1986) *Pursuing Quality.* London: IDC.

Jackson, R. (1991) Will care survive? *British Journal of Mental Subnormality, 37,* 123–9.

Jawed, S., Krishnan, V., Sansom, D. and Butler, C. (1993) First 99 residents of a new mental handicap hospital: a ten-year follow-up study. *British Journal of Developmental Disabilities, 39,* 3–16.

Jay, P. (1979) *Report of the Committee of Enquiry into Mental Handicap Nursing and Care.* London: HMSO.

Jones, G. and Tutt, N. (eds) (1983) *A Way of Life for the Handicapped – New Developments in Residential and Community Care.* London: Residential Care Association.

Jones, K. and Fowles, A. (1984) *Ideas on Institutions: Analysing the Literature on Long-term Care and Custody.* London: Routledge and Kegan Paul.

Keene, N. and James, H. (1986) Who needs hospital care? *Mental Handicap, 14,* 101–3.

Kiernan, C. and Moss, S. (1990) Behaviour disorders and other characteristics of the population of a mental handicap hospital. *Mental Handicap Research, 3,* 3–20.

King's Fund Centre (1980) *An Ordinary Life: Comprehensive Locally-Based Residential Services for Mentally Handicapped People.* London: King's Fund Centre.

King's Fund Centre (1984) *An Ordinary Working Life: Vocational Services for People with Mental Handicap.* London: King's Fund Centre.

King's Fund Centre (1988) *Ties and Connections: An Ordinary Community Life for People with Learning Difficulties.* London: King's Fund Centre.

Knapp, M., Cambridge, P., Thomason, C., Beecham, J., Allen, C. and Darton, R. (1992) *Care in the Community: Challenge and Demonstration.* Aldershot: Ashgate Publishers.

Korman, N. and Glennerster, H. (1990) *Hospital Closure: A Political and Economic Study.* Milton Keynes: Open University Press.

Krishnan, V., Upadhyay, B. and Londhe, R. (1993) New long-stay patients in an urban and a rural hospital for people with mental handicap: a comparative study. *British Journal of Developmental Disabilities, 39,* 17–30.

Leighton, A. (1988) *Mental Handicap in the Community.* Cambridge: Woodhead-Faulkner.

Letts, P. (1992) Unfit to plead? *Community Living, 5* (3), 10–11.

Lister, T. and Ellis, L. (1992) *Survey of Supported Employment Services in England, Wales and Scotland.* Manchester: National Development Team.

Locker, D., Rao, B. and Weddell, J. (1983) The impact of hostel care on mentally handicapped adults. *Mental Handicap, 11,* 100–1.

Locker, D., Rao, B. and Weddell, J. (1984) Evaluating community care for the mentally handicapped adult: a comparison of hostel, home and hospital care. *Journal of Mental Deficiency Research, 28,* 189–98.

Long, M. (1988) Delivering a balanced service. *Community Care,* 28 January, 26–7.

Longhorn, F. (1988) *A Sensory Curriculum for Very Special People: A Practical Approach to Curriculum Planning.* London: Souvenir Press.

Lowe, K. and de Paiva, S. (1990) *NIMROD – An Overview: A Summary Report of a Five-Year Research Study.* Cardiff: Mental Handicap in Wales Applied Research Unit.

Lowe, K., de Paiva, S. and Humphreys, S. (1987) *Clients' Views.* Cardiff: Mental Handicap in Wales Applied Research Unit.

McCarthy, M. (1987a) The debate on community care. *Social Work Today,* 21 September, 17–19.

McCarthy, M. (1987b) Community care debate continues. *Social Work Today*, 28 September, 14–15.

McConkey, R. and McGinley, P. (eds) (1991) *Innovations in Leisure and Recreation for People with a Mental Handicap*. Chorley: Lisieux Hall Publications.

McGee, J., Menolascino, F., Hobbs, D. and Menosek, P. (1987) *Gentle Teaching: A Non-Aversive Approach for Helping Persons with Mental Retardation*. New York: Human Sciences Press.

McGrath, M. (1988) Inter-agency collaboration in the All-Wales Strategy: initial comments on a vanguard area. *Social Policy and Administration*, *22*, 53–67.

McGrath, M. and Grant, G. (1992) Supporting needs-led services: implications for planning and management systems – a case study in mental handicap services. *Journal of Social Policy*, *21*, 71–97.

Maher, J. and Russell, O. (1988) Serving people with very challenging behaviour. In: Towell, D. (ed.) *An Ordinary Life in Practice*. London: King Edward's Hospital Fund.

Malin, N. (1983) *Group Homes for Mentally Handicapped People*. London: HMSO.

Malin, N. (ed.) (1987) *Re-Assessing Community Care*. London: Croom Helm.

Malin, N., Race, D. and Jones, G. (1980) *Services for the Mentally Handicapped in Britain*. London: Croom Helm.

Mansell, J., Felce, D., Jenkins, J., de Kock, U. and Toogood, S. (1987) *Developing Staffed Housing for People with Mental Handicaps*. Tunbridge Wells: Costello.

Martin, J. (1984) *Hospitals in Trouble*. Oxford: Blackwell.

MENCAP (1985) *Day Services Today and Tomorrow*. London: MENCAP Publications.

Mills, J. (1988) An uncaring community. *New Society*, 12 February, 20–1.

Mitchell, F. (1990) Respite care services for adults with mental handicap. *Mental Handicap*, *18*, 33–4.

National Association of Teachers of the Mentally Handicapped (1985) *Towards Tomorrow: Day Services for Mentally Handicapped People*. Manchester: NATMH.

National Development Group for the Mentally Handicapped (1977) *Day Services for Mentally Handicapped Adults*. London: National Development Group/HMSO.

National Development Team (1988) *The Development of a Contraction Strategy for the Brockhall/Calderstones Unit in Lancashire*. Manchester: NDT.

National Development Team (1990a) *Better Lives: A Review of the Quality of Life of the People Living in Borocourt Hospital*. Manchester: NDT.

National Development Team (1990b) *Policies with Values and Vision for the 1990s*. Manchester: NDT.

National Development Team (1990c) *Promises to Keep: Making Community Care for People with a Mental Handicap into a Reality in the 1990s*. Manchester: NDT.

Noonan-Walsh, P. (1988) Handicapped and female: two disabilities? In: McConkey, R. and McGinley, P. (eds) *Concepts and Controversies in Services for People with Mental Handicap*. Dublin: St. Michael's House.

Norris, D. (1982) *Profound Mental Handicap*. Tunbridge Wells: Costello.

Norris, D. (1988) *Have You Tried . . . ? A Handbook of Activities and Services for Profoundly Retarded People*. Tunbridge Wells: Costello Education.

O'Brien, J. (1987a) A guide to personal futures planning. In: Bellamy, G. and Wilcox, B. (eds) *A Comprehensive Guide to the Activities Catalogue: An Alternative Curriculum for Youth and Adults with Severe Disabilities*. Baltimore: Paul Brookes.

O'Brien, J. (1987b) Discovering community: learning from innovation in services to people with mental retardation. In: Kugel, R. (ed.) *Changing Patterns in Residential Services for Persons with Mental Retardation*. Washington, D.C.: President's Committee on Mental Retardation.

O'Brien, J. and Lyle, C. (1987) *Framework for Accomplishment: A Workshop for*

People Developing Better Services. Lithonia, Georgia: Responsive Systems Associates.

O'Brien, J. and Lyle, C. (1991) *Members of Each Other: Perspectives on Social Support for People with Severe Disabilities*. Lithonia, Georgia: Responsive Systems Associates.

O'Brien, J. and Lyle, C. (eds) (1992) *Remembering the Soul of Our Work*. Madison, Wisconsin: Options in Community Living.

O'Connor, N. and Tizard, J. (1956) *The Social Problem of Mental Deficiency*. Oxford: Pergamon Press.

Oliver, M. (1989) *The Politics of Disablement*. London: Macmillan.

Oliver, M. (1992) *Social Work: Disabled People and Disabling Environments*. London: Jessica Kingsley Publishers.

Open University (1986) *Mental Handicap: Patterns for Living*. Milton Keynes: The Open University.

Open University (1990) *Mental Handicap: Changing Perspectives*. Milton Keynes: The Open University.

Oswin, M. (1984) *They Keep Going Away*. London: King Edward's Hospital Fund.

Perske, R. (1988) *Circles of Friends*. Nashville, Tennessee: Abingdon Press.

Perske, R. (1991) *Unequal Justice?* Nashville, Tennessee: Abingdon Press.

Phillips, D., Booth, T., Berry, S., Jones, D., Lee, M., McGlade, A., Matthews, J., Melotte, C. and Pritlove, J. (1988) Group homes and their residents: a comparison of independent living schemes for people with a mental handicap or mental health problem. *Social Services Research, 5*, 14–20.

Pilling, D. and Midgley, G. (1992) Does PASS measure up? Evaluating a measure of service quality. *Clinical Psychology Forum, 39*, 25–8.

Pithouse, M. (1980) The CUSS group home. In: Walton, R. and Elliott, D. (eds) *Residential Care: A Reader in Current Theory and Practice*. Oxford: Pergamon Press.

Pittock, F. and Potts, M. (1988) Neighbourhood attitudes to people with a mental handicap: a comparative study. *British Journal of Mental Subnormality, 34*, 35–46.

Porterfield, J. and Gathercole, C. (1985) *The Employment of People with Mental Handicap: Progress Towards an Ordinary Working Life*. London: King's Fund Centre.

Potts, M. and Fido, R. (1991) *A Fit Person to be Removed: Personal Accounts of Life in a Mental Deficiency Institution*. Plymouth: Northcote House Publishers.

Puddicombe, W. (1991) *Days: In Search of Real Alternatives to the Adult Training Centre*. London: Values Into Action.

Rawlings, S. (1985a) Behaviour and skills of severely retarded adults in hospital and small residential homes. *British Journal of Psychiatry, 146*, 358–66.

Rawlings, S. (1985b) Lifestyles of severely retarded non-communicating adults in hospitals and small residential homes. *British Journal of Social Work, 15*, 281–93.

Raynes, N. (1986) Getting out and about in the community. *Community Care*, 9 October.

Raynes, N. and Sumpton, R. (1987a) Training needs for community staff. *Mental Handicap, 15*, 95–7.

Raynes, N. and Sumpton, R. (1987b) Implications for training. *Senior Nurse, 7*, 47–8.

Raynes, N., Sumpton, R. and Flynn, M. (1987) *Homes for Mentally Handicapped People*. London: Tavistock.

Richardson, A. and Ritchie, J. (1986) *Making the Break: Parents' Views about Adults with a Mental Handicap Leaving the Parental Home*. London: King's Fund Centre.

Richardson, A. and Ritchie, J. (1989a) *Developing Friendships: Enabling People with Learning Difficulties to Make and Maintain Friends*. London: Policy Studies Institute.

Richardson, A. and Ritchie, J. (1989b) *Letting Go*. Milton Keynes: Open University Press.

Rose, J. and Adamson, N. (1990) Investigating the problem of noise in a day centre: are buildings designed as industrial units suitable for education and training? *British Journal of Mental Subnormality, 36*, 118–24.

Russell, O. and Ward, L. (eds) (1983) *Houses or Homes? Evaluating Ordinary Housing Schemes for People with Mental Handicap*. London: Centre on Environment for the Handicapped.

Ryan, J. and Thomas, F. (1987) *The Politics of Mental Handicap*. London: Free Association Books.

Saxby, H., Felce, D., Harman, M. and Repp, A. (1988) The maintenance of client activity and staff–client interaction in small community houses for severely and profoundly mentally handicapped adults: a two-year follow-up. *Behavioural Psychotherapy, 16*, 189–206.

Scally, H. and Beyer, S. (1992a) Gear up for change. *Community Care*, 5 March, 16–17.

Scally, H. and Beyer, S. (1992b) Design for living. *Community Care*, 12 March, 20–2.

Schneider, J. (1992) Can friendship be fostered? *Community Living, 5* (4), 14–15.

Schwartz, D., McKnight, J. and Kendrick, M. (1987) *A Story that I Heard: A Compendium of Stories, Essays and Poetry about People with Disabilities and American Life*. Harrisburg: Pennsylvania Developmental Disabilities Planning Council.

Sebba, J. (1988) *The Education of People with Profound and Multiple Handicaps: Resource Materials for Staff Training*. Manchester: Manchester University Press.

Segal, S. (ed.) (1990) *The Place of Special Villages and Residential Communities*. Bicester: AB Academic Publishers.

Shaddock, A. (1988) The occupational status of staff in community residences for people with intellectual handicaps. *British Journal of Mental Subnormality, 34*, 86–96.

Shaw, I., Williamson, H. and Parry-Langdon, N. (1992) Developing models for day services. *Social Policy and Administration, 26*, 73–86.

Shearer, A. (1983) *An Ordinary Life: Issues and Strategies for Training Staff for Community Mental Handicap Services*. London: King's Fund Centre.

Shearer, A. (1986) *Building Community: With People with Mental Handicaps, Their Families and Friends*. London: Values Into Action/King Edward's Hospital Fund.

Sholl, A., Saunders, M. and Radburn, J. (1991) Relief care for children and adults with a mental handicap: an examination of carers' views. *Mental Handicap, 19*, 161–4.

Simons, K., Booth, T. and Booth, W. (1989) Speaking out: user studies and people with learning difficulties. *Research, Policy and Planning, 7*, 9–18.

Sines, D. (ed.) (1988) *Towards Integration: Comprehensive Services for People with Mental Handicaps*. London: Chapman and Hall.

Sines, D. and Curry, C. (1987) Hospital or community? *Nursing Times*, 25 March, 44–5.

Sinson, J. (1990) Micro-institutionalisation? Environmental and managerial influences in ten living units for people with mental handicap. *British Journal of Mental Subnormality, 36*, 77–86.

Sinson, J. (1992a) A sixth form college for mentally handicapped adolescents: Wentwood Education. In: Gunzburg, H. (ed.) *Despite Mental Handicap: Learning to Cope with Adult Daily Life*. Stratford-upon-Avon: British Society for Developmental Disabilities.

Sinson, J. (1992b) *Group Homes and Community Integration of Developmentally Disabled People – Micro-institutionalisation?* London: Jessica Kingsley Publishers.

Social Services Committee of the House of Commons (1985) *Community Care with*

Special Reference to Adult Mentally Ill and Mentally Handicapped People. London: HMSO.

Social Services Inspectorate (1989) *Inspection of Day Services for People with a Mental Handicap.* London: HMSO.

Spink, K. (1990) *Jean Vanier and L'Arche: A Communion of Love.* London: Darton, Longman and Todd.

Stainton, T. (1992) Big talk, small steps. *Community Living, 6* (1), 16–17.

Steele, D. (1993) Stop wasting money on futile training. *Community Living, 6* (3), 18.

Sugg, B. (1987) Community care: the consumers' point of view. *Community Care,* 22 January, 6–7.

Summerfield, D. (1988) Discharge prospects of a mental handicap hospital population: a survey of nursing perceptions. *British Journal of Mental Subnormality, 34,* 78–85.

Sumpton, R., Raynes, N. and Thorp, D. (1987) The residential careers of a group of mentally handicapped people: the influence of early residential experience. *British Journal of Mental Subnormality, 33,* 3–9.

Sutcliffe, J. (1990) *Adults with Learning Difficulties: Education for Choice and Empowerment.* Leicester: National Institute of Adult Continuing Education.

Sutcliffe, J. (1992) *Integration for Adults with Learning Difficulties: Contexts and Debates.* Leicester: National Institute of Adult Continuing Education.

Szivos, S. (1990) Attitudes to work and their relationship to self-esteem and aspirations among young adults with a mild mental handicap. *British Journal of Mental Subnormality, 36,* 108–17.

Taylor, D. (1987) Useful role for the day centres. *Social Work Today,* 2 February, 28–9.

Thomas, D. (1985) Putting normalisation into practice. In: Karas, E. (ed.) *Current Issues in Clinical Psychology, No.2.* New York: Plenum Press.

Thomas, T. (1989) The mentally handicapped offender: rights and responsibilities. *British Journal of Mental Subnormality, 35,* 108–14.

Thompson, M., Pilkington, F. and Seed, P. (1988a) *Day Services for People with Mental Handicaps.* London: Jessica Kingsley Publishers.

Thompson, M., Pilkington, F. and Seed, P. (1988b) *Day Services for People with Severe Handicaps.* London: Jessica Kingsley Publishers.

Tonkin, B. (1987) Voices in the wilderness. *Community Care,* 15 January, 26–9.

Towell, D. (1984) *Developing Community-Based Residential Services for People with Mental Handicap.* London: King's Fund Centre.

Towell, D. (1985) Residential needs and services. In: Craft, M., Bicknell, J. and Hollins, S. (eds) *Mental Handicap – A Multidisciplinary Approach.* London: Bailliere Tindall.

Towell, D. (ed.) (1988) *An Ordinary Life in Practice: Developing Comprehensive Community-Based Services for People with Learning Disabilities.* London: King Edward's Hospital Fund.

Towell, D. (1990) *Achieving Strategic Change in Opportunities and Services for People with Learning Difficulties: A Principled Agenda for the 1990s.* London: King's Fund College.

Towell, D. and Beardshaw, V. (1991) *Enabling Community Integration: The Role of Public Authorities in Promoting an Ordinary Life for People with Learning Disabilities in the 1990s.* London: King Edward's Hospital Fund.

Tyndall, P. (1987) Community-based respite care for adults with mental handicaps. *Mental Handicap, 15,* 156–8.

Tyne, A. (1987) Some practical dilemmas and strategies in values-led approaches to change. In: Ward, L. (ed.) *Getting Better All the Time? Issues and Strategies for Ensuring Quality in Community Services for People with Mental Handicap.* London: King's Fund Centre.

Tyne, A. (1992) Normalisation: from theory to practice. In: Brown, H. and Smith, H. (eds) *Normalisation: A Reader for the 90s*. London: Routledge.

Tyne, A. and Williams, P. (1987) *The Relocation of People from Calderstones into Ordinary Housing in Burnley District: Report of the PASS Evaluation*. Trowbridge: Community and Mental Handicap Educational and Research Association.

Vanier, J. (1979) *Community and Growth: Our Pilgrimage Together*. Toronto: Griffin House.

Vanier, J. (1982) *The Challenge of L'Arche*. London: Darton, Longman and Todd.

Vanier, J. (1990) A wound deep in man's heart. In: Kelly, B. and McGinley, P. (eds) *Mental Handicap: Challenge to the Church*. Chorley: Brothers of Charity.

Wagner, G. (1988) *Residential Care: A Positive Choice*. London: National Institute for Social Work and HMSO.

Walker, A. (ed.) (1982) *Community Care: The Family, The State and Social Policy*. Oxford: Blackwell.

Walker, P and Naylor, G. (1990) The quality of life of severely mentally handicapped patients in hospital. *Psychiatric Bulletin of the Royal College of Psychiatrists, 14*, 4–6.

Walton, R. and Elliott, D. (1980) *Residential Care: A Reader in Current Theory and Practice*. Oxford: Pergamon Press.

Ward, A. (1993) *Working in Group Care*. Birmingham: Venture Press.

Ward, L. (1982) *People First: Developing Services in the Community for People with Mental Handicap*. London: King's Fund Centre.

Ward, L. (1985) Training staff for 'An Ordinary Life': experiences in a community service in South Bristol. *British Journal of Mental Subnormality, 31*, 94–102.

Ward, L. (1987a) After induction, then what? Providing on-going staff training for 'An Ordinary Life'. *British Journal of Mental Subnormality, 33*, 131–42.

Ward, L. (ed.) (1987b) *Getting Better All the Time? Issues and Strategies for Ensuring Quality in Community Services for People with Mental Handicap*. London: King's Fund Centre.

Ward, L. (1988) What price ordinary life? *Health Service Journal, 98*, 276–7.

Ward, L. (1989) For better, for worse? In: Brechin, A. and Walmsley, J. (eds) *Making Connections: Reflecting on the Lives and Experiences of People with Learning Difficulties*. London: Hodder and Stoughton.

Ward, L. and Wilkinson, J. (1985) *Training for Change: Staff Training for 'An Ordinary Life'*. London: King's Fund Centre.

Welch, B. (1991) Social services in the 90s. *British Journal of Mental Subnormality, 37*, 130–6.

Welsh Office (1983) *The All-Wales Strategy for the Development of Services to Mentally Handicapped People*. Cardiff: Welsh Office.

Welsh Office and Social Services Inspectorate (1989) *Still a Small Voice: Consumer Involvement in the All-Wales Strategy*. Cardiff: Welsh Office.

Wertheimer, A. (1987) Towards a normal working life: new directions in day services. *Community Living, 1* (1), 8–9.

Wertheimer, A. (1988) Where people come first. *Community Care Supplement*, 27 October, ii–iv.

Wertheimer, A. (ed.) (1992) *Real Jobs: A Report of a Conference of Supported Employment Agencies*. Manchester: National Development Team.

Whiffen, P. (1984) *Initiatives in In-Service Training: Helping Staff to Care for Mentally Handicapped People in the Community*. London: Central Council for Education and Training in Social Work.

Whittaker, A., Gardner, S. and Kershaw, J. (1991) *Service Evaluation by People with Learning Difficulties*. London: King's Fund Centre.

Whittaker, J. (1991) Segregation still rules on the college campus. *Community Living, 4* (3), 18–19.

Whittaker, J. (1992) Can anyone help me to understand the logic of Snoezelen? *Community Living*, 6 (2), 15.

Williams, P. (1986) Evaluating services from the consumer's point of view. In: Beswick, J., Zadik, T. and Felce, D. (eds) *Evaluating Quality of Care*. Kidderminster: BIMH Publications.

Williams, P. (1987) *Data on the Performance of Service Groups on PASS*. Trowbridge: Community and Mental Handicap Educational and Research Association.

Williams, P. (1991) Village communities. *Community Living*, 5 (1), 10–11.

Williams, P. (1992) *Evaluation of the NIMROD Project with PASS*. Trowbridge: Community and Mental Handicap Educational and Research Association.

Williams, P. (1993) There's no place like an ordinary home. *Community Living*, 6 (3), 10–11.

Willis, P. and Kiernan, C. (1984) *A New Way Evaluated*. London: MENCAP.

Willmott, P. (ed.) (1986) *The Debate about Community*. London: Policy Studies Institute.

Wing, L. (1989) *Hospital Closure and the Resettlement of Patients*. Aldershot: Avebury.

Wolfensberger, W. (1975) *The Origin and Nature of Our Institutional Models*. Syracuse, New York: Human Policy Press.

Wolfensberger, W. (1989) Human service policies: the rhetoric versus the reality. In: Barton, L. (ed.) *Disability and Dependency*. London: Falmer Press.

Wolfensberger, W. (1990) A most critical issue: life or death. *Changes*, 8, 63–73.

Wolfensberger, W. (1992) Deinstitutionalisation policy: how it is made, by whom and why. *Clinical Psychology Forum*, 39, 7–11.

Wolfensberger, W. and Glenn, L. (1975) *Programme Analysis of Service Systems: Handbook and Field Manual*, 3rd edition. Toronto: National Institute on Mental Retardation.

Wolfensberger, W. and Thomas, S. (1983) *Programme Analysis of Service Systems' Implementation of Normalisation Goals*. Toronto: National Institute on Mental Retardation.

Woolrych, R. (ed.) (1989) *Developing Day Services*. Ross-on-Wye: Bridges (Association of Professions for Mentally Handicapped People).

6   Services to families

Jill Manthorpe

In recent years within the UK the rather simplistic notion that services easily fitted the needs of families governed professional and policy-maker opinion alike. Critiques of services' adequacy and appropriateness have challenged such views. In this chapter there are three main areas of discussion. The first section outlines the complex notions around the ideas that families need services. The second places families within the new *discourse* of formal care and discusses ways in which the needs of families with members who have learning disabilities have been conceptualised. In the third section, the focus is on the delivery of services, the complex process of access and involvement and families' perceptions of the process and their influence.

DO FAMILIES NEED SERVICES?

In asking whether families need services we focus our analysis on what families both say they need and what professionals in the name of the state deem to be their needs. In many ways families who have a member who has learning disabilities are simply families with their own individual needs and their own resources. At certain times, like other families, they are offered services which they may use (such as advice from health professionals) or which they are virtually obliged to use (such as education). In the UK, the state has declared that certain agencies have legal responsibilities for protecting children at risk in particular; here the services offered may well be considered not to be needed by the child or parents alike.

Such a perspective pulls out the difficult notion of need (see Biehal *et al.*, 1992) and poses the question of what is the appropriate boundary between state and collective provision and the individual and his or her family. In the second part of this chapter we shall comment on how the unity of individual and family has been seen as an unproblematic concept; here we focus on the dichotomy between the domestic, private domain of the family and the state or its agents.

At this macro level there are perhaps four questions. These can be identified as who should do what, to whom should 'it' be done and who should pay the cost. The history, in chronological or developmental terms, of services to families with members who have learning disabilities centres around these points.

In broad terms the role of an industrial, capitalist state in welfare has often been seen as combining to maintain and promote an efficient labour force, to control social unrest and to provide a safety net of provision to reduce individuals' fears of insecurity and isolation (Oliver, 1989 and Alcock, 1987). In the UK, the development of the Poor Law and patchy employer or insurance-based financial systems is well documented (Thane, 1982). It is against this backcloth that the piecemeal development of interactions between the state and certain families, such as those with disabled or sick members, can be seen.

McIntosh and Alaszewski (1994) point out that people with learning disabilities have only been visible in policy terms since the beginning of this century. To use Blumer's model of social problem construction (1971) they emerged as problems for the newly developing state educational system, in industrial areas where family members worked outside the home and in urban industries based in factories. Such a social context combined with medical eugenic beliefs that degeneracy was a key societal problem. The focus of this emerging social problem was not simply individuals, for notions of re-generacy and moral or mental defectiveness centred around perceived family behaviour. People with learning disabilities, or mental deficiency, were viewed as the products of innate family dysfunction. The acceptance of a hereditary base for mental deficiency put the family at centre stage. Families were perceived to be variously irresponsible, sexually overactive, poor and criminals, with the views of the Wood Committee (1929) representing the peak of the UK eugenic scare (see Proctor, 1988 for a European perspective).

In his discussion of the Wood Report, Stainton (1992) notes that the thrust of the eugenics movement was four-fold; but euthanasia and marriage regulations were not as acceptable nor as feasible as were segregation and sterilisation. Both segregation and sterilisation were explicit attempts to control actual and potential families and, as sex-segregated colonies or institutions developed, enforced segregation restricted the perceived need for sterilisation. The preliminary effects of intervention on the lives of families with members who had learning disabilities were therefore legally based removals and incarceration under the cloak of social protection, coupled with assessment, supervision and bureaucratic regulation.

Naturally, there were large numbers of people whose lives were only marginally influenced by these interventions. The Wood Committee itself envisaged that for every one person living in an institution such as a colony, there would be two others living at home with their families. Services for the latter were patchy in the extreme, unless they came to attention of the authorities as needing control or accommodation.

The voices of people involved in such processes have been rarely heard. David Barron's (1977) account illustrates the grim nature of his contact with 'services' available at the time of the Second World War, while the anthology of prose, poetry and art, edited for the Open University (Atkinson and Williams, 1990), suggests how institutionalisation put immense strains on people's ideas of personal and social identity. In this anthology the editors comment on the range and diversity of relationships between people. As we shall discuss later, relating the broad experiences of families at certain times misses the variety and individuality of people's lives.

The first 'services' provided for families were therefore those which saw families with disabled members as general problems and people with learning disabilities as being specific problems, if they trangressed certain boundaries. The common Victorian solution to social problems was the institution and policies became concentrated on institutions to the neglect of family relationships. However, the historical legacy of the control and incarceration function of services still has the potential to affect deliverers and recipients alike.

The Development of Services

The neglect of families (despite their role as major providers of care and assistance) can be traced through various reports on welfare provision following the Second World War period. The report of the Royal Commission on the Law Relating to Mental Illness and Mental Deficiency (HMSO, 1957), for example, noted that many hospital patients could live 'in the general community with relatives or friends' (p. 592) with the authorities offering a safety-net of alternative accommodation. Community services were left unspecified and resources were not addressed. The expense of institutional services promoted questions about their necessity (Ryan and Thomas, 1987) while family costs were taken for granted.

Services are hard to describe accurately for the institutional legacy exists both physically and in records. We still need more details of the reality of life for families some of whom might have touched on official systems, but many of whom would have been self-reliant or assisted through voluntary, charitable and religious organisations. It is often overlooked that the 1913 Mental Deficiency Act required local authorities to provide occupation, training and supervision for 'mental defectives' who lived with their families (Atkinson, 1988).

Local authorities' role in providing domestic assistance initially was permissive. The National Health Service Act (1946) permitted local authorities to provide domestic help to households where it was required, including those which had members who were 'mentally defective' (Section 29). It is clear that this power was used more for families with young children and older people rather than other groups, but the power existed and was used. The mandatory provision, introduced by the Health Services and Public Health Act 1968, put a duty on local health authorities to provide domestic assistance or home help to families where members were handicapped by illness or congenital deformity (Section 13).

Dexter and Harbert (1983) report that 10,000 families with a mentally handicapped member received a home help in 1978 but point out that this is probably an underestimate as the recipients might well have been classed under headings of 'elderly' or 'maternity'. Nonetheless, the service was by no means comprehensive and exemplifies neglect of families.

We address here one of the key issues in relation to a discussion of services, the question of who receives the service. This is a question with academic but also practical relevance. As Twigg (1992) notes, most services are aimed at the person with disability or handicap but the close inter-relationships existing domestically means there are various models that agencies use, subconsciously or consciously, in their allocation processes.

Domestic assistance typifies such complexities, particularly for families with an adult member who has learning disabilities. On the one hand, domestic or domiciliary assistance may be involved in teaching domestic skills and promoting independence. On the other it may be crucial in supporting the family as a whole in managing domestic tasks that are inherently difficult in terms of labour or difficult because of the decreasing ability of anyone to carry out such tasks. Care of laundry is a clear example of a task that might need practical assistance particularly if there are few resources available and/or if other family members acquire relevant disabilities or illnesses.

Support and advice

Subsidised domestic assistance was and continues to be allocated on the basis of assessment of families' needs. Such assessments often contain within them ideas of support and advice. Nurses, teachers and social welfare staff have a role in interpreting and explaining to families how service systems work and what is truly available and relevant to their situation. Elements of the complexity of this are raised in the White Paper *Better Services for the Mentally Handicapped*: 'Each handicapped person should live with his own family as long as this does not impose an undue burden on them or him, and he and his family should receive full advice and support' (DHSS, 1971). We shall discuss some of the issues of dual focused services later in this chapter. Hornby (1991) draws attention to the variety of support tasks needed at various times and important distinctions between family members who affect and are affected by disability collectively and individually.

The support process has often been narrowly interpreted and focuses on issues of 'gatekeeping'. It has also been seen as most pertinent to the needs of families with young disabled children where services developed in a fragmented piecemeal fashion. The Warnock Committee (1978) recommended a 'Named Person' to fulfil a co-ordinating role for services that were so confusing. Despite this, Glendinning (1986) lists some nineteen groups that a family with a disabled child might come into contact with.

Advice and support services for families were the focus of the research project described by Glendinning (1986). A resource worker was employed to establish regular contact with families, to act as a point of first contact (a 'single door') on a broad range of matters and to liaise with other agencies.

Innovatory schemes such as this frequently have a limited life-span (Leat, 1992), despite families' repeated pleas for information and emotional support. The voluntary sector in many ways attempts to fill this gap through self-help groups, information, publicity, links with professionals and one-to-one contact. There is wide variation geographically and uneven spread, particularly in class and ethnic terms (see Baxter *et al.*, 1990) within the voluntary sector. Nonetheless many groups and individuals offer a unique source of support to parents. As Ayer and Alaszewski (1984) note: 'Most mothers we talked to found out about the services from other mothers.' Ironically, services which attempt to co-ordinate or make sense of the service world are themselves frequently haphazard.

Attempts to offer assistance to families in a more rational way have been various. The development of Community Mental Handicap Teams, as multi-disciplinary groupings of professional staff working at local level, has moved from the arena of work with children to adults (see Grant *et al.*, 1986) but is threatened by recent changes under the NHS and Community Care Act 1990. This legislation, together with the Children Act 1989, establishes new divisions in health and social services agencies along the lines of purchasers and providers in both sectors. It also confirms divides between adults and children in social services where services remain separate despite mutual dependence (Sutcliffe, 1990). This particular organisational divide appears to be particularly significant at school leaving age when the transition from child to adult status is made in organisational terms. Hubert (1991) describes how the transition from children's services in short-term residential care to adult units is traumatic and distressing for the young people and their parents alike: 'Parents feel that as their children become adult they need increased help and support, whereas the provision of services seems to become haphazard and uncoordinated' (p. 74). This is despite the legislative requirement of the Disabled Persons (Services, Consultation and Representation) Act 1986, where Sections 5 and 6 promote the identification and assessment of disabled school leavers to avoid service dislocation and to develop long-term perspectives of individual and family needs.

Services to families at such stages and ages may be particularly influenced by systems of caremanagement advocated by the Griffiths Report (1988) and the White Paper *Caring for People* (Department of Health, 1989). For families with members with learning disabilities, the principles of sound assessment, individuality, choice, monitoring and review appear a logical improvement to services. The principles of competition, targeting and contracts may be viewed with more disquiet, particularly if resources continue to be limited.

Later parts of the life-course have been put on the policy and research agendas. Previous 'options' of institutional care in hospitals have diminished, alternative residential facilities are in limited supply and the independent sector (both voluntary and commercial) has tended to accept placements where substantial capital or income has been attached as 'dowries' to former hospital patients (Booth *et al.*, 1990).

Services to families with adult members who have learning disabilities are therefore still focused on traditional day care, with innovation from developments in supported employment, educational programmes and care packages that are not centre-based. The Individual Programme Planning system will need to merge into systems of caremanagement to plan for the needs of ageing parents and their adult children. As Grant's survey (1986) in North Wales showed long-term and continuing professional involvement may be appropriate but is rarely possible given other priorities, organisational boundaries and the passive relationships existing within traditional day-care services.

In this section the history of developing services has been shown to be patchy and uneven. Much development has been the by-product of services that have a universal base, rather than a specific focus on people with learning disabilities. Special or specific services have inherited an institutional legacy which stunted the growth of individual support systems. The neglect of families' needs has only recently begun to be addressed systematically as institutional alternatives to families have been found to be inadequate, expensive and inappropriate.

FROM FAMILIES TO CARERS

The current favouring of the term carers has probably confused many families. It represents a change in policy makers' and professionals' views of the relationships involved in what is variously described as community care or informal care. It has also to be seen in the context of growing concern about the quality of care provided in domestic settings, with abuse, mistreatment and neglect assuming new relevance for service professionals.

In the area of service provision for people with learning disabilities, the new conceptualisation of caring has had impact in four main areas. It has highlighted the similiarities between people who provide 'care' for others without payment. Great similarities have been found, for example, in discussions about what is particularly burdensome or rewarding and how services may exacerbate or ameliorate problems. The problem of maintaining continence is one example of this, while issues of legal safeguards have shown similar debates over issues of risk and protection (Alaszewski and Manthorpe, 1991).

At another level, differences between carers have been reconceptualised. We have been reminded of how different experiences are negotiated through other contexts, so that whether one is black or white, female or male, middle class or working class, living in urban or rural settings, part of extended or restricted family networks, has a major external influence on the services that are available (see Atkin, 1993) and are worth the 'cost' of accepting.

The third main area is the reworking of the boundaries between services to carers and services to the individual with a disability. Twigg and Atkin (1993) have added to their models of professional/carers relationships a fourth dimension, the notion of the *superseded carer* (p. 64). In this model one element is that service professionals may aim to maximise or 'free' the disabled person from dependence on carers; another element mirrors this by seeking to assist carers by releasing them from caring tasks. As they point out, the area of learning disabilities has been highly influential in providing evidence for such a model, and we saw it illustrated earlier in this chapter in the extract from the (DHSS) 1971 White Paper.

The last area of impact of caring is allied to the 'discovery' of the family as a potentially abusive setting for adults. Definitions of abuse or mistreatment are numerous and various, but the clear message from research in this area is that not all family care is superior to institutional care from the view point of the disabled person or the carer. Some people with disabilities may require protecting from family members or their carers may need to be 'released' from their responsibilities. In the context of child care, where abuse and neglect have been the objects of attention for many years, new research is indicating that disabled children may be 'in special danger of being abused' (Watson, 1992, p. 113).

In the area of work with adults who have learning disabilities, the categories of abuse or mistreatment which are often applied to older people are equally relevant. The case of Beverley Lewis sadly illustrates this. Beverley Lewis had cerebral embryopathy and was born deaf–blind. She died aged 23, in 1989. In the opinion of Sense, the National Deaf–Blind and Rubella Association: 'She starved to death because her mother did not feed her properly and she could not feed herself' (Sense, 1990, p. 4). In her sister's view, Beverley's neglect was not simply because of their mother's possible chronic schizophrenia but because Beverley 'was not considered as a separate individual with her own needs, which were separate from my mother's needs' (P. Webb, Letter, *The Sunday Times*, 19 November 1989).

For people with learning disabilities other types of mistreatment, such as financial abuse, sexual abuse and deliberate inappropriate use of medication are not confined to domestic or institutional settings. They illustrate the vulnerability of individuals who have severe problems in communicating, in being taken seriously and in receiving good quality care. For families, the policy moves to community-based care as exemplified in the White Paper, *Caring for People* (Department of Health, 1989), run the risk of labelling all family care as superior when it is not even sustainable.

DIRECT SERVICES: INITIAL REACTIONS

It is within such contexts that we can now move to analyse the range of services that are available for families. Many descriptions start with services that are encountered by new parents who have a child with suspected

disabilities. In fact we need to consider this chronology as starting precon-
ceptually as one frequently overlooked service is that of genetic counselling
for families who suspect that there may be hereditary problems. For adults
with learning disabilities themselves, services are often vigilant about their
prospects as parents (Dowdney and Skuse, 1993).

Reproductive technology and learning disabilities have, as subjects, been
closely associated. The influence of the eugenics movement has cast a shadow
over the debates which cover ethical and moral decisions. For many women,
reproductive technology has a sinister element (Rowland, 1993) while for
others the right to choose an abortion is a fundamental freedom, albeit made
in difficult and painful circumstances. Issues surrounding legislation in the
area of abortion in the UK are clearly set out by Phillips and Dawson (1985)
who note that any destruction of a foetus has to be capable of being justified
on the basis of prolonged or significant suffering:

> It is not considered justifiable to abort a foetus for social convenience, for
> example because the birth coincides with a planned holiday, but only if
> the birth presents a threat to the physical or mental health of the mother,
> or if there is a risk that the child, if born, will suffer serious physical or
> mental handicap.
>
> (Phillips and Dawson, 1985, pp. 46–7)

Abortion, then, is available to some families where it is suspected the child
may have severe 'mental handicap'. We are only just beginning to hear the
opinions of disabled people about this issue, mainly from those with physical
handicaps, but as Brown and Smith (1992) illustrate there are undoubted
tensions over abortion within the service worlds and between families and
individuals. Women who in retrospect would have chosen an abortion, say
Brown and Smith, are not 'evil' but:

> they are the ones who get up in the night and do the washing, the ones who
> try to balance the needs of their children with handicaps against those of
> their other children and their parents whilst mediating between genera-
> tions, professionals and neighbours.
>
> (Brown and Smith, 1992, p. 165).

Diagnosis of learning disability is a difficult task and an upsetting process.
Much research has focused on the professional–parent conversations, with
the aim of making disclosure as least difficult as possible. Parents reveal that
this is handled as well as possible by some individual professionals but that
others lack sensitivity, or are embarrassed or fail to provide support (Nursey
et al., 1991).

Abbott and Sapsford's (1987) interviews with two groups of families
provide illustrations of the varied reactions of parents to the news of their
children's disabilities. In essence, the families had to come to terms with
three separate impacts – changed expectations for the child, altered perspectives for the future, and acknowledgement of being a 'different family'.
Service provision therefore is only one part of a general status change.

The great majority (98.5%) of children with disabilities are now living with their own families (Bone and Meltzer, 1989) or in alternative family settings. This compares with 80 per cent of children with severe disabilities who lived at home in the surveys conducted for the White Paper *Better Services for the Mentally Handicapped* (DHSS, 1971, p. 4).

The transfer of care for children away from hospital settings had its origins in debates about the limits of institutional care, with characteristic segregated and poorly resourced facilities. Stainton (1992) argues that the impact of research was minimal until political interest was awakened by the series of hospital scandals (see Martin, 1984) around long-stay care generally. Interestingly, the report into the ill-treatment of residents at Ely Hospital (Howe Report, 1969) gives as a case-study the example of 'Osbert' whose parents placed him in hospital while they went on holiday. The Howe Report into the conditions at Ely describes their reactions to his unrecognisable condition on their return a fortnight later.

The closure of long-stay hospitals has been gradual, but in terms of provision for children, the impetus was quicker. In part this can be explained by continued pressure. The Campaign for the Mentally Handicapped (CMH) and other groups, such as the parents' pressure group, The Spastics Society (under the campaigning name of Exodus), focused on the 8000 children in hospital in the mid-1970s. CMH vividly describe their concerns: 'The mentally handicapped child in hospital is among the most deprived in Britain' (CMH, 1975, p. 9).

Their solutions were various but included residential care (in small domestic units), fostering and domiciliary services. These should form a network of support for families, but could also become the main providers of care if that was preferred. This legacy can be seen in the outcome of the hospital closure programme for children (Leonard, 1991) which resulted in a varied pattern of provision for a particular cohort of children.

For those families, the vast majority, whose children enter neither residential nor hospital care, the service world is composed of services available to children and services available to children and their families on a universal basis together with those that represent efforts to target resources on particular characteristics or circumstances. If we adopt current organisational boundaries to analyse such services we can identify providers at both levels.

Universal services

The impact of any child upon the income of a household has been seen as dramatically lowering the pool of available income. The higher costs associated with disabilities have not in the UK been ameliorated by extra child allowances (as in several EC countries), despite the calls of the Royal Commission (the Pearson Report, 1978), and researchers (e.g. Baldwin, 1985) who focus on the financial impact of disability. At a universal level, parents of children are entitled to child benefit. Other financial help is either related to the family's income and capital, or to the assessed severity of the disability.

In terms of the family's own resources, evidence from a variety of research reports notes that families with a disabled child may be more likely to be headed by a single parent, to be low wage-earners, and to have limited opportunities for overtime and job mobility (Parker (1990) summarises these findings).

The main services provided to families in general with preschool children come from the medical/nursing professions, initially through organised surveillance programmes offered through health visitors but also based around paediatric services. Research evidence shows variations in the level of support offered and seen as acceptable and appropriate by parents. The thread of variability extends into provision of services such as nursery and other forms of child-care, informal play-group provision, the availability of aids and adaptations, respite and transport.

It is not until the education service becomes involved that many parents perceive that the arbitrary nature of the service world begins to assume some coherence. A statutory right to an educational service exists from the age of 2 until a person with disabilities is 19. For many people, contact with the educational services continues for many years after. The 1981 Education Act gives the right to have a professional assessment and to have an agreed statement of need. Ideally, following the Warnock Report (1978), special needs should be catered for in mainstream education, though this is still not possible for many children. Hall (1992) outlines the processes involved for the family as the educational service attempts to meet the needs of the child in the ways its professional advisers deem appropriate and feasible.

The health service, benefits system and educational system are therefore universal services which give particular acknowledgement to the perceived special needs of families with disabled children. Early reactions from services were to offer group solutions; organised care from certain health care settings, particular benefit categories from the benefits systems and special (segregated) schooling from the educational service. In recent years this blanket approach has been diluted by arguments about individual need and calls for flexible, pluralistic services.

This means that traditional health care services for disabled children may be met instead by a variety of providers, including the voluntary sector and local authority social services departments. Examples of these are respite care, play-schemes and home-based therapeutic regimes. As with many health services provided for people with long-term disability, traditional medical and nursing services are now provided within the home, particularly by community nurses. Respite is no longer seen as something needing professional input – it can in many circumstances be provided by other trained families (see Stalker, 1990).

Devising individualised benefits is clearly problematic and so much of the benefits system is still tightly controlled, with little discretion. For families with disabled children, the Family Fund (Bradshaw, 1980) is an indi- vidualised attempt to provide financial help for families whose needs are for items of equipment or other one-off expenses. In other respects the fragmented benefit system responds to families' financial needs with a range of payments in respect of the child, the non-availability for work of the carer or perceived extra allowances through income support or housing benefit if families' incomes are below certain (different) thresholds.

New provisions for the care of children by local authority social services departments (SSDs) under the Children Act 1989, do not really alter the picture. The impact of the new Register for all children 'in need' may well be tokenistic if resources are not forthcoming. The calls for SSDs to work in partnership with parents of children with learning disabilities appear rather rhetorical and predictable. There is little evidence that the attitudes of social workers and policy makers are changing in the area of raising the profile of supportive work with families. Under Section 17 of the Act, SSDs can provide accommodation and financial help to meet the needs of disabled children; the use of such resources may well depend on the redrawing of boundaries by the health and educational services, rather than any needs advanced by parents independently.

Services to families with adult disabled members

In order to discuss the range of services available to families we can adopt three classifications:

- services delivered to the home;
- services provided by a facility;
- services based in a residential setting.

Clearly there are other configurations, based around service functions, provider types and traditional and innovative services.

Services delivered to the home, as described earlier may well be restricted by the presence of a family member, who is seen as capable and 'willing' to provide supervision, practical assistance and emotional support. All this at no cost! For many parents, their main services may well come from the voluntary sector in terms of reliable social or leisure provision attended by the disabled person alone, or accompanied by a family member. Nally and Steele (1992) discuss how involvement in community networks can be an important support for families, although such activity may still confine the individual's restricted social networks to other disabled people. In many ways such artifical networks may partially compensate for the difficulties families with disabled members have in making and keeping friends. As Willmott (1986) notes friends have a community of interest and friendship is important in people's lives. It does not and perhaps in essence cannot provide services in the same ways as organisations.

Other practical services available to families within their own homes may include sitting or respite provision, provision of equipment, housing adaptations and assistance with administering medication. Less tangibly, professionals from a variety of backgrounds may visit to accomplish medical procedures, to offer advice about problem behaviour or coping strategies, or the unbiquitous 'support'. In respect of adults, the introduction of care-management through the gradual implementation of the NHS and Community Care Act 1990 will be highly significant.

Each of the stages of caremanagement, although with local variations, is part of a process of assessment, delivery and review. For the first time 'private' carers will have the right to an assessment if they wish and if the person they are assisting, falls into that category. In terms of service delivery, the assembled package of services is meant to offer families and individuals reliability, consistency and accountability. The notion of a key worker, common in many adult training centres, has been broadened and expanded into that of the care manager. It will be their role to assist in the creation and maintenance of an appropriate care system, subject, of course, to resource considerations.

For many families with members with learning disabilities, the implementation of the new legislation offers the potential for improved services. Lessons have been learned from the planning processes of Individual Programme Plans and the slow move from traditional, large-scale day care. Concerns exist however about two main areas. Firstly, the ability and responsibility of the family and individual to pay for services are subjects which will appear as charges become more widespread in social care. A multitude of service providers may well have several charging bands, from which families may be asked to 'choose'. Secondly, the emphasis of the care management system is on directing resources to those in greatest need. This will have a major impact on families where services, such as they are, no longer are offered as their need is not 'great enough'. Notions of prevention are hard to equate with such resource concentration.

CONCLUSION

Families with members who have learning disabilities are varied. Services had their origins in first blaming then neglecting families. Families were later 'rediscovered' but their needs were met by complex and confusing organisational structures. Currently, families are being divided in two categories, on the one hand those who need extensive support to continue caring for people with profound and multiple disabilities to avoid expensive institutionalisation. On the other hand are groups of families who face restricted access to services in the future as their need is not seen as a priority. Families' alliances may therefore be important influences in re-addressing age-old issues about the delivery of services.

REFERENCES

Abbott, P. and Sapsford, R. (1987) *Community Care for Mentally Handicapped Children*, Open University Press, Milton Keynes.

Alaszewski, A. and Manthorpe, J. (1991) Literature review: measuring and managing risk in social welfare, *British Journal of Social Work*, 21, pp. 277–90.

Alcock, P. (1987) *Poverty and State Support*, Longman, Harlow.

Atkin, K. (1993) Similarities and differences between informal carers, in Twigg, J. (ed.) *Carers: Research and Practice*, HMSO, London.

Atkinson, D. (1988) Residential care for children and adults with mental handicap, in Sinclair, I. (ed.) *Residential Care: The Research Reviewed*, HMSO, London.

Atkinson, D. and Williams, F. (eds) (1990) *'Know Me as I Am': an Anthology of Poetry, Prose and Art by People with Learning Disabilities*, Hodder and Stoughton, London.

Ayer, S. and Alaszewski, A. (1984) *Community Care and the Mentally Handicapped*, Croom Helm, London.

Baldwin, S. (1985) *The Costs of Caring: Families with Disabled Children*, Routledge and Kegan Paul, London.

Barron, D. (1987) Locked away, *Community Living*, 1 (2), July, pp. 8–9.

Baxter, C., Ward, L., Poonia, K. and Nadirshaw, S. (1990) *Double Discrimination*, King's Fund Centre, London.

Biehal, N., Fisher, M., Marsh, P. and Sainsbury, E. (1992) Rights and social work, in Coote, A. (ed.) *The Welfare of Citizens: Developing New Social Rights*, Rivers Oram Press, London.

Blumer, H. (1971) Social problems as collective behaviour, *Social Rights*, 18 (3), pp. 298–306.

Bone and Meltzer, H. (1989) Report No. 3 *The Prevalence of Disability among Children*, OPCS, HMSO, London.

Booth, T., Simons, K. and Booth, W. (1990) *Outward Bound: Relocation and Community Care for People with Learning Disabilities*, Open University Press, Milton Keynes.

Bradshaw, J. (1980) *The Family Fund: An Initiative in Social Policy*, Routledge and Kegan Paul, London.

Brown, H. and Smith, H. (1992) (eds) *Normalisation: A Reader for the Nineties*, Routledge, London.

Campaign for the Mentally Handicapped (1975) *Whose Children?* CMH (now Values Into Action), London.

Department of Health (1989) *Caring for People: Community Care in the Next Decade and Beyond*, Cmnd. 849, HMSO, London.

Department of Health and Social Security (1971) *Better Services for the Mentally Handicapped*, Cmnd. 4683, HMSO, London.

Dexter, M. and Harbert, W. (1983) *The Home Help Service*, Tavistock, London.

Dowdney, L. and Skuse, D. (1993) Parenting provided by adults with mental retardation, *The Journal of Child Psychology and Psychiatry and Allied Disciplines*, 34 (1), Jan., pp. 25–48.

Glendinning, C. (1986) *A Single Door: Social Work with the Families of Disabled Children*, Allen and Unwin, London.

Grant, G. (1986) Older carers, interdependence and the care of mentally handicapped adults, *Ageing and Society*, 6, part 3, Sept., pp. 333–52.

Grant, G. Humphreys, S. and McGrath, M. (eds) (1986) *Community Mental Handicap Teams: Theory and Practice*, British Institute for Mental Handicap, Kidderminster.

Griffiths Report (1988) *Community Care: Agenda for Action*, HMSO, London.

Hall, L. (1992) Severe learning difficulties: educational provision, in Thompson, T. and Mathias, P. (eds) *Standards and Mental Handicap*, Baillière Tindall, London.

HMSO (1957) *Royal Commission on the Law Relating to Mental Illness and Mental Deficiency 1954–1957, Report and Minutes of Evidence*, Cmnd. 169, HMSO, London.

Hornby, G. (1991) Counselling family members with disabilities, in Brown, R. and Robertson, S. (eds) *Rehabilitation Counselling*, Chapman and Hall, London.

Howe Report (1969) *Report of the Committee of Inquiry into Allegations of Ill-treatment of Patients and Other Regularities at the Ely Hospital, Cardiff,* Cmnd. 3975, HMSO, London.

Hubert, J. (1991) *Home-Bound,* King's Fund Centre, London.

Leat, D. (1992) Innovations and special schemes, in Twigg, J. (ed.) *Carers: Research and Practice,* HMSO, London.

Leonard, A. (1991) *Homes of Their Own: A Community Care Initiative for Children with Learning Difficulties,* Avebury, Aldershot.

McIntosh, A. and Alaszewski, A. (1994) Families and care of children with learning disabilities, in Malin, N. (ed.) *Implementing Community Care,* Open University Press, Milton Keynes.

Martin, J. (1984) *Hospitals in Trouble,* Basil Blackwell, Oxford.

Nally, B. and Steele, J. (1992) Policy, organisation and practice in the provision of community services for people with an intellectual disability, in Thompson, T. and Mathias, P. (eds) *Standards and Mental Handicap,* Bailliere Tindall, London.

Nursey, A., Rohde, J. and Farmer, R. (1991) Ways of telling new parents about their child and his or her mental handicap: a comparison of doctors' and parents' views, *Journal of Mental Deficiency Research,* 35 (1), pp. 48–57.

Oliver, M. (1989) Disability and dependency: a creation of industrial societies?, in Barton, L. (ed.) *Disability and Dependency,* Falmer, Brighton.

Parker, G. (1990) *With Due Care and Attention,* Family Policy Studies Centre, London (2nd edition).

Pearson Report (1978) *Royal Commission Report on Civil Liability and Compensation for Personal Injury* Cmnd. 7054, HMSO, London.

Phillips, M. and Dawson, J. (1985) *Doctor's Dilemmas: Medical Ethics and Contemporary Science,* Harvester Press, Brighton.

Proctor, R.N. (1988) *Racial Hygiene: Medicine under the Nazis,* Harvard University Press, Cambridge, Massachusetts.

Rowland, R,. (1993) *Living Laboratories: Women and Reproductive Technology,* Cedar, London.

Ryan, J. and Thomas, F. (1987) *The Politics of Mental Handicap,* Free Association Books, London.

Sense (1990) *Talking Sense,* The National Deaf–Blind and Rubella Association, London, February.

Stainton, T. (1992) A terrible danger to the race, *Community Living,* 5 (3), Jan., pp. 18–20.

Stalker, K. (1990) *Share the Care,* Jessica Kingsley Publications, London.

Sutcliffe, J. (1990) *Adults with Learning Disabilities: Education for Choice and Empowerment,* National Institute of Adult Continuing Education, Leicester.

Thane, P. (1982) *The Foundations of the Welfare State,* Longman, Harlow.

Twigg, J. (ed.) (1992) *Carers: Research and Practice,* HMSO, London.

Twigg, J. and Atkin, K. (1993) *Carers Perceived,* Open University Press, Milton Keynes.

Warnock Report (1978) *Report of the Committee of Enquiry into the Education of Handicapped Children and Young People,* Cmnd. 7212, HMSO, London.

Watson, G. (1992) The abuse of disabled children and young people, in Stainton Rogers, W., Hevey, D., Roche, J. and Ashe, E. (eds) *Child Abuse and Neglect: Facing the Challenge,* Batsford/Open University, London.

Webb, P. (1989) Let nobody die like my sister Beverley, letter in *The Sunday Times,* 19 November.

Willmott, P. (1986) *Social Networks, Informal Care and Public Policy,* Policy Studies Institute, London.

Wood Report (1929) *Mental Deficiency Committee Report, Part III, The Adult Defective,* HMSO, London.

7 Education and assessment services

Glenys Jones

INTRODUCTION

Since the first edition of this book, there have been several important pieces of legislation which have profound implications for the education of all pupils, and so for pupils with learning disabilities. The 1981 and 1988 Education Acts have introduced changes in terminology, assessment, funding and the curriculum of schools. At present, major changes are occurring in all LEAs and schools as a result of the implementation of Local Management of Schools (LMS), where responsibility for managing educational resources is increasingly being passed from LEAs to individual mainstream schools. Alongside this reform, also introduced by the 1988 Education Act, has been the introduction of a National Curriculum for all pupils. Another significant shift in emphasis in recent years has been the increasing role given to parents in their children's education.

Guidelines for the implementation of these changes are still being produced and LEAs are responding differently to these requirements. It is not possible in this chapter to write in detail about these, but references to other publications are given which discuss the potential and actual effects of the legislation. This chapter begins with details of the changes in terminology and perspective introduced by the 1981 Education Act, and discusses the prevalence of special needs and the relativity of this concept. Different forms of assessment are then described, followed by details of assessments which may occur at different stages of a child's life, including the formal assessment procedure introduced by the 1981 Education Act. The range of educational provision available to pupils with learning disabilities is then presented, followed by a section on the implications of LMS and the National Curriculum for these pupils.

THE 1981 EDUCATION ACT: CHANGES IN TERMINOLOGY AND PERSPECTIVE

The 1981 Education Act came into force on 1 April 1983 and was based on the recommendations of the Warnock inquiry (DES, 1978) which dealt solely with the education of children with special needs. As such, it had several implications for children previously described as having a mental handicap – not the least of these being a change in terminology. Children who had been described as mildly or severely educationally subnormal (ESN(M) or ESN(S)) were instead referred to as children with moderate or severe learning difficulties. The categories of handicap specified in the 1944 Education Act were abolished and replaced by the concept of 'special educational need'. According to the 1981 Education Act, a child has special educational needs if they have a learning difficulty which requires educational provision which is additional to, or otherwise different from, the educational provision made generally for children of that age in schools maintained by the LEA concerned. These children were to be referred to as having learning difficulties, irrespective of the type of problem they had (be it sensory, physical or cognitive). They were defined as having more difficulty in learning than other children of the same age – or as having a disability which prevented them using some or all of the facilities normally provided in mainstream schools.

The change from the categorisation of handicap to the concept of special educational need was designed to move away from the notion that children with the same diagnosis (e.g. Down's syndrome; visual impairment) had the same special educational needs and required the same educational provision. Instead, each child was considered as an individual, not as a member of a particular category, with the acknowledgement that a range of factors, not just the diagnosis, would determine the most appropriate educational provision. Thus, there was a move away from viewing learning disabilities as being wholly within the child to viewing needs as a result of the interaction between the nature of the child's disabilities and their environment (i.e. the child's needs varied depending on their context).This was a necessary and desirable move as it became clear that children who ostensibly had similar disabilities did not always require the same educational provision. However, this change in perspective has made for difficulties for both professionals and parents in identifying and defining the special needs population and in planning provision accordingly.

PREVALENCE OF SPECIAL EDUCATIONAL NEEDS

The Warnock Report (DES, 1978) predicted that as many as one in five children (20 per cent) were likely to need extra help at some point during their school career, but that for the majority of this group (18 per cent), the type of help necessary would be available within the existing resources of mainstream schools. It was predicted that the remaining 2 per cent would need resources over and above those usually available, and that these children should be formally identified and assessed, the details of which should be written in a statement of special educational needs.

Whereas previous legislation defined difficulties in terms of the characteristics of individual children, the 1981 Education Act defined special needs in terms of the educational provision required to meet the child's needs. Linking the definition of special educational needs with the nature of educational resources ordinarily available to the child, has meant that whether a child is considered to have special needs is dependent on what the *usual* resources of the mainstream school are and on the nature of the demands made on the child within the school. If a school is well resourced and staff are skilled in teaching children with a wide range of abilities, then fewer children on roll will be deemed to have special needs than in a school where staff are used to teaching children within a rather narrow ability range, with a focus on cognitive, academic skills. Inappropriate teaching materials and techniques may generate or exacerbate the range of learning difficulties experienced by children (Roaf and Bines, 1989). So Warnock's predicted one in five prevalence will not apply to all schools or LEAs – in some cases, there will be more than 20 per cent of pupils with special needs and in other situations far fewer, depending on the teacher's skills, the tasks set, the resources available (Solity, 1992), and on the catchment area of the school.

The concept of special educational need is therefore a relative one – and this is reflected by the figures obtained nationally, where in 1985 in some LEAs, less than 1 per cent of all pupils attended a special school and in others as many as 5 per cent did so (Dessent, 1987).

CRITERIA FOR FORMAL ASSESSMENT

Another significant factor which has given rise to different proportions of children being formally assessed from one LEA to another is that no clear criteria were given to LEAs on when and for whom a formal assessment should be initiated. The advisory Circular 1/83 suggested that there were three groups of children for whom the Secretary of State expected LEAs to produce a statement:

1 those pupils attending a special school
2 those pupils in special units attached to mainstream schools
3 those pupils who have severe and complex learning difficulties which require the provision of extra resources in mainstream schools

(DES, 1983)

Some LEAs though, have chosen only to produce a statement for pupils attending separate special provision and not for the pupils with special educational needs who are placed elsewhere, even if they are receiving extra help. Other LEAs have extended the range of children for whom they produce a statement by including all pupils who are receiving additional resources, including those in mainstream schools. The Audit Commission (1992a) found that the likelihood of a child being statemented depended more on the LEA's interpretation of the 1981 Education Act than on the proportion of children with special needs in the LEA. Not only was there a lack of consistency between LEAs, there was also a lack of consistency within individual LEAs. A study of statements issued showed that statemented pupils had widely differing levels of need. LEAs admitted that factors which had no bearing on the level of need were influential in the decision to issue a statement and also on how quickly this was processed – the most significant factor being the determination of the school or parent.

Since the introduction of the 1981 Education Act and the statementing procedure, LEAs have been constantly trying to establish clear and objective criteria for those children they should statement and those they should not. The Audit Commission (1992a) has recommended that guidance should be produced by the DFE on the criteria to take into account when determining which children should be assessed and for which children LEAs should issue statements. This will be a very difficult task and it remains to be seen whether these criteria increase the consistency and reduce the variation in statementing rates between LEAs.

METHODS OF ASSESSMENT

Before discussing the formal assessment and statementing procedure introduced by the 1981 Education Act, some of the main methods of assessment will be described, followed by details of the type of assessment which may occur at different stages of a child's life. There are several reasons for assessing a child, the three main ones being:

1 To diagnose – is there a problem and if so, what is the nature of it and what are the implications for the child's education?
2 To plan appropriate help – how can the needs identified be met?
3 To evaluate – has the child made progress on the aims and objectives within their educational programme?

A range of assessment instruments has been developed in the last two decades to help determine the skills and abilities of children and adults, in order to plan and evaluate appropriate teaching programmes and provision. Hogg and Raynes have edited a book which describes the particular functions and limitations of many of these tests. They identify four different approaches to assessing people with learning difficulties:

a norm-referenced
b assessment of adaptive behaviour
c criterion-referenced
d behavioural observation

(Hogg and Raynes, 1987)

A particular test or instrument may have features of more than one of the above categories.

Norm-referenced tests

The main function of norm-referenced tests is to assess how well an individual performs in relation to other people from a similar population (e.g. is this child doing as well as other children of his age?). Some of these tests are used to obtain a measure of intelligence and have been used for many years to identify people with learning difficulties (e.g. Wechsler Intelligence Scale for Children (WISC), Wechsler, 1974; Wechsler Adult Intelligence Scale (WAIS) Wechsler, 1981; Bayley Scales of Infant Development (Bayley, 1969). Tests which produce a reading age are also an example of this type of test, whereby teachers can assign an age level to the child's current functioning. The results of these provide an idea of the severity of the problem and have been used in some areas as a screening device to select children most in need of extra input from support teachers.

Assessment of adaptive behaviour

Hogg and Raynes (1987) state that adaptive behaviour and its assessment have become a major focus of interest in the field of learning difficulties. These measures focus on a functional assessment of an individual's competence over a number of domains giving a profile, thus allowing staff to select broad areas it would be useful to work on. Examples of this type of instrument are the Adaptive Behaviour Scale (Nihara *et al.*, 1969) and the Vineland Adaptive Behaviour Scales (Sparrow *et al.*, 1984). Information provided by these scales has been used to aid decisions on appropriate programmes and service provision and to measure change in competence.

Criterion-referenced tests

Neither the norm-referenced tests nor the adaptive behaviour scales above are particularly useful in programme planning. Criterion-referenced tests are better suited to this. These tests usually consist of lists of skills (criteria) in different areas of development which represent achievements and could become teaching objectives (e.g. can do up easy buttons). The criteria are functionally related and usually arranged in the likely order of their acquisition. They are often linked to instructions on which materials to use, how to present these and the response requirements that determine whether or not the pupil has met the criteria. Examples of criterion-referenced tests are the Portage Checklist (Bluma *et al.*, 1976), and the Behaviour Assessment Battery (Kiernan and Jones, 1982).

Behavioural observation

Behavioural observation, as the name implies, concerns the observation and recording of the behaviour of people in everyday situations, acknowledging the importance of the effect of their environment on their behaviour. Such observation is usually done to determine the levels of a specific behaviour before, during and/or after a behavioural programme designed to modify the behaviour (Murphy, 1987). It can be useful in assessing the extent to which behaviours and skills have generalised to other settings beyond those in which they are directly addressed or taught.

ASSESSMENT OF CHILDREN

All children are routinely assessed at different stages during their lives whether or not their development or behaviour is causing concern. This section discusses these assessments and some of the procedures followed for children who are thought to have difficulties or delays in their development.

Prenatal and neonatal assessment

An increasing number of techniques have been developed over recent years for identifying factors (e.g. biochemical, genetic, social) prior to conception and birth which may be associated with later learning disabilities. For example, research has shown that smoking during pregnancy can reduce the birth weight of the baby and that low-birth-weight babies have an increased chance of delayed development or learning disabilities. Women over the age of 35 years may be offered an amniocentesis during pregnancy which can detect some abnormalities prenatally. This test may also be given to younger women where there are prior indications (e.g. family history) of the possibility of a chromosomal abnormality, metabolic problems or of a sex-linked condition, such as haemophilia. If the foetus is found to have a defect, then the parents can decide whether or not to terminate the pregnancy.

Every newborn child is given a physical examination and rated on the ten-point APGAR scale within minutes of being born and is screened for phenylketonuria – a condition which if not treated by a special diet leads to severe disabilities. A baby who is suspected of having a metabolic disorder such as thyroid deficiency or galactosaemia or a chromosomal abnormality may be given further biochemical and genetic tests. It is extremely difficult, if not impossible in most cases, to assess whether a newborn child will have learning disabilities later on. Some children may be considered 'at risk' of having learning disabilities though, because of adverse prenatal, birth or neonatal factors. Children considered to be 'at risk' or those with obvious problems at birth are normally referred to a paediatrician or hospital consultant for assessment and review at regular intervals for as long as necessary. Research continues into the causation of disorders leading to learning disabilities and it is likely that other techniques for identification and diagnosis will be discovered in the future. However, for two-thirds of the current population of people with learning disabilities, it is not possible to establish a cause for their problems or to give a diagnosis.

Assessment of children under five years

Before the age of five, it is likely that personnel in health and social services will be the main people involved in the initial identification and assessment of disabilities (e.g. GP, community health team, paediatrician, clinical psychologist or nursery staff). After the age of five, LEA employees (teachers, educational psychologists and special needs staff) are usually the key professionals concerned.

Much has been written about the benefits of early intervention in helping children with learning disabilities (Gulliford, 1975; Wedell and Raybould, 1976). It is therefore important to be able to identify those children with disabilities at an early age in order to arrange appropriate support and education. In an effort to do this, the developmental screening of total preschool populations has been suggested. In most areas, however, comprehensive screening of all children has been confined to the biochemical testing of the newborn and medical screening for auditory and visual defects (Griffiths, 1973). Screening total populations is costly in terms of time and money and, instead, Lindon (1961) suggested the registration by local health authorities of all children considered to be 'at risk' of inheriting or acquiring a handicapping condition. These children would then be seen more regularly for check-ups. By screening 'at risk' cases only, he maintained that 70 per cent of defects could be detected early and that one was therefore in a good position to take preventive action. Before the 'at risk' concept had been evaluated, most local health authorities had implemented schemes for the establishment and maintenance of risk registers. Risk factors often included were low birth weight, birth problems and siblings with disabilities. The risk registers, however, failed to fulfil their aims (Hamilton, 1968; Knox and Mahon, 1970) for a variety of reasons. Some children who were included on the registers were found to have no significant problems so resources were allocated to children who were not in need of help, whilst others in need, who were not on the registers, were often overlooked. Secondly, the number of risk factors included were often so great that almost the entire child population could be placed on the register, and thirdly, because of the danger of the self-fulfilling prophecy, it was possible that one further risk factor was added to the others that the child already had (Davie, 1975). Using data from the National Child Development Study, Butler (1969) found that the majority of individual pregnancy and labour risk factors were poor predictors of later problems. A small number of factors were better predictors if combined with each other or with factors such as birth order and socio-economic background. On the basis of the evidence and the criticism of the 'at risk' system, the Court Report (1976) recommended that the use of risk registers be discontinued.

The Court Report (op. cit.) also suggested that a programme of health surveillance be carried out by each health authority involving a schedule of interviews or screening tests between health care staff, the child and his parents to aid the early identification of children with special needs. They proposed that after their neonatal examinations, all children should be checked either at the clinic or at home at about the ages of six weeks, seven months, eighteen months, two-and-a-half to three years and four-and-a-half to five years. At present most local health authorities in England and Wales have the facilities to carry out regular developmental checks on the total pre-school population, but not all under-fives are regularly and systematically assessed as some parents do not use the services available. Preschool assessment is mainly conducted by the primary health care team which includes clinic doctors, health visitors and general practitioners. This team may be based in the child health clinic, the health centre or group practice surgery.

These child health clinics endeavour to assess every preschool child at regular intervals. Records are usually kept on the child's movement, posture, vision, eye–hand co-ordination, hearing and speech and social behaviour. A variety of standardised tests and observation techniques using charts and schedules have been devised to assess the behaviour and performance of young children (e.g. Griffiths Mental Development Scales (Griffiths, 1970); Stanford–Binet Intelligence Scale (Terman and Merrill, 1967); Bayley Scales of Infant Development (Bayley, 1969)). The type and depth of assessment carried out vary from one authority to another, but there has been an increase in the number of developmental interviews used. The main purpose of assessment is to detect physical and sensory defects and developmental delay and then to provide appropriate intervention to reduce the effect of these problems on the child's overall development. Where a specific problem is detected such as a visual or hearing impairment, the child may be referred to a specialist for more detailed assessment. If the child is developmentally delayed, he may be referred to a multi-disciplinary child development centre for detailed observation and assessment. Preschool children may also be referred to the educational psychology service for asssessment by professionals or parents concerned about the child's development.

Assessment at school

The 1981 and 1988 Education Acts give schools considerably greater responsibility than in the past for identifying, assessing and making recommendations about provision for children with special needs. A problem which may not have been apparent at home may become obvious when the child starts to attend a nursery or school and different demands are made of the child. Teachers, nursery nurses and playgroup leaders who are in daily contact with children are in an excellent position to identify problems. Research by Chazan *et al.* in 1980, however, suggested that there was often very little systematic observation and recording of children's progress by staff in mainstream schools and classes. A factor which probably contributed to this was the shortage of suitable assessment materials for them to use. There are a number of developmental schedules and charts available derived from standardised tests of infant development (e.g. PIP Developmental Charts

(Jeffree and McConkey, 1976), the Effectiveness–Motivation Scale (Sharp and Stott, 1976) and the Primary Progress Assessment Charts (Gunzburg, 1973)), but these are rarely used by teachers in mainstream schools.

However, since the Warnock Report (DES, 1978), which recommended that staff should improve their methods of assessment and identification, many staff have discussed possible ways of doing this, consulted commercial checklists and schedules and then developed their own to suit their particular children, using language that is meaningful to themselves and to the child's parents. Where the school offers boarding facilities to pupils, care staff have often been involved in the construction of the checklist and will use it for recording behaviours observed outside school hours. These schedules may have taken months, years in some cases, to develop and the discussions held between staff during their development can be extremely useful.

The Warnock Report recommended that school staff should follow a series of stages when assessing a child, before requesting a formal assessment.

Stage 1: the teacher identifies and assesses the problem and designs and implements a programme of help

Stage 2: if the teacher remains concerned they inform the child's parents and may involve a specialist teacher for advice

Stage 3: following this, if necessary, a referral may be made to the LEA or other agency for advice on designing a programme of help

Stage 4: if, after this advice, it is thought that the school needs extra resources to meet the child's needs, then the formal multi-disciplinary assessment procedure would be started and carried out

Stage 5: this may then lead to a formal statement of needs and the provision necessary to meet these

(Department of Education and Science, 1978)

There is a strong case for teachers carrying out their own assessment of children, not only because of the shortage of time available from the outside agencies who have traditionally carried out this role (e.g. speech therapists, psychologists), but more importantly because such assessment will help the staff to understand the child's difficulties and needs and to plan appropriate programmes of help. Trying out different teaching approaches with a child is an assessment in itself, as staff attempt to determine the most effective method to use by observing and measuring the child's response to tasks. The progress made by a child with learning disabilities can be very slow and it is therefore important to keep regular records of observations so that changes which otherwise might go unnoticed can be detected.

FORMAL ASSESSMENT AND STATEMENTING PROCEDURE UNDER THE 1981 EDUCATION ACT

At present, any parent or professional who believes a child may need different or extra resources over and above those that the local mainstream school would usually provide has to make out a case to the LEA for a formal assessment to be initiated. They therefore need to produce evidence on the nature and extent of the child's disabilities together with information on the effect of programmes or interventions tried to date.

If the LEA agrees formally to assess the child, then the child must be assessed by a medical officer, an educational psychologist and the teaching staff (if they attend school). In addition, other professionals involved with the child are asked to write reports giving details of their assessments and work. These reports may include the results of standardised tests such as the Wechsler Preschool and Primary Scale of Intelligence (Wechsler, 1955), the Reynell Developmental Language Scales (Reynell, 1969), the Derbyshire Language Scheme (Knowles and Masidlover, 1982) and the British Ability Scales (Elliott *et al.*, 1978). Results of these tests are but a small part of the reports on a child. Information gained from observation, parents' reports and staff reports are of equal importance. The child's parents are invited to contribute, if they wish, by writing or dictating their own report or submitting independent evidence about their child (e.g. from a voluntary organisation or private practitioner).

All the reports are collated and submitted to the LEA for discussion by senior staff. A decision is then made as to whether it is considered the child's needs can be met from within the usual resources of the local school. If it is felt that the child's needs can be met from within the resources normally available to the school, then a draft statement will not be produced. If, however, the pupil does require provision additional to or different from those usually available, a draft statement of special educational needs will be prepared, and sent to the parents, together with the completed assessment reports. The Education (Special Educational Needs) Regulations 1983 state that this statement of special educational needs must specify:

1 the LEA's assessment of the child's special educational needs
2 the provision the LEA thinks appropriate to meet these needs
3 the type of school the LEA thinks would be appropriate
4 any non-educational provision the child should receive

The parents are invited to comment on the reports and recommendations and can appeal to a local appeals committee if they disagree with any aspect of the draft statement, and ultimately can appeal to the Secretary of State. If there are no objections, then a final statement is produced and signed by the parents and the LEA. This is then legally binding. The provision recommended has to be provided and the parents are legally obliged to send their child to the school concerned. The Audit Commission's report (1992a), however, has said that parents of statemented children should have rights, within limits, to state a preference for their child's school and to change their child's school if they wish. The nature of the provision remains the same for 12 months, when it is reviewed at what is known as the annual review, unless there is a need to review provision earlier than this.

Theoretically, assessment should not simply be conducted with a view to fitting the child into existing or available provision and parents have the right to ask for provision which the authority may not have. If appropriate special provision is not available within the child's LEA then they may be placed in a school or unit elsewhere, paid for by their own LEA. However, in practice, for most children the provision recommended is usually available within the authority. LEAs are required to provide suitable provision for the child and not necessarily the best possible provision.

The Audit Commission (1992b) estimated that there was a total of 1.2 million pupils in England and Wales with special educational needs in 1990. Fourteen per cent (168,000) had a statement (2.1 per cent of the total school population), and of these 106,000 (63 per cent) were attending special schools.

The value of statements

Opinions vary enormously about the usefulness of statements. There are positives and negatives associated with the procedure. On the positive side, it has provided parents with much more written information on their child than they have had previously and has acknowledged the value of the parents' own contribution to the assessment. Both the Warnock Report (DES, 1978) and the 1981 Education Act stressed that parents should be partners with the LEA in this assessment. Parents have the right to be consulted at every stage of the process and to be notified of appeals procedures. Full details of parents' rights under the Act are given in a booklet produced by the Advisory Centre for Education (Newell, 1983). But the extent to which parents are involved varies from one authority to the next and also within LEAs depending on the priorities and practice of the professionals concerned. A survey of 65 of the 104 LEAs conducted by the Centre for Studies on Integration in Education found that half these authorities failed to give parents important information or to involve and consult them adequately (Rogers, 1986).

A major criticism and difficulty of the statementing process is the time it takes to conduct and complete the procedure. When statements were first introduced, a maximum time for completion of six months was recommended, but they have often taken much longer than this – over a year in some cases. In future, the government proposes to introduce statutory time limits for each stage of the process, and LEAs will be penalised if they overrun this, without good reason, possibly being asked to fund an alternative assessment body to do the assessment instead.

Other criticisms are that statements and appeals are costly and time-consuming to complete, taking resources and professionals away from other special needs work. Many educators are very concerned that statements only relate to about 2 per cent of the child population and yet discussion of special needs is often dominated or revolves around those who have a statement, to the possible detriment of the majority of children with special needs – the 18 per cent (Gipps *et al.*, 1987). If the number of formal assessments was reduced, there would be more money available for the provision itself.

When statements were first introduced, the help required was not often expressed in a way which was helpful to staff to plan programmes and it was not possible to use this information to assess whether the help was being delivered or not. The reports often contained descriptions of the child's strengths and weaknesses with perhaps a description of the type of educational arrangements that would be appropriate (e.g. small group; some individual teaching) but very few specific teaching points were made. Some argued that because the statements often took almost twelve months to produce, teaching aims would be out of date by the time the statement was issued. There are also staff who prefer to make their own assessment of the child once they have spent time observing and working with them and who might not refer to previous reports on the child when devising an educational programme.

Many statements for pupils in mainstream schools have been vague in that they have not specified the actual number of hours support time the child needs and so they have not been able to protect a specific level of provision. Teaching hours from support staff may be reduced and neither staff or parents would have grounds for redress. A major reason why LEAs have not been more specific is that they have not felt able to offer guarantees that the finance for this would be available long-term. In addition, because the statement is a legal document, any future decision to reduce the amount of time, for educational reasons, would be time-consuming to renegotiate if the reduction was contested by either parents or staff.

Unfortunately, the statement procedure introduced by the 1981 Education Act has led some teachers and parents to view the formal assessment of children as a potential means to secure more resources (usually extra staff) and much professional time, particularly that of educational psychologists, has been spent discussing whether there were sufficient grounds for initiating a formal assessment. This has been made more difficult in the absence of clear criteria for such decisions, as mentioned earlier.

Annual reviews

In addition to the initial formal assessment, the 1981 Education Act also requires LEAs to review annually all those children who have a current statement of special educational needs whether they attend a mainstream or a special school. This annual re-assessment of the child's needs was welcomed as a positive move. Quite often in the past, children have remained in schools and classes which were no longer appropriate to their needs as there was no official structure for reviewing their placement. However, even with the introduction of the annual review system, it is still the case that once a child is placed in a special school, they usually remain within special provision for the rest of their school career. The Warnock Report (DES, 1978) had envisaged that special schools would take children for short periods of time for intensive work before returning them to mainstream school. But a survey of 85 special schools showed that less than 2 per cent of pupils annually moved into mainstream schools (Audit Commission, 1992a). Some special school headteachers explained this very low figure by saying that mainstream schools were not able or willing to take children with special needs; headteachers of mainstream schools thought that some special school staff were over-protective with the children.

A potential failing in the review system may stem from the fact that very often the annual review is a wholly within school affair. Parents and professionals are invited to the review, but are not obliged to attend. Educational psychologists and other professionals who support the work of special school staff are often pressed for time and so few will attend annual reviews on a routine basis. The educational psychologist may attend if they feel there is a significant need to do so (e.g. a possible change of placement or increase in support), but how are they alerted to this need? School staff are knowledgeable about their own provision but do not often have information on alternatives and are therefore limited on what they might consider and recommend. The Audit Commission Report (1992b) recognising this deficiency, however, has recommended that educational psychologists should attend a child's annual review at least once every two years in order to monitor the success of the school in meeting needs. This may lead to greater movement of pupils between placements in the future.

Schools also vary in how much opportunity they offer to parents to take a full and significant role in the annual review. Some schools send parents the reports before the review and may ask them to submit their own report together with any items for discussion. In other schools parents may listen to the staff and be given the report at the end of the review and then asked for their comments. This gives them less chance for considered comment. There are some professionals who would argue that it is essential for staff and parents to discuss teaching objectives and to agree these, particularly in the area of self-help and independence training, to encourage a committed and consistent mutual response to the child's difficulties and therefore maximise the potential for progress (Borg, 1992). If the staff or parents are concerned about a particular child at the review, a full multi-disciplinary re-assessment can be requested and carried out if the request is considered reasonable by the LEA.

In addition to the annual reviews, pupils with a statement have a legal entitlement to be fully re-assessed between the ages of thirteen and a half and fourteen and a half years, unless the child has been assessed within the last twelve months. This assessment is usually identical in form to the initial assessment but should also include a member of the careers service, generally with responsibility for pupils with special needs. A new statement is produced and all the reports are submitted to the parents. This assessment is designed to assess the pupil's current attainments and functioning with a view to planning for his future needs during his school years and beyond.

EDUCATIONAL PROVISION FOR PUPILS WITH LEARNING DISABILITIES

LEAs have had quite a degree of freedom on how and what to provide for a pupil with special needs so that what is available in any particular area varies and is dependent on the philosophy and practice of the policy makers and planners. In the past, when the type of problem was used to determine the provision, a number of separate special schools designated for particular handicaps were set up (e.g. for the blind, deaf). Now that needs are not seen as solely derived from the type of problem, and that children with a particular disability are perceived to have more in common with normally developing children than with children having the same disability, some of these separate units and schools have been closed or have been moved on to mainstream campuses so that the children can spend some or most of their time with their normally developing peers.

As a result, throughout Britain, there are many different types of placement and ways of meeting the educational needs of children with learning disabilities. Twenty years ago, the children who were not able to manage in mainstream schools without extra support would be placed in separate special provision in schools for children with moderate or severe learning difficulties (ESN(M) and ESN(S)). Now, whilst these schools still exist, the majority of LEAs have tried to limit the numbers of children attending them, particularly for children with moderate learning disabilities. Some LEAs still send a small number of children with special needs to independent schools or schools run by other LEAs outside their own authority. Such placements militate against the development of a body of knowledge and skills within the LEA for dealing with that particular group of children and the schools are difficult to monitor because of the distances involved. Children are also separated from their families, often only spending time with them during school holidays. As a result, many LEAs have been trying to reduce the numbers of children they place at schools outside the LEA.

A range of provision has developed on a rather *ad hoc* basis to meet the different special educational needs of children with learning disabilities. This ranges from total segregation on a residential basis to full integration in a mainstream school. The Warnock Report (DES, 1978) described ten forms of provision which it believed would be needed in the future for children with special educational needs. They were as follows:

1 Full-time education in an ordinary class with any necessary help and support
2 Education in an ordinary class with periods of withdrawal to a special class or unit or other supporting base
3 Education in a special class or unit with periods of attendance at an ordinary class and full involvement in the general community life and extra-curricular activities of the ordinary school

4 Full-time education in a special class or unit with social contact with the main school
5 Education in a special school, day or residential, with some shared lessons in a neighbouring school
6 Full-time education in a day special school with social contact with an ordinary school
7 Full-time education in a residential special school with social contact with an ordinary school
8 Short-term education in hospitals or other establishments
9 Long-term education in hospitals or other establishments
10 Home tuition

(DES, 1978, para. 6.11, p. 69)

There are examples of each of these forms of provision in the majority of LEAs (see Booth and Statham, 1982; Hegarty *et al.*, 1981), but so far, the extent to which children in the special schools and units have contact with mainstream school children is often very limited.

Educational provision for preschool children with learning disabilities

The provision available to children under five with learning disabilities ranges from day nurseries, child minders and playgroups to nursery and infant classes in mainstream and special schools. There is great variation between one local authority and another in terms of what is available and it is often historical accident rather than need which determines the existing preschool provision in an area (Blackstone, 1971).

For a child with learning disabilities, placement in a preschool group can offer a wide range of play opportunities, lessen the child's dependence on his parents and provide the family with support. Because preschool placement is often beneficial to children with special needs it has been the policy of some local authorities to give priority to these children.

Day nurseries

Social Services Departments are responsible for the organisation and running of most day nurseries. Other day nurseries run by voluntary or private groups must be registered with the local social services department. Most day nurseries are open all year round from 8.30a.m. to 5.30p.m. and can take children from a few weeks old to five years of age. They were set up for normally developing children but also admit children with special needs. Children with learning disabilities may be referred from a variety of sources (e.g. parents, health visitor, district nurse, GP, paediatrician). The staff are generally qualified nursery nurses.

A criticism of day nurseries in the past has been that the emphasis was on the physical health and care of the child and not on their intellectual development (Laishley and Coleman, 1978). However, many day nurseries have changed in this respect and nursery staff have developed methods of observing and recording children's development and planning ways of enhancing their skills (e.g. in communication, play, social skills, self-help skills). Having said this, there remains a need for training staff and continued support from other professionals involved with children having special needs (e.g. from speech therapists, physiotherapists, psychologists). Children with learning disabilities often do not learn very much if left to direct their own play and often need skilled guidance from an adult or direct adult involvement if they are to benefit from an activity (Ravenette, 1973). But without specialist help staff may be unsure about the implications of a particular disability and may not match the activities given to the abilities of the child.

Playgroups

The playgroup movement began in 1961 to fill the gaps in existing statutory preschool provision for all children. Playgroups are run under the auspices of social services departments and accommodation varies from purpose-built premises to church halls. They may be run by a committee of local parents or a private body and although most cater for children between the ages of three and five years, some playgroups will accept children from the age of two. Playgroup staff are not generally qualified although some parents may have had relevant training and experience prior to becoming involved with the group. The Preschool Playgroups Association (PPA) is a national voluntary organisation designed to advance the education of children below compulsory school age. It runs training courses for staff and has a sub-committee with responsibility for children with special needs which advises, supports and registers playgroups working with this group of children.

Generally, there are three different types of playgroup and a child with learning disabilities might attend any one of these. They are the ordinary playgroup, the opportunity group and the special playgroup. The latter two groups were devised specifically for the child with special needs – the opportunity group catering for children with special needs together with their brothers and sisters and the special group catering solely for children with special needs. Playgroups range from fairly informal groups where parents meet and talk and children play to more structured sessions supported by speech therapists, physiotherapists or psychologists. As playgroups are parent run and parent focused, it is possible for a parent who has a child with quite severe learning disabilities to attend and stay with the child – thus enabling the child to be with normally developing peers which might not otherwise be possible. Several children with learning disabilities who later attend separate special schools have started off in the mainstream setting of an ordinary playgroup.

The PPA encourages the attendance of children with special needs at ordinary playgroups and this was endorsed by the Warnock Report (DES, 1978). It is very difficult to estimate the numbers of children with learning disabilities currently attending ordinary playgroups. In some LEAs there are many playgroups, as other forms of preschool provision are scarce, whereas in other authorities there are few playgroups because the local schools offer nursery places from the age of three years.

Mainstream nursery classes

Many infant and primary schools administered by LEAs have nursery classes for children between the ages of three and five years, most of whom attend on a part-time basis. They are free of charge, unlike playgroups and day nurseries, and are staffed by trained teachers and nursery nurses. In areas where nursery provision is in short supply, priority may be given to children with special needs.

Parents of a child with learning disabilities may approach the nursery themselves to discuss the placement, or a professional involved with the child might consult the headteacher. The acceptance of a child with learning disabilities is at the discretion of the headteacher and the governors, who have to assess the needs of the child in relation to the resources of the school and the needs of other children in the group. Advantages of placement in a mainstream school are that the child can attend his neighbourhood school with siblings and there are other normally developing children to observe and model. They, in turn, learn to understand and accept children who are different from themselves. Some drawbacks to this type of placement are that the staff may not have any special expertise in teaching these children, the adult–child ratio may be less favourable than in special provision, appropriate materials and resources suited to the child's developmental level may not be available and support from other agencies may not be adequate. Chazan *et al.* (1980) found that preschool staff were often very willing to accept children with special needs but lacked the knowledge to devise programmes of help and received infrequent support from other agencies to help them to do so. This situation is improving in some LEAs where experienced teachers from local special schools work on an outreach basis to support staff in mainstream settings.

Special provision for preschool children

The separate, segregated education of slow learning children officially began with the elementary Education (Defective and Epileptic Children) Act in 1899. This Act gave statutory recognition to the need to make special educational provision for children it considered unable to benefit from that provided in mainstream schools. But this Act did not include those children with very severe learning disabilities. This group of children were deemed ineducable and therefore not entitled to educational provision. It was not until

1970 that these children were given the right to education. Even now, Britain is one of only a few countries where this group of children is entitled to education (Ware, 1990). The 1970 Education (Handicapped Children) Act transferred responsibility from Mental Health Departments to Education Departments. The former Junior Training Centres for children with severe learning disabilities were therefore renamed schools for the educationally subnormal (severe), and came under the auspices and administration of LEAs. Their premises were often inadequate for teaching purposes and the staff were not qualified to teach. Over the last two decades therefore there has been a process of retraining and re-staffing and transfer into purpose-built premises.

Until relatively recently, preschool provision in special schools and units was made only for children with particular sensory or physical handicaps, but many special schools for children with moderate or severe learning disabilities also now have nursery provision.

Peripatetic preschool teachers

In many LEAs there is a team of teachers who work with preschool children and their families before the child is placed in a group or school. They generally visit the child at home on a weekly basis. Some LEAs have Portage schemes (see Cameron and White, 1982) where parents and children follow Portage activities with weekly or fortnightly advice from a support teacher. Their aim is to develop the child's skills, to reduce their level of need and, if possible, to enable their attendance at a mainstream school.

Educational provision for children with learning disabilities between 5 and 16 years

Placement in a mainstream school

The majority of school-age children with learning disabilities (i.e. more than 90 per cent of Warnock's 20 per cent) will be educated in mainstream schools, with or without extra support, for the whole of their school career. A small percentage of these will have statements and extra adult help will usually be provided specifically for them on a part or full-time basis. This help is usually from a nursery nurse or from an unqualified person who is dependent on advice from the school staff or from a visiting advisory teacher. For the vast majority of children with special needs in mainstream schools, help will be provided by their classteacher(s). The classteacher(s) may have some support from other staff within the school who have responsibility throughout the school for these children. In addition, some LEAs have set up schemes where teachers from local special schools work on an outreach basis to support their mainstream colleagues.

Under LMS, some LEAs have chosen to disband their peripatetic services and to allocate this money directly to the schools to appoint their own support staff. This move should suit some headteachers as the Audit Commission (1992a) found that many headteachers preferred to appoint their own staff. Reasons given were that this gave them more flexibility in timetabling, support staff could more easily hold discussions with the class-teacher and the system was seen as more cost-effective, in terms of the reduction in travelling time. Possible disadvantages in headteachers appointing their own support staff are that these staff are less likely to have previous experience of working with children with special needs, and as they are directly managed by the headteachers, they may have less autonomy to make decisions on who they support and how they do this.

If speech therapy or physiotherapy is required, it is likely that the child will have to attend clinic sessions outside the school. The provision of paramedical services such as speech therapy has caused concern to head-teachers of both special and mainstream schools (Audit Commission, 1992a). All twelve LEAs reported problems in obtaining speech therapy for pupils they considered required this. Some of the difficulties arise because therapists are employed by the health authorities and not the LEAs, so the latter do not have the authority to determine how therapy is allocated.

Effects of legislation on the progress of integration of children with learning disabilities

The 1981 Education Act reaffirmed the principle first stated almost fifty years ago in the 1944 Education Act that wherever possible children with special educational needs should be educated in mainstream schools. However, LEAs are not obliged to integrate children with special needs in all cases. The 1981 Education Act advises that integration should only occur if this is compatible with the parents' wishes, and the child's special needs can be met within the mainstream school in a cost-effective way without detriment to other children or staff. Many mainstream schools do not feel ready to accept pupils who would previously have been in separate special provision. They not only believe that are they under-resourced in terms of staffing and materials and therefore other children will lose out, but feel ill-prepared in terms of staff attitudes and their willingness to spend time modifying the curriculum.

Currently, 1.3 per cent of the total school population are educated in separate special schools and they spend little or no time being educated alongside their normally developing peers. Pro-integrationists argue that this percentage is still too large and that a greater number of children could and should be taught in mainstream schools. They are concerned that moves to integrate children have not gathered pace in most LEAs in recent years.

Despite repeated recommendations that integration should occur wherever possible (1944 Education Act; 1970 Education (Handicapped Children) Act; Warnock Report (DES, 1978)) , there has been little incentive for mainstream schools to provide for children with moderate or severe learning disabilities. The 1988 Education Act, whilst restating the desirability of integration may not effect much change in practice and some would even say that it has threatened the development of integrationist practices. The introduction of the National Curriculum and the possibility of published results being used to assess the worth of a school and staff, the introduction of teacher appraisal, the implementation of LMS and the increase in teacher–pupil ratios have all contributed to create a situation in which the ability and willingness of schools to admit or maintain the placement of children with learning disabilities who are time-consuming and often challenging is severely tested.

The Audit Commission and HMI (1992b) made a number of recommendations for the development of appropriate mainstream provision for special needs and said that, 'LEAs should increase the capability of ordinary schools to provide for pupils with special needs' (p. 23). Many mainstream teachers are concerned, however, that such re-allocation may not happen. Although the proportion of children integrated in mainstream schools has not increased significantly, the ability of mainstream schools to support these children has improved in many LEAs. Gipps *et al.* (1987) in their study of six LEAs after the 1981 Act, argued that the Warnock Report (DES, 1978) and the 1981 Act created a climate within which LEAs and schools protected their special needs services and made cuts elsewhere – and that many changes were made to the way in which support to mainstream schools and children was organised and delivered – increasing the support and effectiveness of this for the 18 per cent of children with special needs in mainstream schools and so potentially allowing them to meet the needs of more of the special needs population. This finding was supported by the studies of Goacher *et al.* (1988). However, these increases in support have not resulted in a corresponding increase in the proportion of children being integrated (Swann, 1988).

Dessent (1987) and Swann (1988) have attempted to explain this by arguing that alongside the development of skills in meeting a wider range of needs, staff have also increased their ability to identify needs and increased their awareness of the extent of separate special provision. This has seemed to deskill and demotivate mainstream teachers who believe that someone else has the expertise and responsibility for special needs.

Arguments for integrating children with learning disabilities in mainstream schools

There are several arguments put forward by those who feel that more pupils with special needs could and should be in mainstream schools. Firstly, there may be little difference between a child with moderate learning difficulties attending a special school and the special needs of some of the children attending mainstream schools. This anomaly exists within LEAs as well as between LEAs. Factors which contribute to this situation include the beliefs of teachers and other professionals as to how a child's special educational needs are best met, the availability of special provision, the attitudes of the headteacher and the wishes of the parents.

Secondly, there is a common assumption that children with moderate learning disabilities will make better progress if they attend a special school or unit than if they remain in a mainstream school. In fact, little research has been done to test this. The results of the few studies that have been done, though, have not found any significant difference between the attainments of the two groups (Galloway and Goodwin, 1979; Ghodsian and Calnan, 1977; Hallahan *et al.*, 1988).

Thirdly, Dessent (1987) argues that a system based on special schools is in principle inequitable, and that although special schools provide large amounts of resource for some children, this is at the expense of children who experience difficulties in mainstream. Similarly, Barton and Smith (1989) argue that, 'in human rights terms, the right to education within the community, the right to education alongside non-handicapped peers and the right to access to the mainstream curriculum are rights which cannot, by definition, be met in segregated education (p. 83).

Fourthly, the nature of the educational experience provided for children in special provision is often characterised by narrowness of opportunity (Ainscow, 1989). The National Curriculum should serve to broaden this, however. Currently, many special schools are lacking in facilities and expertise in science, technology and foreign languages and the quality of education in some special schools does not support them becoming centres of excellence (Audit Commission, 1992a). The HMI report, 'Standards in Education 1988–89' noted that while there were continuing improvements in special needs provision, LEAs, schools and teachers need to plan, manage and evaluate the work undertaken much more effectively and consistently.

Special school provision

Despite the views of the pro-integrationists, the Warnock Report (DES, 1978) felt that separate special provision would still be needed for three groups of children with special needs and a continuation of special provision was also supported by the recent Audit Commission's report (1992b). This stated that, 'Special schools continue to be required not only for those pupils for whom mainstream schools can not provide, but also to provide choice for parents' (p. 7). They went on to recommend though that all LEAs should review their special school provision because of falling rolls, surplus accommodation and the requirement to deliver the National Curriculum.

The three groups defined in the Warnock Report for whom special school provision might be required were as follows:

i   those with severe or complex physical, sensory or intellectual dis-
     abilities who require special facilities, teaching methods or expertise
     that it would be impracticable to provide in mainstream schools;
ii   those with severe emotional or behavioural disorders who have
     very great difficulty in forming relationships with others or whose

behaviour is so extreme or unpredictable that it causes severe dis-
ruption in a mainstream school or inhibits the educational progress of
other children;

iii   those with less severe disabilities, often in combination, who despite
special help do not perform well in a mainstream school and are more
likely to thrive in the more intimate communal and educational setting
of a special school.

(DES, 1978, para. 6.10, p. 68)

There are many who agree with this viewpoint and are in favour of retaining
special schools, for a number of reasons. The general advantages cited for
special school provision are that staff are trained to teach children with
special needs, there is a good adult–child ratio, better access to specialist
materials and resources and more frequent support from other professionals
than in mainstream schools. Not all of these are true for all special schools
though and some of the support provided in mainstream schools is of high
quality. Some disadvantages of separate, special school attendance are that
the children may be isolated from their neighbourhood peers, have little or
no contact with normally developing children and may have a long journey
to and from school, making home–school liaison difficult.

The two main types of special placement for children with learning
disabilities are either a school or unit for children with moderate learning
disabilities or a school or unit for children with severe learning disabilities.
Some special schools have children with moderate and severe learning
disabilities on roll. The majority of special schools have their own campus and
are separate from mainstream provision. Other special placements for children
with learning disabilities are observation classes within mainstream schools
and assessment units which are usually on the campus of a special school.

Special units and schools

As stated earlier, at the present time an average of 1.3 per cent of the total
school population still attends special schools or units. There are 1,300 special
schools run by LEAs in England and Wales with 95,000 children on roll. A
further 11,000 pupils attend independent schools for children with special
needs, where LEAs fund places, often on a residential basis. In the Audit
Commission's study of twelve LEAs, they found that 52 per cent of the special
school population attended schools for moderate learning difficulties; 24 per
cent were in schools for severe learning difficulties; 8 per cent were in schools
for emotional and behavioural difficulties and the remaining 16 per cent
attended other types of school (Audit Commission, 1992a).

Schools for children with moderate or severe learning difficulties generally
cater for children up to the age of 16 or 19 years. The number of children on
roll can vary from 30 to over 150. The adult–child ratio is more favourable
than in mainstream schools and will vary within a school from one group to

another depending on the abilities and needs of the children and the type of activities followed. The children may be grouped according to age or developmental level or be part of a family group. Two groups of children with learning disabilities who in the past have been treated differently in the schools for children with severe learning disabilities are the hyperactive, disruptive children (often referred to as those with challenging behaviours) and those children with multiple needs. The latter children may be separately defined and accommodated within the school (e.g. as the 'special care' group), although many headteachers are trying to integrate them into other classes throughout their school. In the past, this group of children were often placed in hospital schools. One of the recommendations of the Warnock Report (DES, 1978) was that wherever possible, children should be educated at a school outside hospital. Several hospital schools on the sites of mental handicap hospitals have now closed and schools for children with severe learning disabilities are taking a greater proportion of special care children.

Observation classes and assessment units

These classes and units are generally for children of primary age and are often part of a mainstream primary school. Their main function is to make a detailed assessment of a child's special educational needs over a period of time in order to determine the most appropriate educational provision. The period of assessment can range from one term to two or three years. Regular case reviews are normally held with other professionals to determine and discuss the child's development and future placement.

Educational provision for pupils over the age of 16 with learning difficulties

In the past, many pupils attending special schools left at the age of 15 or 16 years. The 1981 Education Act entitles education to all those who want to continue up to the age of nineteen years. An increasing number of special schools are therefore offering facilities and an appropriate curriculum for pupils beyond sixteen. Pupils may stay on at schools provided that schools can meet their needs – otherwise they can transfer to a school or college that can. Many colleges of further education now have link courses which pupils may attend on a sessional basis to prepare them for full-time courses when they leave.

For pupils with a statement, the reports written for the re-assessment at ages thirteen and a half to fourteen and a half are sent to social services. During the pupil's last year at school, social services personnel assess and plan for the future needs of the pupil, following guidelines introduced by the Disabled Persons Act (1986). They make a judgement as to whether the person is to be regarded as disabled. It is estimated that about one-third of pupils with a statement will meet the criteria. For young people without a statement, they and their families should be informed of the Disabled Persons Act and if they consider they might qualify for disablement, then an assessment by social services can be arranged.

Colleges of further education are now out of LEA control. Applications are made to the Further Education Funding Council (FEFC), if necessary, for funding the additional resources thought to be required to enable a pupil with special needs to attend a further education college. On leaving school, people with learning disabilities may join a training scheme, attend a Social Education Centre, a sheltered workshop or a college of further education or secure a job in open employment. Staff working with school leavers are often uncertain as to where the pupils will transfer which makes preparation for leaving and planning appropriate programmes of help very difficult.

At the present time, careers guidance for pupils with special needs is still far from adequate, but the recommendations of the Warnock Report (DES, 1978) do seem to have had an effect in certain respects. The report suggested that there should be a teacher responsible in both mainstream and special schools to advise youngsters with special needs on future careers and to liaise with colleges of further education, social education centres, industrial training centres and potential employers to arrange visits and work experience. Secondary schools and special schools vary a great deal as to what they provide as a leavers' programme for children with special needs. As yet, there is certainly no guarantee that a well-designed programme of advice and experience is available at all mainstream and special schools, but there are exceptions where a great deal of work has been done by staff and local colleges in developing link courses and work experience. The Warnock Report also recommended that the Careers Service be involved with the formal re-assessment at 13 or 14 years of age, but again, partly due to large caseloads, in many LEAs the input from the Careers Service does not happen automatically. The Specialist Careers Officer may interview all leavers at a special school, but this is often in isolation from other agencies involved with the child. Many professionals would argue that there is a need to improve the liaison between school staff and the professionals involved in the schemes to which school leavers transfer.

THE 1988 EDUCATION REFORM ACT AND LOCAL MANAGEMENT OF SCHOOLS (LMS)

Local Management of Schools is one of the major changes introduced by the 1988 Education Reform Act that will crucially affect the future of LEAs and has major implications for the resourcing of children with learning disabilities. Under LMS, financial resources are delegated from the LEAs to the governing bodies of individual mainstream schools. The essence of delegation is that schools should manage their own resources, including those for children with special needs. The rationale underlying LMS was that the quality and efficiency of education would improve if there was increased competition between schools and if their governing body, rather than the LEAs, determined how resources were to be allocated. At present, LMS applies only to mainstream schools but it will be extended to special schools (LMSS) by April 1994.

The Audit Commission (1992a) recommended that LEAs and schools should adopt a 'client/contractor' relationship, whereby schools, as the contractors, should be given full responsibility for providing for pupils with special needs. However, although the LEA can recommend the amount of money to be used for a specific purpose, it has no control over whether it is actually spent in this way. The task for LEAs will increasingly be to find ways of ensuring that appropriate provision is made for special needs whilst having little managerial control over those who will be providing it (Audit Commission, 1992a). At present, LEAs continue to pay for statutory responsibilities such as educational psychologists and education welfare officers, but they are under increasing pressure to delegate as many of their resources to schools as possible and many have already delegated at least some of their funds for advisers and inspectors and other elements of their support services. Schools are now able to buy in services from organisations other than the LEA (e.g. from voluntary groups and private practitioners).

In terms of resources for children with special needs, LEAs have had to decide how much money will be allocated to each mainstream school for their special needs population. Different methods of doing this have been implemented by LEAs. As schools vary in terms of size and catchment area, the amount of money allocated to each school has to be worked out separately. Some LEAs have created a formula based on objective criteria. The formula weights schools differently using information about possible indicators of the likely level of need of each school (e.g. the number of free school meals or clothing voucher applications) to arrive at what can be viewed as a fair figure for all. As each LEA creates its own formula, there are likely to be significant differences in practice from one LEA to another. Some LEAs may choose to use test results in their formula and would have a choice as to whether to reward a school having good results (on the grounds that this is a good use of money) or to support and enhance those schools with poor results. However, the latter method might be viewed as supporting bad practice in some schools.

A number of LEAs have asked each school to provide data on the actual incidence of special needs children on roll. Some of these LEAs have asked the schools to band the children according to level of need, placing their pupils with statements in the top band. This method has been supported by the Audit Commission as a way of calculating fair resources for each school. Their handbook *Getting the Act Together* (1992b) which gives details of the practice which schools and LEAs should implement, states that, 'it is quite practical for LEAs to develop systems which record the actual incidence of pupils with special needs in each school and use these as a basis for the distribution of funds for pupils with special needs without statements' (p. 2).

Clearly, there are risks that schools may over-identify to secure more resources. The Audit Commission suggests that the LEA has a system for checking the figures supplied, perhaps by an educational psychologist, but this is likely to bring its own problems and to be a difficult and time-consuming exercise. A lack of clarity on the basis on which competing requests are dealt with may lead to frustration and anger amongst schools. A small number of LEAs have grouped headteachers from families of schools together and asked them to discuss and agree on the allocation of resources for each school to reduce the potential for misunderstanding and grievance.

There are concerns that LMS may work against the best interests of children with special needs. Some LEAs may retain money to allocate resources to children with statements, so schools might refer more children for a formal assessment in order to obtain more funds. This would increase the total costs of producing a statement in addition to increasing the time spent on deciding whether there was a case for initiating a formal assessment. Each LEA has to seek approval from the Secretary of State for the way in which it plans to delegate funds for pupils with statements and has to publish the principles, rules and methods by which it determines the allocation of funds to schools for these pupils.

Other schools may try to avoid admitting children with learning disabilities if they are likely to require expensive additional resources and are unlikely to do well on Standard Assessment Tasks (SATs), although it is not yet clear how the attainment results of children with statements will be reported. Schools which have opted out are free to determine their own admissions policy and may choose to exclude children in their area who have special needs. However, if a maintained school is specified on the statement, the school will be obliged to admit the child. One way of encouraging main-stream schools to admit and maintain the placements of children with special needs would be to offer financial incentives to those who admit such children or to those schools which do not exclude them.

THE NATIONAL CURRICULUM

In addition to the introduction of LMS, the 1988 Education Reform Act introduced a National Curriculum. The National Curriculum forms the basis of what *all* children are to be taught and is seen as an 'entitlement curriculum'. It is not possible here to cover the National Curriculum in detail and guidelines are still being produced by the DFE. A recent book by Daniels and Ware (1990) considers the implications of the National Curriculum for pupils with special needs. One of the main purposes of the National Curriculum was to produce nationally comparable and publicly reportable assessment data. Although the National Curriculum prescribes the areas of the curriculum which all schools must include, there are difficulties in using it as a basis for planning programmes of work. Solity (1992) maintains that at best, it provides a general framework in which teachers have to work. He argues that the statements of attainment are frequently ambiguous, that they need to be translated into realistic objectives for children's learning, and that no clear rationale has ever been given for the curricular sequences offered.

All maintained schools, except hospital schools have to comply with the requirements of the National Curriculum as they are introduced. All schools are required to have a curriculum document showing the main curriculum areas and aims and teaching objectives within these. This allows teachers to assess, programme plan, record and evaluate progress. The child's progress has to be continuously assessed by the teacher and then formally using the national Standard Assessment Tasks at certain key stages (at 7, 11, 14 and 16 years of age). The government has claimed that these key stage assessments are essential to giving parents information about the respective worth of different schools. The early pilots of SATs, however, were found to be very time-consuming. They have since been modified but are now less related to classroom activities and therefore not viewed as likely to yield reliable and valid results about a school's effectiveness (Solity, 1992).

When guidelines for the National Curriculum were introduced, it appeared that little or no thought had been given to children with special needs. In the National Curriculum document, *From Policy to Practice* (DES, 1989), which was given to all schools (special and mainstream) to introduce the new mandatory requirements – there were just three pages on children with special needs. Sections were added to subsequent documents giving guidance on how staff should accommodate these children within the National Curriculum.

Ware (1990) writes that initially, those involved with children with special needs felt that the National Curriculum was unlikely to be applied to schools for children with severe learning difficulties, but that as it is now being viewed as an entitlement curriculum, thought has to be given to how these children can be included within it. She concludes that it is not at all clear that the National Curriculum can be implemented in any real sense for all pupils with severe learning difficulties (particularly the most severely handicapped and those with challenging behaviour) or that it can be implemented in its entirety for any of them. However, many schools for pupils with severe learning disabilities have welcomed and embraced the challenge of finding ways of including their pupils within the National Curriculum framework in meaningful ways. Teaching the full range of subjects under the National Curriculum, though, is likely to be a problem for small special schools with limited numbers of staff.

It is possible for a child to be exempted from parts of the National Curriculum but the DES Circulars (5/89 and 15/89) suggest that such modifications and exemptions should be quite rare. How these modifications and disapplications will be determined and how they will be incorporated in statements have not yet been clarified. Some special educators see the proposals to allow the exclusion of some children with special needs from the National Curriculum as a negation of the principles of integration and entitlement which formed the basis of the 1981 Act (Wedell, 1988).

CONCLUDING REMARKS

The education provided for all children is undergoing major change primarily as a result of the introduction of LMS and a National Curriculum which applies to all maintained schools both special and mainstream. The full impact of these measures on the education of children with learning disabilities remains to be seen, but one can speculate on some of the likely effects.

The intention of the 1981 Education Act was that statements would clarify and record the needs of a small percentage of children with severe and complex needs – typically the needs of those children who were attending special schools at the time the Act was drafted. The system of assessment and drafting of statements is too time-consuming and expensive in administrative costs to be an appropriate mechanism for targeting resources for the majority of pupils with special needs (Warnock's 18 per cent). However, in some LEAs, additional resourcing for special needs is only available via a statement. The procedure is currently under review to clarify criteria for ascertaining which children should be formally assessed, to reduce the time taken to complete the procedure and to improve the system of annual reviews.

In order to enhance the provision for all children with special needs, all schools (both special and mainstream) need to further differentiate the methods and materials used and to make available special resources with which these pupils can help themselves (Audit Commission, 1992b). Special school teachers are likely to work more closely with colleagues in mainstream education in future, providing support or working collaboratively on joint curriculum initiatives (Ainscow, 1989). If special schools are successful in this outreach work, then their rolls may fall and some schools may close. Alternatively, success may increase their referrals as parents and professionals are impressed by what is on offer and there may be a greater number of part-time and short-term placements at special schools, with transition to mainstream being supported by staff in both settings. There has always been great variation in the way in which LEAs have responded to legislation. Now that much of the decision-making has been passed from the LEAs down to the individual schools level, one can anticipate an even greater degree of variation in the provision for children with learning disabilities in the future.

REFERENCES

Acts of Parliament

Education Act (1944), London: HMSO.
Education Act (1981), London: HMSO.
Education (Handicapped) Children Act (1970), London: HMSO.
Education Reform Act (1988), London: HMSO.

General references

Ainscow, M. (ed.) (1989) *Special Education in Change*, London: Fulton.

Audit Commission (1992a) *Getting in on the Act*, London: HMSO.

Audit Commission (1992b) *Getting the Act Together: Provision for pupils with special educational needs*, London: HMSO.

Barton, L. and Smith, M. (1989) Equality, rights and primary education, in Roaf, C. and Bines, H (eds) *Needs, Rights and Opportunities in Special Education*, London: Falmer.

Bayley, M. (1969) *Bayley's Scale of Infant Development: Birth to two years*, New York: Psychological Corporation.

Blackstone, T. (1971) *A Fair Start: The provision of preschool education*, Harmondsworth: Penguin.

Bluma, S. M., Shearer, J., Frohman, A. H. and Hilliard, J. M. (1976) *Portage Guide to Early Education*, Wisconsin: Cooperative Educational Service, Agency 12.

Booth, A. and Statham, J. (1982) *The Nature of Special Education*, London: Croom Helm.

Borg, M. (1992) Model for treatment and training, paper presented at Autisme Europe conference in May, 1992.

Butler, N. R. (1969) *Concern*, 3, 8.

Cameron, R. and White, M. (eds) (1982) *Working Together: Portage in the UK*, Windsor: NFER.

Chazan, M., Laing, A., Shackleton-Bailey, M. J. and Jones, G. E. (1980) *Some of Our Children*, London: Open Books.

Court Report (1976) *Fit for the Future*, London: HMSO.

Daniels, H. and Ware, J. (1990) *Special Educational Needs and the National Curriculum*, London: Kogan Page.

Davie, R. (1975) *Children and Families with Special Needs*, Cardiff: University College of Cardiff.

Department of Education and Science (DES) (1978) *Special Educational Needs (Warnock Report)* Cmnd 7212, London: HMSO.

DES (1983) *Assessments and Statements of Special Educational Needs (*Circular 1/83): Procedures within education, health and social services, London: HMSO.

DES (1989) *National Curriculum from Policy to Practice*, London: DES.

DES (1989a) Circular 5/89.

DES (1989b) Circular 15/89.

Dessent, T. (1987) *Making the Ordinary School Special*, Lewes: Falmer Press.

Elliott, C. D., Murray, D. J. and Pearson, L. S. (1978) *British Ability Scales*, Windsor: NFER.

Galloway, D. and Goodwin, C. (1979) *Educating Slow Learning and Maladjusted Children: Integration or segregation?*, London: Longman.

Ghodsian, M. and Calnan, M. (1977) Comparative longitudinal analysis of special education groups, *British Journal of Educational Psychology*, 47, 162–74.

Gipps, C. V., Gross, H. and Goldstein, H. (1987) *Warnock's 18%: Children with special needs in ordinary schools*, Basingstoke: Falmer Press.

Goacher, B., Evans, J., Welton, J. and Wedell, K. (1988) *Policy and Provision for Special Educational Needs*, London: Cassell.

Griffiths, M. I. (1973) Early detection: developmental screening, in Griffiths, M. I. (ed.) *The Young Retarded Child: Medical aspects of care*, Edinburgh and London: Churchill Livingstone.

Griffiths, R. (1970) *Griffiths Mental Development Scales*, Taunton: Child Development Research Centre.

Gulliford, R. (1975) Enrichment methods, in Wedell, K. (ed.) *Orientations in Special Education*, London: Wiley.

Gunzburg, H. C. (1973) *Primary Progress Assessment Charts*, Birmingham: SEFA Publications.

Hallahan, D.P. *et al.* (1988) Examining the research base of the Regular Education Initiative, *Journal of Learning Disabilities*, 21 (1), 29–35.

Hamilton, F. M. W. (1968) *Medical Officer*, 119, 201.

Hegarty, S, Pocklington, K. and Lucas, D. (1981) *Educating Pupils with Special Needs in the Ordinary School*, Slou h: NFER.

Her Majesty's Inspectorate (1989) *Standards in Education 1988–89*, London: HMSO.

Hogg, J. and Raynes, N. (1987) *Assessment in Mental Handicap*, London: Croom Helm.

Jeffree, D. and McConkey, R. (1976) *PIP Developmental Charts*, London: Hodder and Stoughton.

Kiernan, C. C. and Jones, M. C. (1982) *Behaviour Assessment Battery*, Windsor: NFER.

Knowles, W. and Masidlover, M. (1982) *Derbyshire Language Scheme*, Derby: Derbyshire County Council.

Knox, E. G. and Mahon, D. F. (1970) Evaluation of 'infant at risk' registers, *Archives of Disease in Childhood*, 45, 634.

Laishley, J. and Coleman, J. (1978) Intervention for disadvantaged preschool children, *Education Research*, 20, 216–25.

Lindon, R. L. (1961) Risk register, *Cerebral Palsy Bulletin*, 3, 481.

Murphy, G. (1987) Direct observation as an assessment tool in functional analysis and treatment, in Hogg. J. and Raynes, N. *Assessment in Mental Handicap*, London: Croom Helm.

Newell, P. (1983) *ACE Special Education Handbook: the new law on children with special needs*, London: Advisory Centre for Education (ACE).

Nihara, K., Foster, R., Shellhaas, M. and Leland, H. (1969) *Adaptive Behaviour Scale*, 1st edition, Washington DC: AAMD.

Ravenette, A. T. (1973) Planning treatment programmes: school age children, in Mittler, P. (ed.) *Assessment for Learning in the Mentally Handicapped*, London: Churchill Livingstone.

Reynell, J. K. (1969) *Reynell Developmental Language Scales*, London: NFER.

Roaf, C. and Bines, H. (eds) (1989) *Needs, Rights and Opportunities in Special Education*, London: Falmer.

Rogers. R. (1986) *Caught in the Act*, London: CSIE and Spastics Society.

Sharp, J. D. and Stott, D. H. (1976) *Effectiveness–Motivation Scale*, Windsor: NFER.

Solity, J. (1992) *Special Education*, London: Cassell.

Sparrow, S., Balla, D., Cicchetti, V. (1984) *Vineland Adaptive Behaviour Scales*, Minnesota: American Guidance Service.

Swann, W. (1988) Trends in special school placements, *Oxford Review of Education*, 14 (2), 139–41.

Terman, L. M. and Merrill, M. R. (1967) *Stanford–Binet Intelligence Scale: Manual for the third revision form L–M* , London: Harrap.

Ware, J. (1990) The National Curriculum for pupils with severe learning difficulties, in Daniels, H. and Ware, J. (eds) *Special Educational Needs and the National Curriculum*, London: Kogan Page.

Wechsler, D. (1955) *Wechsler Preschool and Primary Scale of Intelligence*, New York: Psychological Corporation.

Wechsler, D. (1974) *The Wechsler Intelligence Scale for Children* – revised, New York: Psychological Corporation.

Wechsler, D. (1981) *The Wechsler Adult Intelligence Scale* – revised, New York: Psychological Corporation.

Wedell, K. (1988) The new Act: a special need for vigilance, *British Journal of Special Education* 15 (3), 98–101.

Wedell, K. and Raybould, E. C. (eds) (1976) *The Early Identification of Educationally 'At Risk' Children*, University of Birmingham: Occasional Publ. No. 6.

8 Leisure and recreation services

Judith Russell

People with learning disabilities rarely have the opportunity to own leisure in a way that the wider population docs. The factors contributing to this state of affairs are many and complex. Some factors are clearly identifiable and widely recognised, others are not so well documented. Disconcertingly, despite the many benefits that are claimed for leisure, the degree to which opportunities are readily available to people with learning disabilities especially within the wider community context is questionable. What provision is available, is mainly within the specialist, separate provision or limited to structured, planned opportunities through day care or similar services although other examples of integrated opportunities based on freedom and choice are beginning to emerge.

In considering these opportunities, this chapter is less about services and rather more about an exploration of the issues in developing leisure and recreation in the field. Firstly, some of the barriers to leisure opportunity are identified as an important prerequisite to bringing about change. Secondly, there is a review of the profile of leisure within the context of the move to care in the community. Aspects of current leisure research are highlighted in an attempt to provide insights that will enable those who have responsibility for the facilitation of leisure to gain greater clarity on the very real benefits and possible goals. Finally, in recognition of the dynamic changes that are part of services provision in the 1990s, there is an exploration of some of the considerations in taking leisure forward in a purposeful and effective way.

BARRIERS TO LEISURE

Research undertaken in the early 1980s demonstrated that people with learning disabilities spent most of their leisure time engaged in home-based and passive leisure activities (Wertheimcr, 1983; Cheseldine and Jeffree, 1981; McConkey *et al.*, 1981). More recent investigation (Sutcliffe, 1989) suggests that this situation has not changed significantly. On the contrary, the evidence is that it has deteriorated. Sutcliffe found that most leisure time spent outside the home was with other people with learning disabilities rather than with selected friends who shared similar interests. Even among the more independent group of people interviewed, it was found that fewer than 15 per cent went into the wider community for their recreation and that a depressingly negligible degree of integration took place, regardless of whether people lived independently, or in family homes, hostels or hospitals. Sutcliffe found that overall there was a gulf between what people interviewed actually did and the leisure activities they would like to try.

In all the studies cited it is significant to note that the focus is on the individual rather than on the wider organisation and provision of services. Sutcliffe (1989), for example, identifies such individual constraints as lack of confidence, skills, organisational ability and dearth of friends. This approach is echoed by other researchers (Buckley and Sachs, 1987). Such perspectives often fail to take account of the shortcomings of wider society and could loosely be categorised within the medical approach to provision of services for disabled people. In a world so committed to developing leisure, this could provide partial explanation of the reasons for such effective exclusion of people with learning disabilities.

In order to bring about change, one needs first to understand some of the constraints that operate. While acknowledging that there are environmental barriers such as access to transport systems, appropriate equipment and public facilities (Prost, 1992), the greatest challenges to the development of leisure for people with learning disabilities emanate from the attitudes held by non-disabled people, which are reinforced through the practices and procedures of public services. There is a generally held view that disabled people cannot enjoy themselves in the same way as non-disabled people (McConkey and McGinley, 1990). This belief has influenced the development of leisure for people with learning disabilities in many subtle ways.

The majority of staff engaged in the caring professions are women who may have themselves been significantly disadvantaged in terms of leisure. As a result their understanding of the range of possibilities is somewhat limited and largely confined to the belief that leisure activities are simply an antidote to boredom or at best that leisure needs can be met by the odd trip to a local leisure centre or specialist facilities, usually with inadequate support or preparation (Regional Council for Sport and Recreation, 1990).

The attitudes of staff within the educational field have also had an impact on the development of leisure, or rather, the lack of it. The conclusion of the Every Body Active Project (Sports Council, 1991) was that special schools perpetuate the inequalities that disabled children face in leisure and recreation. In a review of eighteen special schools, the project team found that many of the headteachers placed little value on the contribution that physical education could make to the welfare of their pupils. Additionally, the team identified a lack of expertise among teachers, narrow and restrictive programmes of activity and commonly the allocation of just one session a week to the subject. This coupled with an emphasis on recreation rather than education, an absence of extracurricular activities and little evidence of links with community-based recreation provision paints a dismal picture of omission.

For many professionals the boundaries between leisure, therapeutic and rehabilitative approaches remain unclear with the balance still heavily weighted in favour of the latter as evidenced in the inclusion of leisure, albeit still in a limited way, in individual planned programmes within day care services. Furthermore, the insidious diversion provided by attempts to transplant the American therapeutic recreation approaches on to the leisure scene compounds the issue for many carers, struggling to bring about changes in approaches to leisure. With its medicalised perspectives and its language of prescription and programmes it only serves to confuse. As McConkey and McGinley (1990) point out, once an activity is labelled as therapy, things begin to change. The professional takes control, recreation becomes 'treatment' and choices are imposed. Individuals experiencing this have little opportunity to initiate or change activities. That is not to deny that there is therapeutic value in many leisure activities or that a therapist can achieve success with some people that lay persons cannot. But the approach hardly falls into a view of leisure, freely chosen, as the majority own it.

Within the mainstream leisure industry, both statutory and commercial, there is as Barnes (1991) points out widespread apprehension towards people with disabilities. Not only do many believe that any response to the needs of those with disabilities should be provided by the social services department, there is also the belief that the presence of people with disabilities can discourage non-disabled people. Barnes also points to the wide variation, within local authorities particularly, in understanding the needs of disabled people.

The attitudes of those employed in human service organisations have, over the years, led to the establishment and unquestioning acceptance of a number of practices and procedures that mitigate against the accessibility of leisure opportunities for people with learning disabilities. It is these structural barriers (Finkelstein, 1990) that pose a very real threat to any real and lasting improvement in the quality and quantity of leisure opportunities afforded to people with learning disabilities. Even in recent development of services it is possible to detect the legacy of previous eras. Job descriptions and associated work practices serve to maintain the status quo with energies being directed almost solely to daily living skills rather than the broader range that would change the focus to include quality of life issues. Staff working patterns, reflecting the earlier shift systems, take little account of the timing of available leisure opportunities. These and other organisational constraints have been clearly identified by Beardshaw and Towell (1990). They have drawn attention to the fact that existing inflexible services have meant that agencies have found it very difficult to introduce the forms of personal help and support more closely related to a person's needs and preferences and possibly much more supportive of the development of leisure interests and skills.

The interpretation of the principles of normalisation (Wolfensberger, 1975) and the pattern of services that have emerged as a result have varied enormously. The pendulum has swung almost out of sight as many professionals have taken an almost literal interpretation in an effort to bring about much needed change and many important considerations have been overlooked resulting in fewer opportunities rather than more. The need indicated by Russell (1992) to consider the possibilities of hostile environments as a significant problem for people with learning disabilities rather than their own possibly limited experience offers real food for thought.

The personal resources that disabled people have available to support their involvement in leisure can vary enormously. Many people with learning disabilities are dependent for their leisure opportunities on professional carers and/or family. The interest in and commitment of carers to supporting leisure is likely to be of paramount importance. It has been well documented that both parents and carers may in many instances act as gatekeeper to out-of-hours provision. Added to this, the low participation of people with learning disabilities in the labour market and a shrinking benefit system that takes little account of quality of life issues relegate them to a position where resources available for disposal on leisure may well be minimal. This almost certainly dictates whether disabled people can engage in leisure pursuits, if indeed they have access to and personal control over those resources.

The lack of overall direction in the development of leisure is evident across the range of service provision. There is wide variation between and within authorities on the degree to which the leisure needs of those with learning disabilities are recognised and little agreement on what services are trying to achieve (CCETSW, 1992). The question of who provides and how is rarely addressed. One can identify initiatives in leisure provision across community learning disability teams, social services, leisure and recreation departments, the youth and community service and a myriad voluntary agencies; the duplication of effort and complexity further stretches and dilutes the diminishing human and material resources to the detriment of people with learning disabilities. Any attempt to bring about change in this state of affairs is fraught with difficulty. Blocks to interagency co-operation and co-ordination have been documented by McGrath (1991). He outlines organisational defensiveness, professional ideologies, administrative procedures and ineffective procedures for co-ordination, as substantial barriers. Many of these are so entrenched that the inevitable outcome is that each agency continues to work in isolation with limited resources and little hope of providing a coherent service.

CARE IN THE COMMUNITY – THE PROFILE OF LEISURE

Although the Griffiths Report (1988) acknowledged that the needs of those with learning disabilities are largely for social rather than health care, from the moment of publication it was clear that consideration of leisure hardly figured on the agenda of care in the community. The closest the report came to acknowledging leisure needs was a passing reference to support for 'aspects of daily living' and 'suitable' leisure facilities which will improve the quality of life enjoyed by a person with care needs.

In reviewing other documentation a similar picture emerges. In the White Paper *Caring for People in the Next Decade and Beyond* (HMSO, 1989) the requirements outlined for care plans reveal little acknowledgement of leisure need. A subsequent publication *Practice Guidance and Practice Material for Social Services Departments and Other Agencies* (Department of Health, 1991) offers a glimmer of hope with reference to leisure in a section on appropriate arrangements for domiciliary day and residential care. It outlines social and recreational activity as 'low intensity' provision with a flexible approach necessary to accommodate differing client needs and refers to specialist social, recreational and therapeutic services for those with severe disabilities. However, the examples provided in the appendices do little to convince the reader that leisure, other than activities provided through day care and other specialist provision, has been seriously addressed as an important dimension in people's lives.

Care plans from a number of local authorities reflect these omissions. At best one can identify many imprecise and general references to quality of life and social opportunities or in one or two instances, the need to disseminate messages about the benefits of leisure and recreation as part of a health promotion exercise.

The Local Authority Circular *Social Care for Adults with a Learning Disability (Mental Handicap)* (DoH 1992) provides specific guidance on planning services for adults with a learning disability and complements and reinforces the general guidance set out in previous papers. In this circular the leisure perspective is acknowledged and mention made of: 'the move to a personally planned programme of day activities . . . social, educational, vocational and leisure . . . in which skill learning and vocational preparation are prominent', The significant issue is that leisure is again seen as part of day care services and part of a planned programme. This approach clearly reflects the range of issues raised in previous sections, namely the attitudes of non-disabled people, the compartmentalisation of leisure through planned programmes into what might be seen loosely as a therapeutic, rehabilitative view of leisure.

PERSPECTIVES ON LEISURE

It is important to begin to explore further some of the issues underpinning the barriers to developing leisure for people with disabilities and to begin to identify perspectives that will take this area of work forward in a significant way. Whether at the level of policy making, management or support staff, voluntary or statutory sector, it is clear that attitudes and the impact of those attitudes on the provision of services have been extremely restrictive. This has further been compounded by narrow definitions of leisure and limited understandings. What is increasingly clear is that the value of leisure in both the lives of people with learning disabilities and the wider population is rarely recognised or understood by the majority of professionals in human service organisations.

As Driver (1990) reminds us, there is little conclusive scientific knowledge about the benefits of leisure, except for a few specific types of benefit, e.g. health-related benefits of physical activity. Further to that, the study of leisure as it relates to disabled people has largely been neglected (Prost, 1992). Prost points to limited work on physiological and psychological perspectives and others on social integration from a normalisation point of view but identifies that little has been published on what leisure means to people with disabilities. There is much less written on leisure for people with learning disabilities. In the literature reviewed, many far-reaching claims are made on the benefit of leisure for people with learning disabilities. However, much of the support for these claims is anecdotal; well-grounded research is rare. Nevertheless if one begins to explore aspects of leisure for the population at large, there is evidence that permits the strong inference that a wide variety of benefits of considerable magnitude probably exist (Driver, 1990). There is little reason to suppose that research undertaken in the wider sphere cannot help us to understand benefits of leisure as they relate to people with learning disabilities.

Attempts to define leisure are problematic (Prost, 1992). However, while the debate continues, most theorists and researchers argue that it at least has something to do with freedom, discretionary time, self-expression and enjoyment. Earlier definitions tended to focus on the time available outside employment and/or on participation in specific recreational activities (Wilensky, 1961). Recently, this approach has been more and more in question and a re-orientation of perspectives offers new insights for the future.

In recent research Samdahl (1992) challenges the preoccupation of leisure researchers with the rarer leisure activity. She re-orients attention to the more salient opportunities that are available in the course of daily routine and focuses on the prominence of informal social interaction as a common leisure context. Analysis of Samdahl's research shows that leisure is a common occasion throughout the day and week but is more likely to occur in the evening and weekend away from locations and activities associated with work (see also Shaw, 1984). She identified that about half of all leisure situations were characterised by informal social interaction in contrast to formal or task related interactions which were not characteristics of leisure. On this basis, she suggests that leisure may be important because it offers relative freedom from negative judgements allowing individuals to relax from the necessity of matching behaviours to the confining expectations of others. As Kelly (1983) suggests, this quality of leisure may be particularly important for validating important aspects of identity, e.g. affirming and transforming identity (Cheek and Burch, 1976). These views of leisure are endorsed by Haggard and Williams (1992) who suggest that the affirming of identity is an active healthy process associated with self-definition, validation, maintenance and enhancement performed by virtually all individuals and they maintain that leisure may be particularly important in the self-affirmation process. It is however Samdahl (1992) who draws our attention to the fact that in informal social interaction, the self-esteem and basic social interaction skills gained might be critical tools which could enhance or expand leisure opportunity. By opening doors to communication, sharing and trust, individuals might be given the ability to participate in leisure on a frequent daily basis and as she suggests, the starting point of everyday leisure such as informal social interaction may not require unique recreational resources or specific leisure programmes.

Other claims for the benefits of leisure are also illuminating. Limited studies (Hammitt, 1987; Dowell and McCool, 1986; Falk and Balling, 1982) also indicate considerable gains in factual knowledge, recognition, memory, behaviour and skills in leisure participation. The purported value of leisure is further boosted by studies such as those by Buyhoff and Brown (1975) who suggest that, among other things, taking part in leisure activities may lead to an individual becoming more involved as a citizen, learning specific leisure activities and a range of skills. At the level of simple enjoyment Argyle (*Guardian*, 21 September 1991) reminds us that people who participate in active leisure activities are generally happier than those who engage only in passive pursuits.

Certainly, the research reviewed, although undertaken predominantly with non-disabled people does offer some validation for the claims made by writers from the field of learning disability. McKenzie (1990) highlights relationships, insight, perception, confidence and skill as observed gains while McConkey and McGinley (1990) point to self-esteem and expression of emotion reflecting many, if not all, of the benefits identified by writers and researchers in the field of leisure.

THE WAY FORWARD

As Roggenbuck and colleagues (1990) point out, if some of the benefits outlined in the previous section accrue to some individuals or some groups, some of the time, then the learning that occurs would seemingly provide the greatest justification for societal support of leisure. There is certainly strong evidence to support Bas's (1992) view that: 'Leisure is a fundamental requirement for the personal development of the human being. It is the basis for participating in social life' (p. 8). What appears to be indisputable is the fact that the leisure context does make a unique contribution to the quality of life and the development of people with learning disabilities. This presents a challenge to ensure a common commitment to the development of leisure and to see that it is on the agenda in all arenas and all levels of service. In a period of dynamic change in the services to those with disabilities, constraints do operate. It is vital that not just the constraints but also the opportunities are recognised. It is difficult to predict how services and provision will ultimately evolve; it is, however, essential to establish a sense of direction and some clear starting points in the approach to the development of leisure.

The degree to which legislation should be enacted within the field of leisure for those with disabilities is in question. It could be argued that some of the recent legislation has actively worked against the interests of disabled people. The current predominating influence of market economy approaches, reflected in financial constraints in the leisure field in the requirement of compulsory competitive tendering threatened established approaches to leisure provision for non-traditional user groups. Additionally the Education Reform Act (1988) brought about a number of changes in the availability and cost to users of local school premises in out of school hours, in some instances reducing provision, particularly by voluntary organisations. In responding to European initiatives, the British government have not made the level of commitment that others have. An example of this is the European Charter on Sport for All Disabled People (1985) which emphasises the role that leisure plays in enhancing the quality of life for all and endorses the right of disabled people to savour that quality of life for themselves. The Charter maintains that it is the responsibility of government in the social and cultural field to ensure that every person has the opportunity to take part in sport and leisure activities at the level that he/she wants to. While in Italy the right of access is guaranteed through legislation with substantial fines and punitive action for non-compliance (Bas, 1992), the response in England and Wales has been very different. Despite the much publicised report *Building on Ability* (Department of the Environment, 1989), the report of the Minister of Sport's review group, there are no statutory requirements on leisure providers or indeed any substantial additional resourcing. It is doubtful, in the current climate whether statutory or voluntary providers will be either willing or able to make a commitment to expanding leisure for disabled people without being required to do so. The question is can the Government ignore this important dimension in provision, given the many identified benefits?

The inflexibility of service provision in the 1980s and the way in which it has militated against the needs and preferences of people with learning disabilities have already been identified in a previous section. On entering a period where service provision and delivery are in a state of flux, there is a chance for reappraisal of basic principles and associated practice. While the principles of normalisation and social role valorisation (Wolfensberger, 1985) are embedded in a number of publications, documentation and operational policies, and have led to a coherent value base giving services a sense of direction and purpose, there is recognition that the interpretation of the principles and pattern of services that have emerged, have varied enormously. Hogg (1993) alleges that the terms have been used in ways that are often ambiguous, damaging and open to misinterpretation. Certainly, as Ryan and Thomas (1991) point out, a valued service to people with learning disabilities and other user groups has not become generally available and the interpretation of the principles has not aided the development of leisure.

If, as identified, the leisure context can provide one of the greatest opportunities for the development of self-identity and valued social roles, serious thought must be given to future service planning and management. A serious attempt must be made to introduce and evaluate a range of approaches that encompass a stable and reliable framework to capitalise on the complex web of networks and groupings that offer the more common leisure occasion and embody the flexible independent, person-centred approaches that are based on people's hopes and ambitions for their own lives. Only if this can be achieved and provision tailored to the individual, can serious attention be directed to leisure.

There are a number of examples emerging which embody approaches more facilitating of leisure. One such approach is the service brokerage scheme (Nelson, 1991; Salisbury, 1987) where, working in support of the person with a learning disability, the 'broker' operates from a position of independence, free from the bureaucracy of existing services, can acquire in-depth knowledge of local areas and capitalise on community networks. Another approach worthy of investigation is the emerging quality of life concept (Hogg, 1993; Goode, 1989). In reviewing the literature, Goode has developed an essentially ecological model which implies the matching of client need to environmental resources across four domains, i.e. economic, social, political and cultural. (Hogg offers a useful discussion of the concept as it relates to leisure.) These approaches offer a more conducive climate for the facilitation of informal social interaction and the development of leisure skills and opportunities.

Given the plethora of leisure initiatives across a range of statutory and voluntary agencies, the question of who takes lead responsibility is difficult to respond to. What is becoming increasingly apparent is that the traditional role of social services in facilitating access to other services such as leisure and education is unlikely to continue in the longer term. In considering these and other issues, the Minister of Sport's review group recommended that local authority leisure service departments should assume responsibility for the provision of recreation for people with disabilities at local level and advocated a co-ordinated approach encompassing both statutory and voluntary effort. In reviewing the situation, it is clear that no one agency can provide, there is neither the base of experience and skill nor the resources. Statutory and voluntary collaboration and co-operation will be essential to the future development and maintenance of the leisure context for people with learning disabilities.

Although progress is slow, a number of initiatives reflecting voluntary/ statutory collaboration are in existence. Within the Yorkshire and Humberside region there are partnership projects involving local authority leisure and recreation departments and Disport, a voluntary sporting body, for those with learning disabilities, leading to a range of provision in local communities. Projects have included the establishment of a gymnastics club for preschool children in conjunction with staff of a community learning disability team which involved training of staff, negotiation of support and resourcing from several local authority and voluntary agencies and administrative support, the voluntary partner being able to work more easily across departments and access sources of funding more readily. Other instances of co-operation across the region include the establishment of an inter-agency forum within one local authority area, leading to research and eventually to a leisure advocacy scheme for adults with learning disabilities. In the development of leisure, the voluntary agency can often act as an 'honest broker' to bring together and facilitate inter-departmental co-operation and work practice.

In reviewing the provision of leisure for people with disabilities in 1990 the London Borough of Bromley identified uncoordinated, piecemeal provision and deficiencies in key areas of research, policy development, publicity and promotion, information, inter-departmental liaison, and co-operation with the voluntary sector locally and regionally. Although leisure services took the lead, the ensuing 'No Limits' project embraced inter-departmental co-operation, with staff being seconded to the project from social services and leisure departments. The project was designed to ensure successful and effective work was translated into good common practice and that the provision should ultimately become part of mainstream service delivery. The various dimensions of the project included development days, multi-activity days, a pilot 'buddy scheme', 'No Limits' clubs and a broad programme of training and education of sports providers in the public and private sectors, leisure and day centre staff, physical education teachers/professionals, volunteers and coaches in specific sports. In addition to this, a project steering group of people with disabilities was established and a forum of voluntary and statutory agencies. In this instance the leisure services committee took a leading and pro-active role in co-ordinating provision with the ultimate aim of establishing effective inter-departmental communication and partnership.

In developing the leisure context there appear to be two major issues. Firstly, there is the need to educate and involve people with learning disabilities in a range of activities that will develop interests and skills and provide a basis for choice. Secondly, but of fundamental importance is the recognition that people with learning disabilities have the right to own leisure in the way that the population at large owns it, i.e. that leisure is freely chosen, enjoyable and takes place predominantly at evenings and weekends.

There is a need to differentiate between the two aspects of leisure development. Programmes of leisure education need to be developed as a priority across education services, whether that be special and mainstream schools or the further education sector. Access to physical education for pupils with disabilities as designated in the National Curriculum must be seen as a right rather than a concession. Day services can and in some instances do, provide leisure education as part of personal development opportunities. Much greater emphasis does, however, need to be given to high-quality, well-resourced programmes staffed by those with qualifications and experience in the leisure field. The focus, outside formal day-care settings, should be on enabling people with learning disabilities to develop, in settings of their choice, a range of involvements in leisure activities.

In facilitating this, there are a number of considerations for those working in the support role. Of primary importance is the need to ensure that individuals are able to preserve some discretionary time, that the demands of independent living or personal care do not become exclusionary. On the basis of evidence from research, it is possible that the starting point for developing leisure involvement and interests might be somewhat different from what has been generally accepted. The common and fairly routine leisure experience, identified by Samdahl (1992), that is the informal social interactions that are very much part of community life, may well provide an initial focus. Such situations will have to be carefully thought through and facilitated by those supporting individuals with learning disabilities but may form a sound basis for acquiring the critical skills to enhance or expand leisure opportunity.

People's ability to enjoy leisure is closely related to the amount of money they have available to spend (Abercrombie and Warde, 1988; Willis, 1985) and limited resources do impede the freedom essential to leisure. In order to ensure the learning experiences, the development of identity and self-expression that are typical companions of leisure, access to resources needs to be guaranteed. Self-advocates, carers and service providers need to join forces in arguing the case for individual funding that will support leisure involvement and open up a better quality of life.

There is little by way of good practice in establishing a direction that is agreed and owned by all. The philosophy, approach and associated action do need to be established in a public statement of purpose. Work has been undertaken by some voluntary agencies in conjunction with local authority leisure managers which has led to a written statement and a forward plan. For these approaches to fully succeed, however, much broader inter-departmental and inter-agency involvement has to be achieved from the earliest possible point. A shared common vision of leisure and leisure provision among all those who support people with learning disabilities is likely to move the work forward in a much more coherent and effective manner.

At a time of service re-orientation, substantial investment in staff development is essential. Training in the area of attitudes, approaches and leisure perspectives will need to transcend the boundaries of statutory and voluntary agencies. A key area for development is a commonly shared understanding of the role of leisure and the benefits and considerations in facilitating leisure as an essential component of multi-disciplinary training schemes. This will need to be accompanied by well-planned and concerted action by professionals from all disciplines.

CONSIDERATIONS IN DEVELOPING PROVISION

1 *Policy makers*

- In order to establish clear starting points and an overall direction in promoting leisure provision for those with disabilities, policy makers need to take the lead by developing a clear statement of intent.
- Decisions are required on who will take the lead in the local area in developing a coherent and well-planned range of opportunities in the field of leisure.
- Attention needs to be directed to establishing flexible service provision that more closely reflects a person's needs and preferences and supports the creation of a climate more facilitating of leisure.

2 *Service managers*

- Managers will need to develop inter-agency co-operation across the statutory and voluntary sectors based on clear agreements encompassing a shared vision, clear practices, procedures, roles and responsibilities in the arena of leisure.
- They will also need to ensure the establishment of a structure and mechanisms that will capitalise on the community networks and groupings that offer the more common leisure occasion.
- Care managers particularly need to ensure that leisure education and leisure participation are integrated into care plans and that these perspectives are translated into adequately resourced individual plans.

3 *Service providers*

- Statutory and voluntary partnerships especially among leisure providers that actively develop and maintain the leisure context in the lives of people with learning disabilities will be essential to capitalise on available expertise and resources.
- Consideration will need to be given to the identification of independent support for people with learning disabilities to ensure participation in leisure activities of their own choice. This may include leisure 'brokerage' schemes and the possible development of leisure advocates. The voluntary sector, if resourced to do so, is well placed to make a significant contribution in this area of work, e.g. building databases of local leisure provision, offering training on disability and leisure issues for a range of personnel.
- Education providers, in both the school and further education sectors need to ensure access to the national curriculum in physical education.
- Additionally, high-quality, well-resourced programmes of leisure education can do much to support those with learning disabilities. These should be developed and staffed by those with qualifications and experience in the field of leisure.
- Multi-disciplinary staff development programmes need to encompass the range of perspectives on leisure.

• An integral part of developing leisure provision for people with learning disabilities will be developmental activities with carers.

CONCLUSION

Much of the development in leisure provision for people with learning disabilities to date has been *ad hoc* and opportunistic. It has been based on limited understandings, has attracted fairly uncritical evaluation and has been influenced by individual and medical perspectives. This situation is likely to continue in the short term. In the economic climate of the early nineties, the establishment of a coherent, well-resourced and planned approach to the development of leisure is unlikely to be assured. Projects are most likely to evolve on the basis of a combination of interested parties and available resources, unless there is an investment in research and a re-direction and re-allocation of funding. The challenge will be to put together strategies that will capitalise on the multitude of social and care networks and build the links between services and groups in the community. Provided it is given the resources for the task, it is likely that the voluntary sector, especially in the disability sporting arena, will play a key role in bringing together and exploiting the available human and material resources.

REFERENCES

Abercrombe, N. and Warde, A. (1988) *Contemporary British Society*, Cambridge: Polity Press.

Barnes, C. (1991) *Disabled People in Britain and Discrimination: A Case for Anti-discriminatory Legislation*, London: Hurst & Co.

Bas, D. (1992) 'Social and cultural tourism', *World Leisure and Recreation* 34, 3: 8–9.

Beardshaw, V. and Towell, D. (1990) *Assessment and Case Management: Implications for the Implementation of 'Caring for People'*, London: King's Fund Institute.

Buckley, S. and Sachs, B (1987) *The Adolescent with Down's Syndrome: Life for the Teenager and for the Family*, Portsmouth: Portsmouth Polytechnic.

Buyhoff, G.J. and Brown, P.J. (1975) 'Social and individual learning benefits from recreational engagements', paper presented at the EDRA 6 Workshop. Lawrence, KS.

CCETSW (1992) *Learning Together – Shaping New Services for People with Learning Disabilities*, London: CCETSW.

Cheek, N.H. and Burch, W.R. (1976) *The Social Organisation of Leisure in Human Society*, New York: Harper & Row.

Cheseldine, S. and Jefferee, D.M. (1981) 'Mentally handicapped adolescents: their use of leisure', *Journal of Mental Deficiency Research* 25: 49–59.

Department of Education and Science (1988) *Education Reform Act*, London: HMSO.

Department of the Environment (1989) *Building on Ability*, Report of the Minister for Sport's Review Group 1988/89, London: HMSO.

Department of Health (1991) *Practice Guidance and Practice Material for Social Services Departments and Other Agencies*, London: HMSO.

Department of Health (1992) *Social Care for Adults with a Learning Disability (Mental Handicap)*, Local Authority Circular (92) 15.

Dowell, D.L. and McCool, S.F. (1986) 'Evaluation of a wilderness information dissemination programme', in R.C. Lucas (compiler), *Proceedings, National Wilderness Research Conference: Current Research* (USDA Forest Service General Technical Report INT-212: 494–500), Ogden, U.T.: Intermountain Research Station.

Driver, B.L. (1990) 'Focusing research on the benefits of leisure: special issue introduction', *Journal of Leisure Research* 22, 2: 93–8.

Falk, J.H. and Balling, J.D. (1982) 'The field trip milieu: learning and behaviour as a function of contextual events', *Journal of Educational Research* 76: 22–8.

Finkelstein, V. (ed.) (1990) *Disability – Changing Practice*, Milton Keynes: The Open University.

Griffiths, R. (1988) *Community Care – An Agenda for Action*, A Report to the Secretary of State for Social Services, London: HMSO.

Goode, D.A. (1989) 'Quality of life and quality of work life', in W.E. Kiernan and R.L. Schalock (eds) *Economics, Industry and Economy: A Look Ahead*, Baltimore: Paul H. Brookes.

Haggard, L.M. and Williams, D.R. (1992) 'Identity affirmation through leisure activities: leisure symbols of the self', *Journal of Leisure Research* 24, 1: 1–18.

Hammitt, W.E. (1987) 'Visual recognition capacity during outdoor recreation experiences', *Environment and Behaviour* 19, 6: 651–71.

HMSO (1989) *Caring for People: Community Care in the Next Decade and Beyond*, London: HMSO.

Hogg, J. (1993) 'Assessment methods and professional directions', in *Community Care for People with Learning Difficulties: Report on C.C.E.T.S.W Conference Series*, London: CCETSW.

Kelly, J.R. (1983) *Leisure Identities and Interactions*, London: Allen & Unwin.

McConkey, R. and McGinley, P. (eds) (1990) *Innovations in Leisure and Recreation for People with Mental Handicap*, Chorley: Lisieux Hall.

McConkey, R., Walsh, M. and Mulcahy, M. (1981) 'The recreational pursuits of mentally handicapped adults', *International Journal of Rehabilitation Research* 4: 493–9.

McGrath, M. (1991) *Multidisciplinary Teamwork*, Aldershot: Gower Publishing Company Limited.

McKenzie, A. (1990) 'Badaguish: adventure holidays in the Scottish highlands', in R. McConkey and P. McGinley (eds) *Innovations in Leisure and Recreation for People with Mental Handicap*, Chorley: Lisieux Hall.

Nelson, S. (1991) 'Fixed up for life', *Community Care* 9 May.

Prost, A.L. (1992) 'Leisure and disability: a contradiction in terms', *World Leisure and Recreation* 34, 3: 8–9.

Regional Council for Sport and Recreation – East Midlands (1990) *Taking Shape – Sport for People with Disabilities*, Conference Report, Nottingham: RCSR.

Roggenbuck, J.W., Loomis, R.J. and Dagostino, J. (1990) 'The learning benefits of leisure', *Journal of Leisure Research* 22, 2: 112–24.

Russell, O. (1992) 'Professional and planning issues in assessment', in N.A. Malin (ed.) *Community Care for People with Learning Difficulties*, London: CCETSW.

Ryan, J. and Thomas, F. (1991) *The Politics of Mental Handicap*, London: Free Association Books.

Salisbury, B. (1987) *Service Brokerage*, Canada: G. Allan Roeher Institute.

Samdahl, D.M. (1992) 'Leisure in our lives: exploring the common leisure occasion', *Journal of Leisure Research* 24, 1: 19–32.

Shaw, S.M. (1984) The measurement of leisure: a quality of life issue, *Society and Leisure* 7: 91–107.

Sports Council (1991) – Research Unit (North West) *Every Body Active Project.*

Sunderland Polytechnic *et al.* Phase Two Monitoring Report – Implementing the Schemes, London: The Sports Council.

Sutcliffe, R. (1989) *A New Direction for the Adult Education and Leisure Integration Project*, London: Mencap.

Wertheimer, A. (1983) *Leisure*, London: Values into Action.

Wilensky, H.L. (1961) 'The uneven distribution of leisure: the impact of economic growth on "free-time", in E. Smigel (ed.) *Work and Leisure*, New Haven: College and University Press.

Willis, P. (1985) *The Social Condition of Young People in Wolverhampton in 1984*, Wolverhampton: Wolverhampton Borough Council.

Wolfensberger, W. (1975) *Programme Analysis of Service Systems*, Toronto: National Institute for Mental Retardation.

Wolfensberger, W. (1983) 'Social role valorisation – a proposed new term for the principle', *Mental Retardation* 21: 234–9.

Wolfensberger, W. (1985) 'An overview of social role valorization and some reflections on elderly mentally retarded persons', in M.P. Janieki and H.M. Wisniewski (eds) *Aging and Developmental Disabilities: Issues and Approaches*, Baltimore: Paul H. Brookes.

9   Empowerment and advocacy

Ken Simons

INTRODUCTION

Empowerment and advocacy are both fashionable words. They are liberally scattered across many texts on services for people with learning difficulties,[1] but what do they mean? Used interchangeably with terms like 'participation' and 'consumerism', there is a danger they will simply become tags to indicate a generalised desire to be progressive. While most people would agree that people with learning difficulties are one of the least powerful groups in society – a group whose views have not only been ignored but, almost by definition, discounted as worthless – there is much less agreement on how to change things.

To have power is to be able to influence events. Although few people feel powerful, most of us have some power: as individuals (by virtue of skills or experience), through our relationships and through the groups and organisations to which we belong. For people with learning difficulties, empowerment means having access to the same kinds of mechanisms, enabling them to gain some influence over the world around them and to have at least some control over their lives.

Advocacy, of all kinds, is about acquiring a voice. It is difficult to imagine being empowered without being heard. Advocacy and empowerment are therefore inextricably linked. However, to behave in ways that are empowering implies a commitment not just to listen to people with learning difficulties, but to act on what they say.

Empowerment is not a process 'by which those in society who have power can dispense some to those who don't have any' (Oliver, 1993). By definition, empowerment implies a process in which people with learning difficulties *take* some control over what is happening. However, that does not absolve professionals from the responsibility to use all the means at their disposal to aid that process.

A STRATEGY FOR EMPOWERMENT

The aim of this chapter is to produce an outline strategy for service providers, designed to focus on different ways in which people working in services can promote empowerment and advocacy. The core of the chapter is divided into four sections. The first highlights a number of underlying messages and recurring themes. The remaining three sections deal in detail with specific elements that form the core of a strategy: section two looks at ways of supporting individuals, section three focuses on the services themselves, while the final section deals with the wider issue of building links.

SECTION ONE: THEMES AND MESSAGES

This section sets out to identify some of the broader issues for service providers to think about, unlike the later sections which represent more of an agenda for action.

There are no simple answers

The empowerment of people with learning difficulties will not lead to a quiet life for professionals. Sometimes they will tell us things we don't want to hear. Supporting service users in their attempts to challenge the system will inevitably create conflicts of interest for professionals. As users become more assertive, some of the tensions inherent in the system will become clearer. Much of what we suggest requires ingenuity and imagination to implement; it is not a simple blueprint. People working in the system are going to have to think long and hard about how they are going to respond to these challenges.

Learning the lessons

For any strategy to have maximum effect there has to be a capacity for the system as a whole to learn some of the general lessons from user involvement. This means a willingness amongst professionals to be self-critical, as well as being prepared to make links, to generalise from specific situations and to draw out the wider implications of events. Users should not have to fight the same battles over and over again.

It will take time to have an impact

Much of what we outline here will not necessarily lead to instant revolution (no matter how much we would sometimes like it to). The impact of the strategy will not fit into some neat timetable. It takes time for people to gain confidence and experience. Many will need convincing that services really do mean business.

Avoid unrealistic goals for people

For people to have some control over their lives does not mean they should have to manage without help. While people with learning difficulties have often shown themselves to be capable of much more than we assumed, many will still need support to achieve their goals. Autonomy should not be confused with self-sufficiency.

The need for structures to adapt to people with learning difficulties

One of the problems that people with learning difficulties face is the erection of 'readiness' barriers; the almost unconscious assumption that people need to be prepared or need to have acquired skills before they can participate, as though participation were a reward rather than a right. If people with learning difficulties find it hard to use a particular structure, then the solution lies in changing the structure, not the people. Involving people with learning difficulties in decision making does not mean 'business as usual' simply with a few users present.

The need for cultural change

Empowerment and advocacy are not optional extras that can be tacked on to a traditional service. They represent a significant change in relationship between users and service providers. Even with good intentions, positive initiatives can be undermined by the subtle signals sent to people with learning difficulties; for example, when professionals insist on 'teaching' service users about self-advocacy (here the sub-text is: 'We are still the experts, we know what is best for you'). Modelling good practice throughout an organisation can send clear messages to users, staff and families about the value being attached to involvement and inclusion. The skills required to help people decide what they want and make informed choices are different to those involved in telling people what their needs are.

Involvement is for everyone

Inclusion should mean inclusion for everybody, not just for the people who we think would benefit from it, or who we think could make the most effective contribution (Rioux, 1992). The real challenge is to find ways of including the people who, in the past, were automatically excluded; the people with severe challenging behaviour, and the people with the most profound disabilities. It also means squarely tackling many of the factors that lead to people being marginalised. These include issues relating to ethnicity, gender, age and sexuality (see, for example, Morris and Lindow, 1993).

The importance of diversity

People with learning difficulties are as diverse as any other group of people. They have widely varying attitudes, skills, experience and interests. Not everybody will want to join a self-advocacy group. A range of options for people to get involved will enable people to find the niche in which they are most effective or with which they feel most comfortable. An effective strategy has to include many different strands and to operate at a number of levels.

Tension over who speaks for whom

In a survey of social services departments Croft and Beresford (1990) found that the reservations about user involvement most frequently expressed by professionals revolved around the issues of 'representation'; who should speak for whom?

As Viv Lindow (1991) has pointed out, users can get caught in the most frustrating of catch 22s. If they are articulate, they are 'not typical' (and can therefore be ignored). If they have difficulty expressing themselves, then their views are by definition seen as valueless.

All people who use services should be listened to and taken seriously. That does not mean they cannot be challenged, but it is up to the professional to justify his or her response (this is after all what being accountable means). If professionals genuinely believe that what is being said does not represent the views of other users, then they should make sure that those who have been left out get a chance to have their say. Professionals should not take it upon themselves to decide what users think.

There are plenty of other people who may try to claim the right to speak for users including their families and carers' organisations. Both have a contribution to make, but it is not as a substitute voice for users. Carers have their own legitimate concerns and user empowerment should never been seen as a reason for ignoring families. There is a sense that user empowerment will not work unless families are also empowered. Inevitably, there will be tensions; some carers remain adamant that people with learning difficulties wouldn't possibly speak for themselves. Setting out to find ways to help users and carers work together is one way of resolving these tensions.

SECTION TWO: A FOCUS ON INDIVIDUALS

Many professionals are most at ease with the notion of empowering individuals; it has clear echoes of the therapeutic tradition which remains strong in the personal social services. Yet, for many people with learning difficulties the reality remains that services, while providing physical support, have undermined them as individuals and left them isolated. The main object of the following suggestions is to create a framework which through encouraging and valuing self-expression, enables people to reassert themselves as individuals, with feelings and aspirations to be respected.

Individual planning

Planning services on the basis of individual need has been a key element in policy over the last decade. The intention was to try and find a mechanism that would make services much more responsive to users. The different models of individual programme planning (IPPs for short) have all been characterised by a number of key aims. They were intended to be:

- a mechanism for reforming and improving services;
- a basis for planning services, ensuring that new developments reflected the identified needs of individuals;
- a way of co-ordinating the delivery of otherwise fragmented services;
- a forum for including the views of users and their families.

The ideas underlying individual planning have gained increasing currency, and indeed underlie many of the current community care reforms (in particular, caremanagement). At the same time there has also been increasing criticism of the way they work in practice. In their review of day services the Social Services Inspectorate (SSI, 1989) describe IPPs in some areas as 'bureaucratic and cumbersome' (one group of users apparently complained they were 'worse than Mastermind'). Low levels of active participation by users in IPPs have been reported both by the Social Services Inspectorate in Wales (WO/SSI, 1989) and by Humphreys and Blunden (1987), while Laws and colleagues (1988) found users and their families regularly excluded from IPP meetings. Simons (1993) reports that users were often critical of the way IPPs work, and many of the same complaints crop up in *Oi, It's My Assessment*, a booklet just produced by London People First (1993).

Arguments about 'need' go to the heart of many of the concerns about IPPs. To involve users and carers in assessment and planning implies a move away from a process in which statements of 'need' are seen as some sort of objective reality to be revealed by professionals, towards one in which they are the outcome of a process of negotiation between users, their families and professionals. However, a recent study of assessment found the views of professionals still dominating (Ellis, 1993). Further, professionals were often defining need solely in terms of the services that were available locally, effectively using the lack of knowledge on the part of potential users to ration the support offered. Indeed, concerns about the advisability of recording 'unmet need' for individuals is threatening to undermine many of the principles of caremanagement (Brindle, *Guardian*, 28 December 1992). Finding ways of ensuring that people with learning difficulties and their families have a chance to say what services they feel they want are crucial in any effective individual planning system.

There are some positive models. Simons reports that users were more positive about IPPs when:

- they were the main focus of the exercise and were being listened to.
- the IPP resulted in action which reflected *their* aims and priorities.

- they had some control over the process. For example, through deciding who should attend the IPP meeting and where the meeting should be, or defining what should be recorded and having responsibility for keeping the notes from IPP meetings.
- users were helped to prepare for their IPP.

(Simons, 1993)

Attempts have been made to make individual planning more accessible. For example, in shared action planning the aim is to set up a process in which the users develop their own plan (Brechin and Swain 1987). This starts by trying to define who the important people are in the life of that individual, and trying to draw them into the process. Nevertheless, the user remains at the centre of the process. Considerable emphasis is placed on helping the user explore possible options. Here, planning is seen as a way of trying to help users take some control, rather than being a management tool reflecting the needs of the organisation.

Many of the ideas underlying shared action planning also underlie the concept of service brokerage (Brandon and Towell, 1990). Service brokers are independent agents who are accountable solely to the user and their family and friends. The role of the broker is to help the individual decide what support they require, then to design (with the approval of the user) a package of services and help negotiate this package with an appropriate provider. As with shared action planning, there is often a strong emphasis on helping people identify and draw on the support of friends, family and other people from the local community.

The independence of the broker from services resolves some of the potential conflicts of interest. By separating out the design of services from concerns about controlling resources (those are resolved in the negotiations with providers and purchasers) the broker is freed from the tensions faced by people who are directly employed by the service provider. The rationing of services becomes much more transparent and open to challenge by the users.

Service brokerage is not without its critics within the disability movement (Davis, 1990). To people who have a clear idea of what they want, service brokerage has sounded suspiciously like yet another instance of professionals telling them what they need. For many in this group, self-assessment and 'being your own care manager' are the key aims (Morris and Lindow, 1993).

Recovering identity

For most of us our past is crucial to our sense of ourselves. Our memories about our life give us a sense of place and belonging. Yet people with learning difficulties are too often treated as though they have no history and no experiences. It is not unusual for someone to have lived in an institution for most of their life, yet end up leaving it with no evidence that they have ever lived there at all, arriving in a new placement with few possessions, and no mementos from their past. Enabling people with learning difficulties to tell their story is one way of helping them reassess the past and, perhaps, to emerge with a much more positive sense of identity. Listening to people with learning difficulties tell their stories is a crucial way for professionals to re-assess the impact of the services they provide.

Techniques for helping people to piece together their experiences include reminiscence work (Potts and Fido, 1990) and helping people produce portfolios (Clare, 1990) or life story books (Frost and Taylor, 1986).

Not all the memories uncovered will be comfortable ones. Sometimes this work will produce revelations with profound implications, for example, uncovering examples of sexual abuse (Brown and Craft, 1992). It is important that staff involved in this kind of work are able to identify when additional support or skills are required.

Labelling

Arguments about labels have been a striking feature of the field of services for people with learning difficulties over the last decade. The debate about the appropriateness of 'mental handicap' and 'learning difficulties' (and more recently, learning disability) has been rehearsed *ad nauseam* and there is insufficient space to do full justice to all the arguments (see Sutcliffe and Simons, 1993 for a fuller discussion). However, there are two relevant points here. First, many people with learning difficulties feel strongly about the labels that are used to describe them. To ignore those views is to effectively tell service users that their views and feelings do not count; scarcely compatible with ideas about empowerment! Second, self-definition can be empowering. Defining oneself through labels can be a way of developing an identity marked by positive potential rather than the negative assumptions of others. For example, the adults with learning difficulties interviewed by Simons (1993) mostly rejected 'mental handicap' because, 'It means the person can't cope on her own and do things ... and she can', whereas 'learning difficulties' (although not universally popular) seemed to imply possibilities: 'If you put "people with learning difficulties" then they know that people want to learn.'

Artists first

'They said, "You should go to a school for backward people." I felt disappointment, and it was like an ending to me.'

These lines are from a member of the Greystoke Poets' Group. Although the group is mainly made up of people from a local day centre, they deliberately meet away from the centre premises, hence the name of the group. Some of the people from the same day centre are also involved in Arts First, a group of people from Avon day centres who have rented their own studio.

Again, the group takes its work seriously. Paintings are carefully framed and mounted and have been exhibited in a number of settings.

Art is a feature of the activities in many day centres, but here it can often be little more than a scheduled activity designed to fill time. Although the end product may be pinned to the wall for a short while, it is not always valued by staff (sometimes it is just thrown away). There is sometimes little effort made to help people develop their own technique or a sense of their own style. But art, poetry and drama are important to people with learning difficulties. When Avon People First organised a conference for their fellow service users, the workshops on these topics were heavily over-subscribed, being far more popular than all the other workshops put together. Subsequently in Avon, some people with learning difficulties have become involved in Artshare, a disability arts network described as a 'celebration and expressions of the concerns of disabled people', while with the support of ACTA (a local arts charity) some have staged a drama festival, presenting their views on topics ranging from crime to independent living.

Developing assertiveness skills

Much of the 'training' that services provide to users is about compliance; from getting people to behave 'reasonably' to behaviour modification. While there is evidence that at least some of the anger and frustration underlying 'challenging behaviour' has been prompted by the lack of control people have over their lives, we respond to that anger by reducing people's autonomy still further. One way to try and break out of this cycle is to help people acquire the skills of asserting themselves without having to resort to aggression. Paradoxically it is often staff that get access to assertiveness training courses, although there are imaginative examples where such opportunities have been set up for users (Winchurst *et al.*, 1992).

SECTION THREE: A FRAMEWORK FOR QUALITY

'Quality', like 'empowerment', is another idea in vogue. It has some similar characteristics; it can mean many different things in different contexts. It is hard to be against having better quality services (it would be like being in favour of sin) but, as Pfeffer and Coote (1991) point out, not everything that falls under the heading of quality assurance actually makes a difference to the lives of users; sometimes it can even be harmful.

Working on the principle that users and their families should have a say in what constitutes a good service, the following elements have a good claim to a place in any framework designed to promote better quality services.

Support for people to complain

The 1990 NHS and Community Care Act specified that all social service departments should have accessible and comprehensive complaints procedures. Complaints procedures sound like a simple idea, but in practice they have proved to be a lot more complicated. Misunderstandings about what constitutes a 'complaint' appear to be widespread.

Just because the complaints procedures exist does not mean that users with a grievance will automatically use them. For example, Simons (1993) found that otherwise confident members of user groups often remain reluctant to pursue formal complaints.

Many users and their families will need encouragement and support from an independent source to make effective use of complaints procedures. There have been examples of user groups successfully helping members to pursue complaints, and a wide variety of other organisations are also beginning to take on this role. For example, both in Hereford and Worcester, and in Avon, the local Citizen Advocacy organisations (see later) have been given funding to provide a complaints advocacy service. The advocates will be local people (not employed by the service providers) who will give short-term assistance to people making complaints.

Keeping it a secret?

Before people can use a complaints procedure they need to know it exists. Although the procedures have been in place for two years, many areas still do not have material prepared specifically for people with learning difficulties. There is a widespread failure to make information of all kinds available and accessible to service users.

If information is power, then any serious strategy for empowerment ought to have at its heart policies which ensure that information is freely available in a form that people can use.

In principle the rules for producing accessible material seem straightforward: stick to everyday language, use a large clear typeface, include the words of people with learning difficulties themselves wherever possible, and take care where text is broken (across a line or page). Although it is sensible to avoid jargon, it may be more empowering for users sometimes to stop and explain words in wide use (the object is not to limit the vocabulary of people with learning difficulties). Above all, the style must not be patronising.

Nevertheless, not all people with learning difficulties will be able to follow text. Producing material that can be used in a group, or read by supporters is one way around this impasse. So is using graphics images of all kinds. For example, in Somerset as part of a project on total communication speech therapists have worked *with* people with learning difficulties to develop a set of symbols that are meaningful and relevant to users. These symbols are widely used throughout the county.

As the technology has evolved it has become easier to consider non-text-based ways of communicating. Audio tapes, videos, and even interactive computer software are all possibilities. Although the technology may sound intimidating, there is no reason that people with learning difficulties cannot be involved in its use. For example, Centre Shot, a project supported by the Joseph Rowntree Foundation, involved people with learning difficulties making videos (see Williams, 1993).

It is not just the form that matters, but also the content. An effective information strategy ought to include letting users know about:

- their rights (see, for example, The Residents' Rights pack – Allen and Scales, 1990);
- what they can expect from a service. Users' charters would fall into this category;
- new ideas or alternative kinds of services (not just what is available locally);
- services as they are and not as professionals would like them (Winkler, 1990). This would have to at least acknowledge some of the criticisms users and carers make about services.

Involving users in training and conferences

One way of ensuring that users get access to new ideas and influences is to include them in opportunities for training and conference-going.

Having users present often changes the nature of events for the better. It forces presenters, trainers and organisers to think about the structure of the event (more participative) and the accessibility of the language used. It also subtly helps change the relationship between users and professionals.

The relationship can be even more dramatically given a jolt by having users as trainers and conference presenters. Having users as the 'experts' reverses the status quo, forcing professionals to revise the way they view users. It also provides an important platform for users to put over their perspective. Several groups now have extensive experience in presenting their own training material, including Skills for People in Nottingham, Advocacy in Action in Nottingham, and People First of London.

Choosing staff

The relationships users have with staff is often very important to them; the quality of that relationship can be a crucial element in determining the way they judge services. People with learning difficulties often greatly value the support of particular professionals, but they also find some thoroughly alienating (see, for example, Simons, 1993).

Tension in the relationship can be a particular problem if the member of staff is someone in whom the user might expect to confide, for example, a key worker or care manager. However, few users have any say in who is assigned to this role for them. As a bare minimum, they ought to have the right to seek a change in key worker or care manager, if they are not satisfied with that relationship.

Ideally, people with learning difficulties should to have a clear role in selecting (and even firing) all staff. It is now not unusual for users to be informally involved in staff appointment, for example, meeting candidates or showing them around the service. Some organisations have successfully involved users in formal interviewing panels. This has two advantages: users get a definite say in appointments, and there is a clear message to potential staff that the views of users matter, and indeed, that they have influence in their employment.

Paradoxically, this involvement has taken a step backwards in some areas because of concerns about equal opportunities. For example, in one county, nobody can be on an interviewing panel unless they have been on an equal opportunities training course (not an unreasonable prescription in itself), but since no users have access to the training, it acts to exclude them.

People with learning difficulties tend to be very concerned about 'fairness' (after all, many are all too familiar with being treated unfairly). Some groups have developed their own equal opportunities practice when they have managed to get funds to appoint workers (Whittaker *et al.*, 1991). Equal opportunities should not be used as an excuse for excluding users.

Seats in the boardroom: involving users in meetings

Involving people with learning difficulties in management groups, planning committees, working parties, and all the other paraphernalia of management, is vital. It can have great symbolic significance, sending the message that people with learning difficulties must be involved in all activities. It also ensures that there is regular contact between users and decision makers. However, for it to have maximum impact steps have to be taken to make the structures more accessible, and more inclusive. Much to the frustration of many users, this message has yet to be heard by many organisations. The members of Advocacy in Action, from Nottingham, now withdraw from meetings that do not adapt to their needs.

Andrea Whittaker has highlighted a number of simple steps that can be taken to improve matters. These include:

- ensuring beforehand there is a real commitment to involve users on the part of existing committee members.
- getting members of the committee to meet users in advance.
- enabling users to observe the meeting beforehand to see if they wish to be involved.
- keeping the language used simple, and avoiding jargon.
- providing individual supporters for people, whose role it is to ensure that the users can get to the meeting, can follow what is happening, and can make an effective contribution.

(Whittaker, 1990)

Depending on the individuals involved, other options to be considered will include: ensuring the venue is physically accessible, documents in Braille, hearing loop systems, language interpreters (including BSL signers).

It will take resources to ensure that users can take part in management and planning of services, but the amounts required are often not so unimaginable. For example, in Clwyd, each local planning group has a small budget to be used to enable participation. Here, user involvement has been reinforced by a policy which made it a condition for access to additional funding available through the All Wales Strategy (Harper, 1988).

Involving users in evaluating and inspecting services

People who use services are the inside 'experts' on the quality of provision; involving them in evaluating and inspecting services is one way of tapping in to that expertise. It is also a way of ensuring that the focus is kept on issues that matter to users.

In Hillingdon, a formal evaluation of services was led by two self-advocates (Whittaker *et al.*, 1991). In other instances, people with learning difficulties have joined non-disabled people in evaluations. For example, users have been involved in PASS teams (evaluations designed to measure the extent that services fit the philosophy of normalisation).

Practice guidance on inspection from the Department of Health and the Social Services Inspectorate is unequivocal: 'the process of inspection should always include the involvement of users' (DH/SSI, 1991). Unfortunately, the guidance manual ducks out of offering detailed models of how this might be done, although it does raise the possibility of having users on both inspection teams and the advisory committees that oversee the work of inspection units.

Three-way contracts

One of the key elements in the recent reforms to both the NHS and social service departments is the idea of the purchaser/provider split. The declared aim of this attempt to set up a quasi-market for social care was to increase choice for users and stimulate innovation. The initial experience has not been positive. An early survey of contracts between local authorities and independent sector providers found little evidence of increased choice and many concerns that the introduction of contracts could reduce innovation (Common and Flynn, 1992). Part of the problem has been the tendency on the part of purchasers to go for block contracts, where they effectively purchase a standard service for a large number of people from a provider with an effective monopoly.

There is little scope for user involvement in block contracts. However, a number of commentators have argued that spot contracts – the purchase of specific services for named individuals – offer many opportunities for users to become much more actively involved in determining the specifications of services. For example, the Association for Residential Care have developed a model three-way contract (Churchill, 1991) which they claim will help make people with learning difficulties become actively involved in defining what is expected of services.

Working together: Quality Action groups

Given that staff, users and families have different perspectives there has to be some kind of forum for them to exchange views if they are to work together effectively. Remarkably, in many services there is no opportunity for the three groups to talk to each other. This is where Quality Action groups come in.

The role of a Quality Action group is to try and improve the quality of a service from the point of view of the people most directly affected: front-line staff, users and families. The groups are designed to bring together the participants and enable them to focus in very concrete terms on a local service. The typical group will work through the following set of tasks:

- deciding what their 'ideal' service might look like;
- looking at how the current service works;
- using a comparison of the two to develop an agenda for change;
- identifying one area and developing a plan;
- putting the plan into action;
- monitoring the effects.

The Norah Fry Research Centre has produced a pack to help support the development of Quality Action groups, based on the experiences of such groups from around the country (Milner *et al.*, 1991).

Consulting users: shutting the stable door?

In the past 'consulting' about plans for services was often the main way that users were involved in developing services. However, all too often the experience of being consulted has not been a positive one for people with learning difficulties. Unless service users have been involved in developing plans and setting the agenda in the first place, and unless the process of consultation is very participative, then the whole exercise can be singularly sterile.

The 1990 NHS and Community Care Act requires social services departments to publish annual plans and to consult widely upon them. To do this effectively means, amongst other things:

- co-opting people with learning difficulties on to planning committees;
- making the plans accessible to people with learning difficulties;
- actively seeking the views of self-advocacy groups;
- providing self-advocates with the resources to make an effective submission;
- responding to the comments of users;
- changing the subsequent years' plans in the light of comments (and acknowledging that influence).

SECTION FOUR: MAKING LINKS

> On its own, a better system of services will *not* [her emphasis] enable people with learning difficulties to be fully integrated and to exercise their citizenship rights.
>
> (Rioux, 1992)

People who are isolated are not empowered. The whole thrust of this section is to identify ways of enabling people with learning difficulties to build links that will increase their influence. As we emphasised earlier, this involves relationships that extend well beyond the boundaries of services. If services are taking empowerment seriously, then they will have to accept that they cannot rely solely on internal processes; being open and accepting an independent element is crucial. As Winn and Quick (1989) comment: 'Suggestions from outside the organisation help to challenge patterns of thought too ingrained to be challenged within.'

Self-advocacy

Self-advocacy is a term which is used in two distinct contexts. At times it is used to describe the process by which individuals become more confident and learn to express preferences and make choices. Much of what was referred to in section two (focusing on individuals) would often be called self-advocacy. However, the term is also commonly used to refer to the activities of the self-advocacy movement; the groups being controlled *by* people with learning difficulties. Self-advocacy, in this context, is about collective empowerment.

Many professionals are uncomfortable with the idea of collective self-advocacy. Yet most of us resort to collective action at some stage; the professional association, the political party, the self-help group, the running club or the church are all ways that people get support from people with common interests or experiences, or try to exert influence in ways that would not be possible as individuals. It is important for professionals to recognise that people with learning difficulties have just as much right as anyone else to act collectively. One of the most liberating experiences for many users is to discover that they are not alone; that there are others in a similar position. There must be opportunities for users to get together, to share experiences, and to learn from each other. Support for the development of vibrant, independent user group movements ought to be the keystone of any strategy for empowerment.

There has been considerable debate about the most appropriate models for self-advocacy. As Steve Dowson has pointed out professionals often set out to shape the form and the agenda of self-advocacy groups; for example, by insisting that they take the form of elected day-centre committees focusing on a relatively narrow range of issues within the centre (Dowson, 1990). Such service-based groups can be of great value, but they inevitably tend to be much less effective than the independent groups (often called People First groups) which draw members from a whole range of services, and which inevitably tend to have much wider horizons than the service-based equivalents.

To be really effective, independent groups need some resources. Some like Clwyd People First have made successful bids for joint funding, and the People First office in London was set up and support workers employed with the support of the Joseph Rowntree Foundation. With this kind of backing these groups (and others like them) have made some substantial achievements, some of them noted elsewhere in this chapter.

Involvement in self-advocacy groups does not, of course, preclude participation in 'mainstream' organisations; churches, women's groups, community action groups can all provide important opportunities for people with learning difficulties to make a contribution to society, as well as being potential sources of support (Hutchison *et al.*, 1992).

Finding allies: citizen advocacy

Even the most articulate of self-advocates can sometimes do with an ally. Citizen advocacy (Butler *et al.*, 1988) represents one way of organising 'allies' for people who are vulnerable or isolated. Both professionals and families can and often do help people with learning difficulties be heard. However, both groups often face genuine conflicts of interest: 'I would fight to the death for my son's rights, but I also recognise he sometimes needs an advocate against me' (the words of Mr Gwyn Davies, from the Bryn-y-Neauadd Advocacy Scheme).

Professionals are usually responsible for more than one service user. They therefore have great difficulty when the interests of a particular individual conflicts with the interests of others. They tend to opt for the solution that delivers the 'greatest good'. This can be a particular problem for people who are seen to be disruptive or who are unpopular. There also tend to be limits to the extent to which professionals will support users in a challenge to the employing agency. Staff who are seen to be supporting such a challenge at best run the risk of being labelled as 'negative'; at worst they may risk their jobs. Few are prepared to do that.

Although families are often genuinely concerned about their relative with learning difficulties here, too, there may be conflicting interests. For example, families may emphasise safety and security, while users may be arguing for the right to take risks.

Designed to overcome these potential conflicts of interest, citizen advocacy involves the recruitment of an unpaid private individual (the advocate) who is matched on a one-to-one basis with a person who is at risk of isolation or exclusion (the partner). The citizen advocate should have no direct connection with the service their partner is using; the only loyalty of the citizen advocate is to their partner. Citizen advocates are usually recruited and matched by independent organisations that themselves try to keep at arm's length from the services. In some cases, where there is no family involved, the citizen advocate may be the only person in the partner's life who is not paid to be there. Citizen advocacy is, by definition, about commitment.

There is still widespread confusion about the term advocate, and the meaning of citizen advocacy. There are still many managers and professionals who have not heard or who discount the arguments about conflict of interest, and for whom the idea of 'professional advocacy' sounds more attractive (and more controllable). Even where citizen advocates have been welcomed it is often on the basis of a partial misunderstanding. For example, there is a widespread belief that citizen advocates are only for those who cannot speak for themselves.

Citizen advocacy can be about any or all of the following:

- helping people decide what they want;
- helping people say what they want effectively;
- helping people be heard;
- providing friendship and emotional support;
- helping people make links with others in the community;
- providing practical support for people to achieve their aims;
- preventing the abuse of isolated or vulnerable people.

As yet users do not have any formal 'rights' to an advocate. The 1986 Disabled Persons Act included a section which gave people the right to have a 'representative' but that section of the act has never been implemented. However, this does not stop agencies adopting policies which make it clear that users can seek the support of an advocate, and that the advocate has an acknowledged role. For example, this is one of the features of some users' charters.

Extending the logic of citizen advocacy, some organisations in the US, Canada, and (more recently) the UK have built 'circles of support' around vulnerable people (Mount *et al.*, 1988). Rather than passively waiting for society to become more accepting, they have attempted to construct 'supportive communities'. Often advocates have played a crucial role in forming and supporting circles. With a strong emphasis on inclusion, and recognising and valuing abilities in people, these organisations are not 'services' in the conventional sense, but independent entities, with many parallels with the citizen advocacy movement.

Politics

Many of the key decisions made about services for people with learning difficulties will be made by politicians who, in all likelihood, will have had little direct contact with service users. Most politicians (whether in local or in central government) will have been lobbied by professionals and by organisations representing families (MENCAP and RESCARE are obvious and effective examples of the latter). So far relatively few people with learning difficulties will have had a chance to make their views known directly to the politicians who represent them. That absence from the political process is undoubtedly one of the reasons why people with learning difficulties (and the services they use) have remained so marginalised. Involvement in the political process is one of the hallmarks of citizenship; if participation means anything then it ought to mean the right to be involved in politics. Encouragement and support for users to vote, along with help for users to discover on what programme politicians are standing (particularly in relation to people with learning difficulties) ought to be an issue for all services. Similarly there ought to be an acknowledgement that people with learning difficulties have the right to lobby, campaign, demonstrate and join political parties – without being labelled as having challenging behaviour.

CONCLUDING THOUGHTS

There is a danger that much of what is argued for here could become just another set of 'sticking plaster' solutions. There are two key factors that are missing: a decent income for disabled people and anti-discrimination legislation. The latter would ensure access to all kinds of new opportunities for disabled people, while the former would enable them to purchase the kind of support *they* want (it is no accident that we equate income with 'purchasing power').

Much to the frustration of the disability movement (see Ford, 1991) attempts to argue for payments direct to disabled people, in order to enable them to purchase their own support, has run foul of earlier legislation; the government has recently confirmed that direct payment of money by service providers to individuals is against the terms of the 1948 Chronically Sick and Disabled Persons Act, and that they have no plans for amending legislation. Likewise a private member's bill incorporating elements of anti-discrimination failed to get government support, and was defeated.

The campaigns for these major changes will no doubt continue. Arguably, even if they were successful, there would still be a place for many of the mechanisms suggested here. In the meantime, there are still some people with learning difficulties who are not even allowed to choose their clothes (WO/SSI, 1989). There is much that *can* be done to ensure that people with learning difficulties are no longer ignored.

NOTE

1 'Learning difficulty' is the preferred term throughout this chapter.

REFERENCES

Allen, P. and Scales, C. (1990) *Residents' Rights: Helping People with Learning Difficulties Understand Their Housing Rights*, Brighton: Pavilion Publishing.

Brandon, D. and Towell, N. (1990) *An Introduction to Service Brokerage*, London, Good Impressions Publishing.

Brechin, A. and Swain, J. (1987) *Changing Relationships: Shared Action Planning with People with a Mental Handicap*, London: Harper & Row.

Brown, H. and Craft, A. (1992) *Working with the Unthinkable*, London: Family Planning Association.

Butler, K., Carr, S. and Sullivan, F. (1988) *Citizen Advocacy: A Powerful Partnership*, London, National Citizen Advocacy.

Churchill, J. (1991) 'Contractual matters', *Community Care*, Supplement, 28 March, iv–v.

Clare, M. (1990) *Developing Self Advocacy Skills*, London: Further Education Unit/ REPLAN.

Common, R. and Flynn, N. (1992) *Contracting for Community Care*, York: Joseph Rowntree Foundation/ Community Care.

Croft, S. and Beresford, P. (1990) *From Paternalism to Participation*, Brighton: Open Services Project/Joseph Rowntree Foundation.

Davis, K. (1990) 'Old medicine is still no cure', *Community Care* 27 September, 14.

DH/SSI (1991) *Inspecting for Quality: Guidance on Practice for Inspection Units in Social Service Departments and Other Agencies*, London: HMSO.

Dowson, S. (1990) *Keeping it Safe*, London, Values Into Action.

Ellis, K. (1993) *Squaring the Circle: User and Carer Participation in Needs Assessment*. York: Joseph Rowntree Foundation/Community Care.

Ford, C. (1991) 'Direct payments: report of a meeting with Virginia Bottomley', *Coalition* June, 3–4.

Frost, D. and Taylor, K. (1986) 'This is my life', *Community Care*, 7 August, 28–9.

Harper, G. (1988) 'Consumer-led service planning', *Community Living*, 1 (6), 18–19.

Humphreys, S. and Blunden, R. (1987) 'A collaborative evaluation of an individual plan system', *British Journal of Mental Subnormality*, 33 (1), 19–30.

Hutchison, P., Beechly, L., Foerster, C. and Fowke, B. (1992) 'Double jeopardy: women with disabilities speak out about community and relationships', *Entourage*, 7 (2), 16–18.

Laws, M., Bolt, L. and Gibbs, V. (1988) 'Implementing change in a long stay hospital using an individual planning system', *Mental Handicap*, 16 June, 74–6.

Lindow, V. (1991) 'Experts, lies and stereotypes', *The Health Service Journal*, 28 August, 18–19.

London People First (1993) *Oi, It's My Assessment*, London: London Borough's People First.

Milner, L., Ash, A. and Ritchie, P. (1991) *Quality in Action: A Resource Pack for Improving Service for People with Learning Difficulties*, Brighton: Pavilion Publishing.

Morris, J. and Lindow, V. (1993) *User Participation in Community Care*, London, Community Care Support Force.

Mount, B., Beeman, P. and Ducharne, G. (1988) *What Can We Learn about Bridge Building?* Conneticut: Communitas Inc.

Oliver, M. (1993) *Disability, Citizenship and Empowerment: Workbook 2, The Disabling Society*, Milton Keynes: The Open University.

Pfeffer, N. and Coote, A. (1991) *Is Quality Good for You?* London: Institute for Public Policy Research, Social Policy Paper No. 5.

Potts, M. and Fido, R. (1990) *A Fit Person To Be Removed*, Plymouth: Northcote House.

Rioux, M. (1992) *Exchanging Charity for Rights: The Challenge of the Next Decade*, paper presented at the October MENCAP Conference in London.

Simons, K. (1993) *Sticking up for Yourself*, York: Joseph Rowntree Foundation/ Community Care.

SSI (1989) *Inspection of Day Services for People with a Mental Handicap: Individuals, Programmes and Plans*, London: Social Services Inspectorate.

Sutcliffe, J. and Simons, K. (1993) *Self Advocacy and People with Learning*

Difficulties: Contexts and Debates, Leicester: National Institute for Adult and Continuing Education.

Welsh Office/SSI (1989) *Still a Small Voice: Consumer Involvement in the All Wales Strategy*, Cardiff: Welsh Office Social Service Inspectorate.

Whittaker, A. (1990) *Involving People with Learning Difficulties in Meetings*, London, King's Fund Centre.

Whittaker A., Gardner, S. and Kershaw, J. (1991) *Service Evaluation by People with Learning Difficulties*, London: King's Fund Centre.

Winkler, F. (1990) 'Consumerism and information', in Wynn, L (ed.) *Power to the People: The Key to Responsive Services in Health and Social Care*, London, King's Fund Centre.

Williams, C. (1993) *Video First*, Bristol, Norah Fry Research Centre.

Winchurst, C., Stenfert Kroese, B. and Adams, J. (1992) 'Assertiveness training for people with mental handicap: a group approach', *Mental Handicap*, 20, 97–101.

Winn, L. and Quick, A. (1989) *User Friendly Services: Guidelines for Managers of Community Health Services*, London: King's Fund Centre.

10 Financial services

Paul Martinez and Andrew Balchin

This chapter provides an introduction to and an overview of social security provision for people with learning disabilities. It is argued that the changes made in recent years in the name of rationalisation and simplification have not resolved the acute difficulties experienced by people with learning disabilities in taking up rights to benefit. These difficulties are examined and described through a brief survey of available benefits and a summary of the main principles underlying the social security system which affect disabled people. There is an account of efforts which have been made to promote the full take-up of welfare benefits followed by a tentative analysis of some of the issues arising out of the social security system in so far as they affect health and local authorities. Perhaps the first and most important question which must be asked, however, is 'Why bother with benefits at all?'

A person with a learning disability may meet a very large number of people who will provide assistance on a voluntary or paid basis. At one time or another contact may be made with volunteer advocates, specialist, generic or hospital social workers, general practitioners, special needs teachers, careers officers, occupational therapists, day centre and residential homes staff. The problem with welfare rights is that none of the individuals, groups or professions on this list have any particular responsibility to ensure that the correct benefits are being received by their clients. This is not to disparage the valuable assistance which is often provided in terms of advice, information and even advocacy. Rather, it is to state the obvious – people in one or other of the different roles are engaged, generally, in discharging that role and welfare rights work, if it is undertaken at all, is done as a voluntary or fringe activity. All too often, people with learning disabilities slip through the net.

It might be supposed, on the other hand, that the Benefits Agency as the main administrative organisation for social security benefits would have a crucial role to play in terms of assisting claimants generally and perhaps claimants with disabilities in particular. Unfortunately, it has become clear over the last decade that the Agency is withdrawing from direct contact with claimants. Home visits and face-to-face interviews have become increasingly difficult to obtain. Furthermore, the information and advice role of the

Agency has been restricted largely to its freephone service. This telephone advice line is not without its uses but is limited, nevertheless, to claimants who (i) have a telephone; (ii) can get through; and (iii) are able to formulate a fairly pointed and specific set of questions. In one particular area affecting disabled people, the Benefits Agency is spectacularly unhelpful. The Attendance Allowance Unit in Blackpool has records and details of thousands of severely disabled claimants. Entitlement to Attendance Allowance can, in many cases be a trigger to entitlement to Income Support which is administered locally, and yet, Attendance Allowance recipients are neither advised of this possibility nor is there any communication with local officers to prompt a claim. That this opportunity is foregone and families left to makeshift as best they can is an indication of the role in which the Benefits Agency has cast itself or allowed itself to be cast.

The virtual absence of take-up initiatives from the Agency places members of the caring professions in something of a quandary. Social workers, for example, are clearly under considerable pressure to deliver some sort of service to clients with welfare rights problems. Research suggests that this sort of assistance is highly valued by clients. The same research also indicates, however, that social workers can be actively hostile to any welfare rights role on the grounds that it is remote from their professional concern, or that it is too complicated or even that it is beneath their professional dignity.[1] Three questions arise from this discussion. Should members of the caring professions become involved in providing welfare rights help and in assisting their clients through the maze of benefits? In a situation of financial restraint and resource rationing is it reasonable for line managers, elected members and management teams to expect their staff to assume some sort of responsibility in this area? Is it necessary, thirdly, to supplement and support the work of individuals who are not specialists by employing welfare rights workers? It is part of the argument of this chapter that the answer to all three questions must be an emphatic 'YES'.

The benefits system is complex and convoluted. It is difficult not to sympathise with the reluctance of a busy day centre worker to engage with the sometimes arcane rules and procedures which govern entitlement to benefits. On the other hand, if members of caring professions find this task daunting, how much more difficult it is for people with learning disabilities and their families. It is important, moreover, to enforce every possible right and entitlement because there are so few of them! In 1981 it was estimated that benefits available to a person with a learning disability fell short of the extra cost of coping with disability by almost £20 per week (Buckle, 1984, 1987). The gap between income – even assuming the maximum take-up of benefits – and necessary expenditure has actually increased along with the increase in poverty in Britain in the last decade (CPAG, 1988). The maximisation of disposable income is an essential component in securing any objective of independent living in the community. It is possible, however, to find social services departments which have produced elaborate individual personal plans which make little reference to benefits or income. Finally, and above all, the 'bother' with benefits is necessary to ensure that real choices are available to people with learning disabilities. There are very substantial amounts of benefit which are not claimed and it has been established that low and inadequate take-up of welfare benefits is a particular problem for people with disabilities (CPAG, 1984). To take some responsibility for ensuring that full entitlements to benefits are claimed is to open up possibilities in terms of enhanced opportunities, improved quality of life and widened choices out of all proportion to the effort involved.

THE BENEFITS MAZE

One of the more forbidding aspects of welfare benefits is their complexity. This is the result, in large part, of the piecemeal introduction and articulation of the social security system. What has been conspicuously lacking in the development of the welfare state is any sort of unified income maintenance scheme for people with disabilities which would be adequate to maintain a reasonable standard of living, which would compensate for the increased costs of disability, which would not discriminate between different types of disablement and which would operate under clear, systematic and readily comprehensible rules. Indeed, it is precisely such a scheme which is being campaigned for by most organisations which represent disabled people (Buckle, 1987). What actually exists is a hodge-podge of overlapping benefits with different criteria of eligibility, conditions of entitlement and principles of assessment. At least three systems can be discerned. The first to be created were benefits associated with the national insurance principle. These comprise benefits such as Unemployment and Sickness Benefit, Invalidity Benefit, Retirement and Widow's Pensions. Entitlement to national insurance benefits is conditioned by prior payment of contributions; the scheme in other words is a sort of collective insurance policy. While it is possible to obtain national insurance 'credits' in certain circumstances, contributions are generally levied on people in full-time employment. Such contributory benefits by their nature cannot assist young people under 16; nor will they assist people with learning disabilities who will never enter the contribution system if they do not obtain employment. Most disabled people are catered for by non-contributory benefits, notably Disability Living Allowance and Severe Disablement Allowance. Most adults with learning disabilities will also claim one or more of the third sort of benefit – means-tested benefits. These are exemplified by the most important: Income Support, which in April 1988 replaced Supplementary Benefit. They do not depend on national insurance contributions but are stringently means-tested. In general terms this means that for every pound of income from some other source (including most other social security benefits) entitlement to benefit is reduced by the same, or a similar amount.

The inherent difficulties in coping with a benefits system which has been introduced over a forty-year period and is based on different and to a large degree contradictory principles are exacerbated considerably by the rate of change to which the system is subject. The 1988 changes to the main means-tested benefits and 1992 disability benefits changes which were introduced to simplify and unify the existing system have actually added further layers of complexity to an already baroque structure. The tempo of rapid change in the benefits system has been inversed still further by the Courts. In recent years major Court decisions have changed the interpretation of the law relating to Invalid Care Allowance, Severe Disablement Allowance and Attendance Allowance.[2]

The paragraphs which follow give a brief introduction to the main benefits which people with learning disabilities may be claiming. It is beyond the scope and intention of this chapter to offer a detailed analysis or a practical guide to such benefits. Even if this were to be attempted it would rapidly become out of date. Excellent handbooks are available from the Disability Alliance and from the Child Poverty Action Group[3] and these guides are strongly recommended. In addition to the annual handbooks there are three journals which provide an up-to-date guide to changes in the law, new developments and articles of interest: *Adviser* (National Association of Citizens Advice Bureaux and Shelter), *Welfare Rights Bulletin* (CPAG) and *Disability Rights Bulletin* (Disability Alliance). It may also be noted that the Benefits Agency produces a series of guides to certain benefits. These guides are free of charge and represent a reasonable introduction to Income Support, the Social Fund and non-means-tested benefits for people with disabilities.[4]

DISABILITY LIVING ALLOWANCE

Disability Living Allowance (DLA) was introduced in April 1992. It is non-means-tested, tax free and entitlement does not depend on having paid national insurance contributions. It is comprised of two components and a person may qualify for one or both components. The Care Component is aimed at people who need help looking after themselves; the Mobility Component is aimed at people who have difficulties in walking.

The Mobility Component is currently worth up to £31.40 per week and the Care Component up to £44.90 per week. These benefits are particularly important to people who are not employed since they do not overlap with or count against other social security benefits. Indeed their relative significance is increasing all the time since they are being used by the Government as 'passports' to other benefits. Thus, for example, the higher rate of Mobility Component confers exemption from road tax. Receipt of either component may qualify a disabled person to receive Severe Disablement Allowance. They also have the effect of increasing an award of Income Support by up to £60.15 per week.

DLA replaced Mobility and Attendance Allowances as benefits for people under 65 while Attendance Allowance has been retained for the over 65s. The introduction of the new benefit has been fraught with difficulties. Complexity has been increased by having a Care Component payable at one of three different rates, each with different disability tests, and a Mobility Component with two different rates. More radically, the much criticised doctor's visit to assess entitlement to Attendance Allowance and Mobility Allowance has been replaced by a self-assessment claim form. Whilst this represented a welcome shift from professional to self-assessment, the form, adding up to 40 pages of questions, presents difficulties to many people with learning disabilities, whilst the rigid question-and-answer format allows little scope for adequate representation of the full range of care and mobility needs of people with learning disabilities.

However, DLA does offer some significant new opportunities to increase benefit entitlement. People with learning disabilities were largely excluded from the single-tier Mobility Allowance. The DLA Mobility Component introduced two amended rates, higher and lower, which whilst limited in scope do represent an important recognition that mobility difficulties can arise from learning as well as physical disabilities. Entitlement to the higher rate of payment is still problematic. This is a result of a decision by the House of Lords to the effect that walking means 'putting one foot in front of the other'.[5] The consequence of this decision is that only people with learning disabilities who are unable to walk at all, who have some other disability which affects the motor ability to move or whose behaviour is very severely disturbed will qualify, whilst those who cannot walk from A to B without assistance or who are in personal danger from traffic because of behavioural problems are confined to the less generous lower rate.

The Care Component comprises three rates of payment: a higher and middle rate payable to people who require personal attention or supervision during the day or night or both; a lower rate for people who require less intensive care or who are unable to prepare a cooked meal (the so-called cooking test). Significantly for younger people with learning disabilities, under 16s are required to satisfy additional criteria or are excluded from entitlement to some rates of DLA.

Despite the move to self-assessment, a successful claim for DLA still requires a degree of good fortune or considerable assistance – probably from a GP, or welfare rights officer, nurse or social worker.

INVALID CARE ALLOWANCE AND SEVERE DISABLEMENT ALLOWANCE

Invalid Care Allowance is a benefit for carers. It is payable to a person of working age who is caring for someone who receives the Disability Living Allowance Care Component at either the higher or middle rate. Severe Disablement Allowance is a long-term benefit for people who are ill or disabled, which replaced the old non-contributory Invalidity Pension. The main condition is that the claimant has been incapable of work for 28 weeks.

Most claimants will also have to demonstrate that they can be regarded as 80 per cent disabled for the same length of time. These benefits are worth £33.70 per week each (1993 rates), are non-taxable and non means-tested. They differ in one critical way from Disability Living Allowance, however. Invalid Care Allowance and Severe Disablement Allowance overlap with other social security benefits. They are counted as income for the purposes of means-tested benefits and also cannot be paid at the same time as other national insurance benefits are paid to or on behalf of the claimant. The DLA Mobility and Care Components are excepted and do not overlap with Severe Disablement and Invalid Care Allowance.

Thus, a woman who receives a Widow's Pension will not be able to claim Invalid Care Allowance or Severe Disablement Allowance. Similarly, it will not increase family income when a woman claims Severe Disablement Allowance if her husband is claiming an increase in benefit for her. What she would gain, he would lose. There is one key exception to this rule, however. Severe Disablement Allowance and Invalid Care Allowance act as 'passports' for premiums added to Income Support. These premiums can still be paid if a person is *entitled* to either allowance but cannot be actually *paid* because of the 'overlapping' rules. The peculiar policy implication of the overlapping benefit rules is that the financial benefits accrue principally to couples where one partner is working, or where the family will usually be enjoying a higher standard of living than that of an unemployed couple. Such restrictions as to entitlement also create significant problems of low take-up.

MEANS-TESTED BENEFITS: INCOME SUPPORT

Means-tested benefits are among the most problematic in terms of take-up. Numerous campaigns have demonstrated that claimants in general and claimants with learning disabilities in particular failed to claim their full entitlement. Take-up is also hampered by frequent changes in legislation, typified by the 1988 replacement of Supplementary Benefit by Income Support.

In comparison with Supplementary Benefit, Income Support is considerably simplified. Supplementary Benefit weekly additions which were supposed to be tailored with some precision to the particular circumstances of the claimant were replaced by a variety of 'premiums' at fixed rates. As far as people with learning disabilities are concerned, the most important premiums will be those related to disability. Entitlement will usually be based on receipt of Disability Living Allowance or Severe Disablement Allowance. As a result of these changes, people with disabilities have lost out in two ways. On the one hand, people with very large extra weekly expenses caused by disability, have found that the fixed-rate premiums are worth less than the extra weekly Supplementary Benefit additions. On the other hand, people who were entitled to small weekly additions of Supplementary Benefit, are not entitled to any Income Support premiums at all.

For claimants who were actually receiving extra weekly amounts of Supplementary Benefit the Government attempted to limit their losses by paying an amount of 'transitional protection'. However, such protection has reduced as Income Support is uprated each year and disappears altogether when Income Support is equal to or above the level of Supplementary Benefit as it was in April 1988.

This complex and convoluted scheme has created two further problems of benefit take-up. Firstly, there are problems associated with ensuring that people with learning disabilities are awarded the appropriate premiums. Secondly, there are many such claimants who would be or would have been better off on the Supplementary Benefit scheme, but only if their Supplementary Benefit entitlement *had been correctly calculated in April 1988*. There will be very considerable numbers of claimants with learning disabilities who should have been entitled to higher amounts of Supplementary Benefit because of their various special needs and the weekly additions which were therefore appropriate. In the late 1980s a number of highly successful campaigns were conducted which succeeded in obtaining retrospective reviews of Supplementary Benefit entitlement resulting in payments of many thousands of pounds in arrears to claimants with learning disabilities. Indeed, so successful were the campaigns that the Government acted to bring in new legislation which now limits reviews of entitlement in most cases to 12 months, effectively shutting the door on any attempt to make up for the under-claiming of the past.

THE SOCIAL FUND

One of the more difficult problems posed by social security provision concerns the Social Fund. The significance of the Fund only emerges if it is placed in context. In 1983, following widespread criticism of the excessive exercise of discretion in the administration of Supplementary Benefit, the Government introduced detailed rules by which the scheme would be operated. Supplementary Benefit was to be both means-tested and 'needs-tested' in that claimants in different circumstances would be guaranteed a minimum income for their (different) day-to-day needs – but no more. Single payments were introduced to pay for all those necessary items for which a Supplementary Benefit recipient could not reasonably be able to budget.

Single payments disappeared altogether in April 1988, to be replaced by Social Fund payments. These represented a retrograde step since the payments are at the discretion of Social Fund officers whose decisions are not subject to appeal but are subject to a cash-limited budget and to the more or less unfettered discretion of the officer. The majority of payments consist of loans which are recoverable from claimants. Not least among criticisms which have been made of the Fund is that it represents a fairly cynical attempt by the Benefits Agency to involve other agencies, notably social services departments, in the assessment of potential eligibility for payments (Stewart and Stewart, 1986). The most acceptable part of the Social Fund Scheme is undoubtedly the provision of 'community care grants' to assist people to move into or re-establish themselves in the community and to help other people to continue to live in the community. Whatever their other defects, community care payments at least have the merit of being grants rather than repayable loans.

Co-operation or collaboration with Benefits Agency local offices in the administration of the Social Fund will probably be fairly uncontroversial as far as area health authorities are concerned. It will require only sufficient knowledge of Social Fund conditions to ensure that any funds available to health authorities to assist people with learning disabilities moving into the community are used to meet needs that are not catered for by the Social Fund. Local authorities on the other hand have been presented with a dilemma. The abolition of Supplementary Benefit Single Payments has ultimately led to an increase of income and debt referrals to social services departments. Local authorities have been faced with three choices. Staff could be encouraged to make use of the Social Fund at the risk of subordinating social services departments as very junior and unequal partners in an income maintenance administrative scheme. On the other hand, local authorities could boycott the scheme altogether, although it would be difficult to do so without making some alternative provision, which could only have significant revenue implications. Finally, and this is perhaps the worst choice of all, social services departments might choose not to formulate any policy. The last choice can only lead to personal choices being made by staff and an extremely uneven and contradictory set of responses to clients from different teams and different individuals. In the face of such a dilemma, many local authorities have opted for a middle way, sometimes known as 'determined advocacy'. Staff will assist claimants in applying to the Social Fund and act as their advocate but will stand short of actively assisting the Benefits Agency in determining the priority of individual needs.

DISABILITY WORKING ALLOWANCE

Disability Working Allowance is a relative newcomer to the stable of means-tested benefits. Introduced in April 1992 it is tax free and is paid on top of low wages or self-employed earnings for people whose disabilities put them at a disadvantage in getting a job. The Allowance is intended to encourage people with disabilities to return to or take up work by topping up low earnings. The key incentive is aimed at people on Invalidity Benefit or Severe Disablement Allowance. To date the rate of take-up of Disability Working Allowance has been appallingly low. This might be attributed to three reasons. First, in common with many benefits it is taken fully into account as income for other means-tested benefits, e.g. Housing Benefit. Second, to get the Allowance you must have 'a physical or mental disability which puts you at a disadvantage in getting a job'. On an initial claim this is generally accepted without question. However, on a reviewed claim made every six months a claimant may be asked to go through a process of detailed self-assessment backed up by the opinion of a professional case worker. Failure to satisfy this 'disability' test will result in loss of benefit, hence there is no guaranteed ongoing financial support for those in low-paid work. Finally, the Allowance might prove more successful if allied to concrete measures to tackle discrimination against people with learning disabilities in the labour market and an improvement in housing and educational opportunities.

TAKE-UP CAMPAIGNS

The failure of the poorest claimants to claim or take up benefits to which they are entitled, has been the subject of growing interest and concern over the last decade. There is an extensive literature which attempts to analyse and explain the reasons for low take-up and, by implication, to suggest ways in which take-up might be improved.[6]

A large number of initiatives have been undertaken mainly but not exclusively by local authorities to promote the take-up of benefits. A number of these initiatives have been directed towards people with disabilities and towards people with learning disabilities specifically. Probably the most expensive in terms of the costs paid to workers, but also the most successful and most systematic has been mounted by Nottingham Welfare Rights Service. Three welfare rights workers interviewed people with learning disabilities and their carers. Following the interviews, claims were made for benefits and support provided for any appeals which were necessary. Over 40 per cent were failing to claim benefits to which they were entitled. As a result of the initiative, 445 people with learning disabilities claimed and were awarded over £1,000 per year on average in extra benefits (James, *et al.*, 1986).

Take-up campaigns have been conducted by interviews with users of adult training or social education centres (Cleveland Welfare Rights Service, n.d.; Bradford Benefits Campaign, 1987) and with attenders of a day centre for people with learning disabilities (Bennett and McGavin, 1980). In a number of places, including Leeds, Sheffield and Birmingham, surveys have been conducted at day centres, claimants' homes, and adult training centres by way of questionnaires. The questionnaires were designed by welfare rights workers to be administered by relatively untrained volunteers. Advice on making claims and follow-up work was done after the questionnaires had been processed by more experienced workers.[7] In Manchester there was a highly successful but limited campaign to increase the take-up of benefits amongst children with learning disabilities who attend special schools. The project discovered that almost half of the young people interviewed were failing to claim significant amounts of benefits to which they were entitled (Owen) Finally, there have been a number of successful exercises where non-specialist workers in contact with disabled people have taken on the task of promoting the take-up of benefits, often with a welfare rights agency providing support and casework backup. In Leicester, health service staff have been encouraged to adopt this approach (Leicester City Council Benefits Campaign, 1987). Occupational therapists and physiotherapists took on this role with considerable success in Islington (Cohen, 1983).

A number of inferences may be drawn from such campaigns. People with learning disabilities are failing to claim significant amounts of benefit to which they are entitled. The Nottingham figures suggest that as many as 40 per cent of people with learning disabilities are under-claiming. This index of under-claiming is not a vague or optimistic 'estimate' but emerges from validated results of claims being identified, submitted, processed and benefit awarded as the result of welfare rights activity. The most successful and rigorous take-up work, however, is relatively time consuming and expensive. It involves face-to-face interviews with people in their homes and extensive casework in support of claims. The take-up exercises demonstrate, further, that successful campaigning is highly dependent on a broad inter-disciplinary approach involving a variety of workers who have contact with people with learning disabilities and their carers and who are trained and supported at least to the point of being able to 'sign-post' benefits and make referrals. Disabled people are not, finally, 'too proud to claim'. What emerges from the campaign reports is that the principal reason for under-claiming is that families are simply overwhelmed by the complexities of the benefits system, or worse, put off by unproductive encounters with unsympathetic staff, incomprehensible procedures, lengthy delays and so forth.

Experience suggests that take-up work is an essential part of service provision for people with learning disabilities. The above considerations might well form an initial element of policy development for social services departments, and perhaps also area health authorities. Geoff Fimister (1986) in his stimulating handbook describes various models that such a service might adopt.

WELFARE BENEFITS AND THE HEALTH SERVICE

At the risk of oversimplification, there is an assumption built into the system of social security that the material as well as the medical needs of patients should be met by the National Health Service. The reduction or withdrawal of benefits which claimants are entitled to receive while they are in hospital is the logical consequence of this premise. Benefits are withdrawn after four weeks (Disability Living Allowance Care Component), reduced after six weeks (Income Support and Severe Disablement Allowance) and reduced further or withdrawn after a year. At first sight, the avoidance of 'double provision' may seem both sensible and straightforward. Difficulties arise, however, as soon as one begins to ponder some of the practical applications of this principle. In what sense, if any, are out-patients 'in hospital'? Are patients 'in hospital' on the days that they are admitted or discharged from hospital? If prior to discharge, there is a period of experimental living, possibly with nursing support but without other medical intervention, in former staff accommodation or purpose-built accommodation in hospital grounds, does this constitute being 'in hospital'? This section reviews some of these questions. It is part of the argument of this chapter, however, that the issues of boundary and borderline may only be resolved in the interests of patients by the development of two strategies within the Health Service: to ensure that the full benefit entitlement of patients is taken up and to ensure that full regard is paid to the implications for the income and benefits of patients when new or different services are being planned.

It seems likely that in the foreseeable future there will be a considerable growth in demand for regular short-term care for both adults and children with learning disabilities. Short-term care poses considerable problems as entitlement to benefit may be severely disrupted. Entitlement to DLA Care Component, for example, is lost for each day spent in local authority care or in hospital, where a 'day' in this context means a day and a night. This rule comes into operation after 28 'days' which are linked together (84 days in the case of children). Periods in care or hospital are linked together unless they are separated by periods of 28 or more days spent not in care or hospital. It may well be, therefore, that people will prefer forms of short-term or respite care which will require considerable flexibility on the part of the Health Service.

A further major consideration for hospital administrators would be to ensure that their patients or residents with learning disabilities make claims for benefits to which they are entitled. This is particularly important in relation to long-term hospital residents who may be preparing to live in the community. Such residents will be likely to be spending periods of days or weeks out of hospital 'on holiday', staying with relatives or trying out proposed living arrangements. Invariably such residents will only be receiving around £14 per week 'hospital pocket money' and the limitation of their cash resources is likely to frustrate more imaginative (and costly) activities outside hospital. Indeed, it is difficult to see how such residents will be able to enjoy external visits and still less how they might familiarise themselves with bills, dealing with day-to-day expenses and so forth. Hospital administrators may be able to make considerable extra sums available to such patients if they ensure that claims for the full daily or weekly awards of Severe Disablement Allowance, Income Support and Disability Living Allowance are made for any period spent out of hospital, including the days leaving and returning to hospital accommodation. In larger units this almost certainly means devoting some extra staff resources to this work, but the arguments for such take-up exercises, which can only be 100 per cent successful, are overwhelming.

LOCAL AUTHORITIES AND WELFARE BENEFITS

Many local authorities are aware of the problematic nature of benefit provision and the consequent low rates of take-up, confusion and demoralisation on the part of claimants. Many have responded by setting up welfare rights units and by mounting take-up campaigns. Indeed, almost all of the campaigns directed towards people with learning disabilities have been run by welfare rights officers employed by local authorities. This section briefly reviews the recent social security changes introduced with Care in the Community, the creation of educational opportunities for young people with learning disabilities and finally the opportunities provided by the new Independent Living Fund.

Under rules in force before April 1993, people entering residential care homes were able to claim their accommodation and living costs from the Benefits Agency by way of Income Support. Limits were placed on the amount claimed depending on the nature of the care provided. People with learning disabilities who were living in residential care on 31 March 1993 can continue to claim the special higher rates of Income Support. However, people entering residential care after 1 April 1993 will come under new community care arrangements. Entry to residential care will first be determined by local authority social services departments who will conduct a needs *and* financial assessment. If they deem residential care to be appropriate, they will pay the home's fees and work out how much a person with learning disabilities can afford to contribute, based on income, including social security benefits and any capital a person may have. Unless a person has other income sufficient to meet the cost of the home, a claim for Income Support will need to be made and is paid at the same rate as if a person is living at home, except it will include a residential allowance of £45 per week (£50 in London). The net effect of this process is to leave residents in care with personal expenses of £12.65 per week. The Disability Living Allowance Care Component is withdrawn four weeks after a person moves into residential care permanently, whilst the Mobility Component will remain in payment. The only exception to these rules applies to people who are meeting the *full* cost of the fees of an *independent* residential care home. They are allowed to retain entitlement to Disability Living Allowance Care Component.

The requirement to conduct a needs assessment prior to any entry to residential care effectively makes local authority social services departments the gatekeepers to financial assistance for people with learning disabilities. In addition, it marks the further extension of means-testing into local authority services and a significant 'hiving off' of central government responsibilities to local authorities. It is not too far fetched to suggest that in the future the Government might be tempted also to offload responsibility for the Social Fund Community Care Grants system to local authorities now that they have lead responsibility in this area.

The adoption of a comprehensive needs assessment has, however, presented local authorities with new opportunities to integrate welfare rights take-up into the care assessment procedures. Since many of the care needs assessed closely match the criteria for Disability Living Allowance, some local authorities are offering systematic benefit checks backed up with casework support by Welfare Rights Units. Some authorities have also mounted take-up campaigns specifically to mitigate the vast effects of introducing charging for services such as home helps.

Over recent years, the education system has been undergoing the same sort of upheaval as that which has affected welfare benefits. Partly as a result of this process there are a number of ways in which the benefits provision for students with learning disabilities gives rise to important opportunities in special needs education through benefit incentives to pursue education beyond school leaving age.

Whether as part of a conscious policy or as an unintended consequence of policy, there is now greater financial support than before for young people with learning disabilities to remain in full-time education. As well as the possibility of Disability Living Allowance, school children with learning disabilities are able to claim Income Support as soon as they reach their sixteenth birthday. The main criteria which they will have to satisfy are that they are not capable of doing an ordinary job or that they are so severely disabled that they would be unlikely to obtain employment within a year, even if they were available for work.[8] There is a pervasive misconception that such young people can only claim benefit when they *leave* school. Families will need considerable support and guidance to ensure that rights to benefit are established. Claims should also be made at the young person's sixteenth birthday for Severe Disablement Allowance. Whilst SDA will be deducted in full from Income Support, it does ensure that the additional Disability Premium is included in overall entitlement. Furthermore, it is important to establish entitlement to SDA before the young person reaches the age of 20 after which there is an additional (and much more stringent) 80 per cent disablement test. Apart from incentives from the social security system, local authorities have a power to pay grants to support further education. These grants, known variously as Educational Maintenance Allowances, Post 16 Awards or Minor or Discretionary Awards are ignored for Income Support purposes for all students aged 16–18. (The grants are, however, counted in full as income for any student who receives Income Support who is aged 19 or over.)

There are certain implications for the format and shape of education provision arising from the rules for Income Support and Severe Disablement Allowance. Firstly, for Income Support purposes, the education should be 'full-time' which in this context means education comprising 12 or more hours per week of classes (young people aged 16–18) or education which is defined as full-time by the Education Authority (students aged 19 and above). The rules for Severe Disablement Allowance are rather different: any young person in education aged 16–18 must not be receiving more than 21 hours per week of education which would be suitable for young people who are not disabled. Courses in special schools will be regarded as 'special education' but problems may arise in respect of young people whose disability is relatively small and who have been integrated into mainstream education. Experience suggests that a difficulty which might appear insuperable in theory is capable of resolution in practice: many young people with learning disabilities will require special support or classes with a high teacher–student ratio.

The availability of financial support for full-time education raises the issue, finally, of the desirability of extending opportunities for disabled people living in the community or offering education as an alternative to day-centre or training-centre provision. Students who are aged 19 and over can be in full-time education and continue to receive Income Support providing they are entitled to a Disability Premium. If people with learning disabilities can return to full-time education without prejudice to their benefit income, this opens up the prospect of using educational provision as part of a determined strategy of development and promoting independence.

Lastly, in this brief survey of the benefits system and local authority services, the role of the Independent Living Fund should be examined. The Fund was initially established as an independent trust that made payments to individuals with severe disabilities to enable them to live independently in the community. It was designed as a temporary replacement for weekly cash help that used to be available to some people with severe disabilities under the old Supplementary Benefit scheme. The Fund ceased to accept new applications in November 1992 and was re-established in April 1993 with a new scheme which provides less cash and less choice over personal care arrangements. Essentially, the Fund provides cash help as a top-up to services provided by the local authority to people in their own homes. To qualify, a person must be aged between 16 and 65, getting Income Support and DLA Care Component at the highest rate and be so severely disabled, physically or mentally, that extensive help with domestic duties or personal care is needed to ensure independent living. Provided the local authority is giving domiciliary services valued at least at £200 per week, and total care needs have been assessed at less than £500 per week, the Fund may pay the difference.

Despite the new restricted criteria and the criticism that the Fund does not have any statutory basis and is managed by a Board of Trustees, its significance lies in the fact that, for once, disabled people can have an amount of income for personal care needs which is under their control. The overwhelming success of the first Independent Living Fund demonstrated that such control is the key to promotion of meaningful care in the community and real independent living.

NOTES

1 The relationship between social work and social security is explored comprehensively in Becker and MacPherson (1986); Stewart and Stewart (1986); Becker and MacPherson (eds) (1988).

2 Respectively: *Drake v Chief Adjudication Officer* (1986) ECJ, The *Times*, 25 June 1986; *Clarke v Chief Adjudication Officer* (1987) ELR, 25 June 1987; *Moran v Secretary of State for Social Services* (1987) CA.

3 Disability Alliance *Disability Rights Handbook*; CPAG *National Welfare Benefits*

Handbook; CPAG *Rights Guide to Non-Means-Tested Benefits*. All available from CPAG, 1–5 Bath Street, London, EC1V 9PV (Tel. 071-253 3406). Prices on application.

4 Benefits Agency booklets: *A Guide to Income Support, A Guide to the Social Fund, A Guide to Non-Contributory Benefits for Disabled People*. Available from Benefits Agency offices and Leaflets Unit, PO Box 21, Stanmore, Middlesex, HA7 1AY.

5 *Lees v Secretary of State for Social Services*, reported as an appendix to Social Security Commissioner's decision R(M) 1/84.

6 For a bibliography of take-up issues see Falkingham (1985).

7 Respectively: Chapeltown CAB (1980); *Sheffield Disablement Benefit Take-up Campaign Report* (1985); Napolitano (n.d.).

8 Regulation 13(2)(b) Income Support (General) Regulations, 1987.

REFERENCES

Becker, S. and MacPherson, S. (1986) *Poor Clients: The Extent and Nature of Financial Poverty amongst Consumers of Social Work Services*, Nottingham: Nottingham University Benefits Research Unit.
—— (eds) (1988) *Public Issues, Private Pain – Poverty, Social Work and Social Policy*, London: Insight.
Bennett, T. and McGavin, P. (1980) *Pyenest Survey Report*, Harlow: Community Services Department.
Bradford Benefits Campaign (1987) *Report*, Bradford: Bradford City Council.
Buckle, J. (1984) *Mental Handicap Costs More*, London, Disablement Income Group.
—— (1987) *Poverty and Disability – Breaking the Link*, London: Disability Allowance.
Chapeltown CAB (1980) *Disability Project Report*, Leeds: NACAB.
Child Poverty Action Group (1984) *Benefits Take-up, Facts, Figures and Campaign Details*, London: Child Poverty Action Group.
—— (1988) *An Abundance of Poverty*, London: Child Poverty Action Group.
Cleveland Welfare Rights Service (n.d.) *Shelton Adult Training Centre Campaign*, Middlesborough: Cleveland County Council.
Cohen, R. (1983) *Able to Claim*, London: Islington People's Rights.
Falkingham, F. (1985) *Take-up of Benefits: A Literature Review*, Nottingham: Benefits Research Unit, Nottingham University.
Fimister, G. (1986) *Welfare Rights Work in Social Services*, London: Macmillan.
James, I., Stafford, P. and Ripon, P. (1986) *Welfare Rights Work with the Community Mental Handicap Team*, Nottingham: Welfare Rights Services.
Leicester City Council Benefits Campaign (1987) *Cut the Cost of Ill Health and Disability*, Leicester: City Council.
Napolitano, S. (n.d.) *A Fairer Deal for Fairways*, Birmingham: Tribunal Unit.
Sheffield Disablement Benefit Take-Up Campaign (1985) *Report*, Sheffield: Sheffield City Council.
Stewart, G. and Stewart, J. (1986) *Boundary Changes*, London: Child Poverty Action Group, British Association of Social Workers.

Part II

Implementing the Community Care Act

11 Professional and planning issues in assessment

Oliver Russell

The challenge is . . . to ensure that we provide a seamless service based entirely around the needs and wishes of users of care and their carers.

(Virginia Bottomley, 1992)

WHAT IS A SEAMLESS SERVICE?

What exactly is 'a seamless service'? How do we recognise one? Many of the community services for people with learning disabilities which I know are far from seamless, indeed some are not only coming adrift at the seams but the fabric is actually falling apart. 'A seamless service' may be a catchy phrase for the Secretary of State to use but does it mirror the reality of community care in the 1990s?

When the White Paper *Caring for People: Community care in the next decade and beyond* (Department of Health, 1989) was published in November 1989 there were hopes that it might herald an era of radical change and innovation in the way that community care was conceived and delivered. The changes outlined in the White Paper were intended to:

- enable people to live as normal a life as possible in their own homes or in a homely environment in the local community;
- provide the right amount of care and support to help people achieve maximum possible independence and, by acquiring or re-acquiring basic living skills, people would be helped to achieve their full potential;
- give people a greater individual say in how they live their lives and the services they need to help them do so.

(Department of Health, 1989, p. 4)

The proper assessment of need and good caremanagement were seen as the cornerstones of the new way forward. Although the Department of Health saw assessment and caremanagement as a continuum, three distinct processes were identified in the draft guidance:

- needs assessment
- the design of a care package

- implementation of the agreed 'package'

(Department of Health, 1990)

It was envisaged that the individual user and any carers should be involved in assessment and that their wishes should be taken into account. It was expected that the assessment and caremanagement process would promote flexible and imaginative responses to care needs (Department of Health, 1990)

In this chapter I consider some of the challenges which may face professionals who are engaged in the assessment process. Although I shall not deal directly with caremanagement there is inevitably much that is common ground. Before considering how assessment and caremanagement are likely to be implemented I shall review some of the more controversial issues which relate to the profound changes in emphasis which the White Paper envisages.

DOES ASSESSMENT NEED PROFESSIONAL SKILLS?

The shift from an emphasis on diagnostic assessment to the assessment of strengths and needs, and the shift from professional assessment to self-generated assessment processes reflects an ongoing change which is taking place in the value base of the caring professions.

In a perceptive paper on the implications of normalisation for those who work as professionals in health and social services David Brandon remarks that 'the heart of professionalism is putting oneself in the shoes of the patient – imagining how it is for him or her' (Brandon, 1991, p. 40). He observes that few definitions of professional skill begin from the viewpoint of service users. Professional skill is usually equated with being 'expert' which in turn often reflects a commitment to the evaluation and treatment of pathology.

Brandon remarks that policies based on normalisation involve shifting the focus of attention away from a study of the pathology of the individual to an exploration of their experiences as a user of services. Assessment procedures look at the nature of the changes required if services are to meet that individual's needs. He recognises five major themes as the foundation of a user-based service:

- good relationships;
- maximising choices;
- effective participation;
- personal development;
- greater mixing.

Brandon (1991) suggests that these five themes provide a complex three-dimensional jigsaw which provides a template for understanding an individual's personal and social needs. The proposals in the White Paper give a strong emphasis to such a user-based service.

HOW TO GO ABOUT ASSESSING NEED

It was Urie Bronfenbrenner (Bronfenbrenner, 1979) who emphasised that we could only fully understand a person's needs when we were able to see the person dealing with their environment. In other words, the person might be having difficulties, not because of any inherent fault in their psychological or bodily function but because they were having to deal with a hostile environment. Bronfenbrenner taught how important it was to consider the person within the setting where they live or work. His view corresponds with the underlying assumptions of the White Paper and subsequent legislation.

WHAT DO WE MEAN BY ASSESSMENT?

We all approach assessment from different backgrounds, from different experiences and perhaps with different prejudices. I shall begin by clearing the decks of some unwanted cargo. As a psychiatrist I have been trained in the use of particular observational skills which enable me to assess a person's behaviour and prescribe appropriate treatment. I use the word assessment to describe what I do when I work in my out-patient clinic. There are, however, other uses of the word 'assessment' and we need to be clear about what we are doing when we say that we are carrying out an assessment.

I suggest that we may find the word assessment used in three different ways:

1 *Diagnostic assessment* – as used in clinical settings where the assessor searches for the signs or symptoms of disease or abnormality.
2 *Assessment of individual strengths and needs* – as used in conjunction with Individual Programme Planning meetings where the assessor is not concerned with illness or disorder but with an individual's intellectual or emotional strengths and with their social and economic needs.
3 *Assessing the strength of community support for an individual* – as used perhaps by a service broker when helping to draw up a plan for individualised funding.

I would like to explore these three concepts in a little more depth.

Diagnostic assessment

In making a diagnostic assessment we ask: 'What is going on inside this person?' We are likely to assess their intellect through psychological tests. We assess their mental state through a psychiatric assessment. We assess their physical disability through a medical examination and we assess their emotional and social functioning through a social work assessment. Through these various procedures we attempt to reach a progressively clearer picture of how the person functions within their environment and of any factors which are interfering with their performance or their quality of life.

As professionals we often bring these findings together at a case conference where we weigh up and consider the different contributions which we have heard. Multi-disciplinary case conferences are particularly fashionable at the moment. Whether they are an effective use of resources is another matter! In services for people with learning difficulties we have Community Learning Difficulties Teams which bring together people from different disciplines.

We are all very used to these modes of assessment. The diagnostic approach still has great value, but on its own we recognise that it provides an inadequate account of an individual's needs. The approach is basically concerned with identifying pathology and, because the assessment is primarily concerned with analysing parts of the whole, the process inherently devalues the person by discounting their own experience. In recent years more attention has been given to an alternative approach – individual planning.

Assessment of individual strengths and needs

In making a diagnostic assessment we asked: 'What is going on inside this person?' In developing an Individual Programme Plan (an IPP) we are much more interested in how the person relates to the social world in which they live than to their disability or impairment. In assessing individual strengths and needs we work with the service user to identify those aspects of their lives where we can agree on some goals which might lead to an enhancement of their lifestyle.

I shall call this approach 'individual planning' but you may recognise the process by another name. The development of individual planning arose from a recognition that the person for whom plans were being made often had little chance to voice his or her views. Individual Programme Planning meetings were introduced as a means to include the person at the centre of the planning process. Assessment became much less concerned with pathology and what the person could not do and much more concerned with the person's strengths and needs and what they could do. The person whose life was being discussed would be involved in the meeting and encouraged to voice her opinion. Strengths and needs lists would be drawn up and goals and objectives would be set. Although professionals continue to play a dominant role in such meetings it is usual to involve only those people who are intimately concerned with the client. Meetings will often involve members of the family and others who occupy key roles in the person's life.

In this context a satisfactory assessment is one in which the professionals use their skills to draw sensitive and positive portraits of the person's life, emphasising the strengths and needs that the person has.

IPPs have been only a partial success. Although professionals lost some of the decision-making power, the client is still far from being in control of their lives. The IPP system still has much to commend it but as an approach it has been found wanting.

Assessing the strength of community support for an individual

In making a diagnostic assessment we asked: 'What is going on inside this person?' It may be more relevant to ask: 'What is going on around this person?'

The development of interest in ways to overcome the inherent problems of the IPP led to the development of ideas such as 'Circles of Support' (Mount, 1987). Circles of Support are created to establish and support a personal vision for an individual and to build community support and action on behalf of the person concerned. Those who are engaged in this approach say that Circles of Support consist of a group of people who wish to help a person realise some of their dreams. The essential difference from the IPP is that the person him/herself has a much greater degree of control over his or her assessment. The professional role is substantially diminished.

Closely associated with the idea of the 'Circle of Support' is the concept of 'Service Brokerage' (Brandon and Towe, 1989) in which processes are provided whereby an individual can be assisted to purchase their own individualised services and to control those services. Service Brokerage has been pioneered in Alberta and British Columbia but is now being piloted in the United Kingdom (Simons and Russell, 1991).

THE INITIAL EXPERIENCE OF LOCAL AUTHORITIES WHICH HAVE BEGUN TO INTRODUCE ASSESSMENT AND CAREMANAGEMENT

In a very helpful overview Beardshaw and Towell draw attention to some common themes that may be found among the diverse models of assessment and case management found in the United Kingdom and abroad (Beardshaw and Towell, 1991). They make the point that investment in existing, inflexible services has meant that agencies have found it very difficult to introduce forms of personal help and support that relate closely to a person's needs and preferences. 'Perverse incentives in funding and planning which have favoured residential care and other established service strategies have compounded the problem' (Beardshaw and Towell, 1991, p. 7).

They conclude their review by stating that there is a need to move forward to a truly holistic model of assessment where the wishes of user and carer are central and where the goal is to identify an appropriate range of supports for the user rather than provide a standard service package of day and residential care. They use an example from a paper by John O'Brien and Beth Mount to demonstrate sharp contrasts in the style and context of assessment.

Two assessments

The first of these assessments was done by a multi-disciplinary professional team as part of a regular case review cycle. The second took place at the suggestion of Mr Davis's day care organiser and was done by Mr Davis, members of his family, neighbours, members of his church and two of his social care workers with the help of an outside facilitator.

1 Mr Davis has a mental age of 3 years, 2 months. His IQ is 18. Severe impairment of adaptive behaviour, severe range of mental retardation. Becomes agitated and out of control. Takes (medicines) for psychosis.

   Severely limited verbal ability; inability to comprehend abstract concepts. Learns through imitation. Has learned to unlock the Coke machine and restock it and to crank a power mower and operate it.

   The family is uncooperative. They break appointments and do not follow through on behaviour management plans.

2 Ed lives with his mother and sister in (housing project). Ten of his relatives live nearby and they visit back and forth frequently. His father spends little time with him, but two of his sisters have been very helpful when there are crises. His family agree that he will live with one or another of them for the rest of his life.

   Ed is at home in his neighbourhood. He visits extended family members and neighbours daily. He goes to local stores with his sister and helps with shopping. He goes to church. Ed dresses neatly, is usually friendly and shakes hands with people when he meets them.

   He is a very big man, with limited ability to speak. When he gets frustrated and upset he cusses and 'talks' to himself in a loud voice. These characteristics often frighten other people who do not know him well. He has been excluded from the work activity centre because he acts 'out of control' there. He has broken some furniture and punched holes in the walls there and scares some of the staff people very much.

   Ed likes people and enjoys visiting the neighbourhood. He loves music, dancing and sweeping. He likes loading vending machines and operating mechanical equipment. He likes to go shopping. He likes to cook for himself and for other people and can fix several meals on the stove at home. He likes to hang clothes and bring them off the line. He likes to stack cord wood and help people move furniture. He prefers tasks that require strength and a lot of large muscle movement.

(O'Brien and Mount, 1991)

I have quoted this story at length because it seems to me to provide a very clear illustration of the contrasts between the traditional professional assessment and gives a glimpse of the alternative assessment processes that need to be introduced if user and carer involvement is going to be taken seriously. Beardshaw and Towell (1991) call attention to the considerable investment in staff time and in training that will be required if local authorities are to engage with users and carers in assessment. The scale of the changes will demand concerted action by professionals from all of the disciplines involved. However, a start on the changes was made by many authorities before the White Paper was even published.

In a perceptive study of ten local authorities in England, Nirmala Rao summarises the major cultural and operational changes needed to give effect to the White Paper's vision of an assessment system which is sensitive to the needs of the service user (Rao, 1991). Kent County Council pioneered caremanagement for elderly people on a pilot basis in 1987 and subsequently extended the approach to people with learning disabilities. Surrey has developed locality-based teams with local care managers responsible for overseeing the assessment of needs and the delivery of individual care plans. Effective asessment will ultimately depend upon the degree to which different agencies can collaborate in the assessment process. Although social services departments are the lead agency, other local authority departments such as housing and education will need to be involved, together with health authorities and Family Health Service Authorities. Rao draws attention to the requirement for:

> the provision of sufficient assessors to ensure a full assessment of each referral; services which are accessible and relevant to minority communities; the provision of packages of care which respond with a wide range of choices for users and carers at times when they need that assistance; and sufficient resources for assessment to enable a speedy and effective response.

(Rao, 1991, p, 45)

The experience of those who were in the vanguard of planning for the introduction of assessment and case management is illuminating and provides some helpful insights into what may lie behind the rhetoric. In another study Virginia Beardshaw worked closely with senior officers from eleven local authorities on the initial stages of implementing the new proposals and reported on their struggles to bring about change within the system (Beardshaw, 1991). This project became known as the MAIN network (mutual aid implementation network). She and her co-workers saw assessment and caremanagement as pivots at the centre of the new service systems. The two processes were seen to mediate between the needs of those who were service users and those who were responsible for purchasing the services. Beardshaw emphasises that assessment and caremanagement are two distinctly different things – 'they are about tailoring services around individual needs and about resource rationing' (Beardshaw, 1991, p. 7). Assessment and caremanagement also reflect a tension between the White Paper's twin objectives of maximising choice and making the best use of locally available services. The service user wishes to exercise more choice from the range available, the purchaser hopes to target the limited resources more effectively. Beardshaw envisaged that well-organised assessment and caremanagement could become the route to a more flexible provision of services and a more sensitive targeting of resources.

Those who participated in the exercise with Beardshaw discovered that it was necessary to move forward on a number of different fronts simultaneously.

As far as assessment and caremanagement were concerned they identified the need for:

• a split between purchaser and provider functions;
• clear-cut criteria for targeting resources to those most in need;
• a move from service-led to client-centred screening and assessment systems;
• a need to involve users and carers.

IMPLEMENTING THE NEW STRATEGY

Bringing about these very substantial changes was not likely to be easy. Two broad approaches were envisaged. The first depended on large-scale systems re-design, the second on what was referred to as a 'virus approach' in which the local authority system was 'infected' through small-scale caremanagement projects. Humberside decided on major restructuring, Hampshire on a 'virus approach'. The MAIN group recognised that whichever approach was adopted there would need to be effective local implementation strategies. These would be characterised by the development of a shared vision about future support to enable people to live in their own homes; building partnerships with users and carers and carrying out a systematic stock taking of the strengths and weaknesses of the assessment processes.

The following list of key issues in implementation emerged from the group's discussions:

1 Moving towards a distinction between purchaser and provider functions within social service departments.
2 Developing clear-cut criteria for targeting services to those most in need.
3 Moving from service-led to client-centred screening and assessment systems.
4 Involving users and carers.
5 Building in quality standards and review procedures as assessment and caremanagement approaches are developed.
6 Devising 'user-centred' information and financial budgeting systems.
7 Ensuring consistency of approach.
8 Staff skills.
9 Working with elected members.

DEVELOPING CRITERIA FOR TARGETING SERVICES TO THOSE MOST IN NEED

It was clear to those who worked on the MAIN project that assessment was a very demanding and time-consuming activity and unless there was agreement on the priorities to be adopted a local authority would quickly find itself unable to cope with the pressure for resources to meet needs. Devon social services undertook extensive consultation to try and target services better and identified three levels of priority.

First priority

Those people who, without the active involvement of the Department, would be in danger of physical and emotional harm.

Second priority

Those people who, without the active intervention of the Department, would be at risk of losing their independence.

Third priority

Those people who, without the active intervention of the Department, would be unable to maintain a satisfactory quality of life.

Devon County Council then undertook pilot studies of a differentiated system of assessment in their seven districts. At the beginning each client received a core assessment, which any professional was equipped to undertake. This could trigger further professional specific assessment where needed. The Devon Core Assessment Guide not only provides a basic assessment instrument for local authority staff, it is also being extensively used by primary health care teams in the county. (The guide is reproduced in Beardshaw, 1991, pp. 17–21.)

CAREMANAGEMENT

Before considering assessment procedures any further it is important to clarify what is meant by 'caremanagement'. Two helpful publications have been produced by the Department of Health, *Care Management and Assessment: Practitioner's Guide* and *Care Management and Assessment: Manager's Guide* (Department of Health Social Services Inspectorate and Scottish Office Social Work Services Group, 1991a, b). These two handbooks provide detailed guidance on the principles and practice of caremanagement and assessment and are invaluable sources of information. The handbooks define caremanagement as follows: 'Care management is the process of tailoring services to individual needs. Assessment is an integral part of care management but it is only one of seven core tasks that make up the whole proceess.' The seven core tasks are:

- publishing information
- determining the level of assessment
- assessing need
- care planning
- implementing the care plan
- monitoring
- reviewing
  (Department of Health Social Services Inspectorate and Scottish Social Work Services Group, 1991a)

The legislative requirement to carry out assessments

Section 47 of the NHS and Community Care Act 1990 places a duty on local authorities to assess the care needs of any person who appears to them to need a community care service and decide in the light of that assessment whether or not they should provide any such service. They are also required to notify other relevant statutory agencies of any community care needs which it appears that other agencies may need to provide.

ASSESSMENT FOR COMMUNITY CARE PLANS

The first priority for local authorities is to establish in negotiation with other care agencies, the assessment arrangements that have to be in place by April 1993. As has already been said, caremanagement makes the needs and wishes of users and carers central to the caring process. The needs-led approach aims to tailor services to meet individual requirements. I shall discuss the importance of establishing assessment as a separate function in its own right which should be monitored against explicit standards of performance.

The importance of separating assessment from care delivery

It is generally agreed that assessment is best achieved where practitioners responsible for assessment do not also carry responsibility for the delivery or management of services arising from that assessment. Assessment should be established as a separate organisational function that is not tied to any services or set of services.

Determining the level of assessment

I do not need to give a detailed account of the levels of assessment envisaged in the new system. The *Practitioner's Guide* (Department of Health Social Services Inspectorate and Scottish Office Social Work Services Group, 1991a) provides an excellent and very clear account of various steps in arranging an assessment. The type of assessment response will normally be related as closely as possible to the presenting need. However, where the person appears to be 'disabled' under the terms of the Disabled Persons (SCR) Act 1986 the local authority is required to offer a comprehensive assessment, irrespective of the scale of need that is initially presented. Table 11.1 briefly sets out the proposed levels of assessment.

The first level of assessment (simple level) is one that could be undertaken by a receptionist or administrative clerk. It might, for example, be concerned with the issue of a bus pass. The second level (limited assessment) might be undertaken by a vocationally qualified member of staff, for example, in relation to the need for basic domiciliary support. The third level involves the same type of staff but perhaps from more than one agency. The fourth

Table 11.1 Levels of assessment of care need

Type of assessment	Needs
Simple assessment	Simple, defined
Limited assessment	Limited, defined, low risk
Multiple assessment	Range of limited, defined low risk
Specialist assessment	
• simple	Defined, specialist, low risk
• complex	Ill-defined, complex, high risk
Complex assessment	Ill-defined, interrelated, complex, volatile, high risk
Comprehensive assessment	Ill-defined, multiple, interrelated, high risk, severe

level will involve specialist staff at an ancillary grade while the fifth and sixth levels will require professional specialist assessment.

It is intended that assessment procedures will be combined into one integrated process bringing together the contributions from all relevant care agencies, so that the needs of the individual are considered as a whole.

CONCLUSION

Is a seamless service an attainable goal? Has it been possible to incorporate assessment and caremanagement into the ordinary routines of social services departments? How will other agencies respond to the demands of this style of working?

My guess is that those local authorities which have successfully achieved a split between their purchasing and providing roles will have little difficulty in taking assessment and caremanagement on board as an effective way of targeting their resources and of making a reality of user and carer involvement. Those authorities which are still struggling with their purchaser/ provider split are not going to get much help from caremanagement until they resolve their underlying structural problems. As Brandon has commented: 'Most organisations are constipated by their own history . . . and facilitate the identification of all the hidden agendas, power games, relationships, which block more user-based strategies. It takes courage to tackle issues which are personally and structurally so full of fear' (Brandon, 1991, p. 51). Let us hope that some of you have the courage to free up the log jam.

REFERENCES

Beardshaw V. (1991) *Implementing Assessment and Care Management: Learning from Local Experience 1990–1991*. London: King's Fund College.
Beardshaw V. and Towell D. (1991) *Assessment and Case Management: Implications for the Implementation of 'Caring for People'*. London: King's Fund Institute.
Brandon D. (1991) The implications of normalisation work for professional skills. In

(ed.) Ramon S. *Beyond Community Care*, London: Macmillan in association with MIND.

Brandon D. and Towe N. (1989) *Free to Choose: An Introduction to Service Brokerage*. London: Good Impressions.

Bronfenbrenner, U. (1979) *The Ecology of Human Development: Experiments by Nature and Design*. Cambridge, MA: Harvard University Press.

Department of Health (1989) *Caring for People: Community Care in the Next Decade and Beyond*. London: Department of Health.

Department of Health (1990) *Caring for People: Community Care in the Next Decade and Beyond. Draft Guidance: Assessment and Case Management*. London: Department of Health.

Department of Health and Social Services Inspectorate and Scottish Office Social Work Services Group (1991a) *Care Management and Assessment: Practitioner's Guide*. London: HMSO.

Department of Health Social Services Inspectorate and Scottish Office Social Work Services Group (1991b) *Care Management and Assessment: Manager's Guide*. London: HMSO.

Mount B. (1987) Personal futures planning. University of Georgia (unpublished manuscript).

O'Brien J. and Mount B. (1991) Telling new stories: the search for capacity among people with severe handicaps. In (eds) Meyer L. H., Peck C. A. and Brown L. *Critical Issues in the Lives of People with Disabilities*. Baltimore: Paul H. Brookes.

Rao N. (1991) Policy issues. In (ed.) Ramon S. *Beyond Community Care*. London: Macmillan, in association with MIND.

Simons K. and Russell O. (1991) Service brokerage in Bristol. *Llais* 20: 17–19.

12 Assessment methods and professional directions

James Hogg

CASE MANAGEMENT FORM AND CONTENT

There can be little doubt that at the service delivery end of the operation, case management has been seen as a means to the effective management of resources. In a sense, case management might be evaluated as standing or falling by whether or not the process delivers with respect to effective resource management. In this, case management bears the stamp of the business orientation and philosophy that has engendered the approach. Some critics, such as Jack (1992), have suggested the essential political aims of case management are ideological, i.e. 'to reduce public expenditure . . . and . . . dismantling the 'inefficient' state monopoly of health and welfare provision'

The concept of a case manager has been introduced as a professional advocate to undertake or arrange individual assessments of need, and to plan and arrange the provision of the most appropriate and economic package of care; co-ordinated monitored and reviewed.

(National Development Team, 1991, p. 5)

Care management is the process of tailoring services to individual needs. Assessment is an integral part of care management but it is only one of seven core tasks that make up the whole process.

(Scottish Department of Health Social Service Inspectorate & Scottish Office Social Work Services Group, 1991, p. 5)

There is no widely accepted definition of case management. Generically case management refers to any method linking, managing or co-ordinating services to meet individual need.

(Beardshaw and Towell, 1990)

Figure 12.1 Selected 'definitions' of assessment in the process of case management
Source: Jack (1992)

(Jack, 1992, p. 5). Thus Jack argues, case management is an ideologically loaded strategy that smacks more of the trade fair than welfare.

But, it can be argued, human values are placed at the heart of this process as represented in that deceptively simple word 'need'. 'Need' is everywhere to be found in discussions of case management:

> The concept of a case manager has been introduced as a professional advocate to undertake or arrange individual assessments of need and to plan and arrange the provision of the most appropriate and economic package of care; co-ordinated monitored and reviewed.
>
> (National Development Team, 1991, p. 5)

To the question 'What is care management?' the Scottish Department of Health Social Service Inspectorate gives need a central place: 'Care management is the process of tailoring services to individual needs. Assessment is an integral part of caremanagement but it is only one of seven core tasks that make up the whole process' (Scottish Department of Health Social Service Inspectorate and Scottish Office Social Work Services Group, 1991, p. 5). Even where definitions of case management are not explicit, 'need' is in evidence: 'There is no widely accepted definition of case management. Generically case management refers to any method linking, managing or co-ordinating services to meet individual need' (Beardshaw and Towell, 1990).

The place of needs assessment may be seen clearly in the cycle of case management i.e (1) publication of service on offer: (2) the preliminary identification of need determines the level of assessment required; (3) assessment of need is then undertaken; (4) followed by case planning; (5) implementation of the case plan; (6) monitoring of its success and, (7) review.

My task here is to focus on assessment as a central component of the process of case management. To do this I should like to begin with some brief reflections on the ideologies that have given such impetus to the familiar components of our present service orientation, ideologies of normalisation and social role valorisation, and the orientation of community care, de-institutionalisation, least restrictive environments and the provision of valued options. I will then move on to suggest that it is in developments in the way in which we look at and assess quality of life that we will find the most unambiguous and broadly based approach to need assessment. With respect to those who use services, I intend to focus on adults with intellectual disabilities and, in order to have a concrete example of services, to consider specifically day and leisure services in particular. However, the principles that I am going to discuss can readily be applied to other populations and types of service provision, and the choice of adults and day and leisure services is simply to give a context to some of the observations I will be making.

QUALITY OF LIFE: BEYOND NORMALISATION

A quality of life (QOL) approach offers us the chance to avoid some of the pitfalls that have emerged in trying to develop our service entirely in the light of normalisation philosophy and its successor, social role valorisation (Wolfensberger, 1985). My own belief is that though these philosophies have had great significance in encouraging important changes in service philosophy and provision, they are in practical terms often ambiguous and open to damaging misinterpretations. In addition, they are too preoccupied with the image of how service settings should appear rather than the substance of people's experiences. Nevertheless, in broad terms, the introduction of the concept of social role valorisation, as an intended clarification of normalisation, placed the issue of value and its nature firmly on the agenda. The concept, while providing a general direction to the way in which services should be developed, however, characteristically overemphasises image and competence rather than taking its starting point in the history, experiences and psychological reality of the people with whom we are concerned. In order to develop services which take into account both objective social values and this subjective reality, we must turn to recent developments in the way in which we think about, analyse and assess QOL in general and in relation to people with intellectual disabilities in particular.

A number of authors have recently come to the conclusion that 'QOL may soon replace normalization, community adjustment and deinstitutionalization as a guiding principle in the design, delivery and evaluation of services for persons with disabilities and their families' (Goode, 1989, p. 337). Goode (1988a, p. 1) also makes the link between the QOL concept and the concept of need which is central to this chapter: 'The importance of the QOL concept as both a needs assessment tool and as a criterion evaluation measure is well documented.' Indeed, 'monitoring', phase 6 of the cycle noted above, clearly entails just such criterion evaluation measures.

However, let us not pretend that the way in which we think about and analyse QOL is a simple matter. The complexity of QOL assessment has been amply illustrated in the excellent *Quality of Life for Persons with Disabilities* study undertaken by David Goode (1988) in the Mental Retardation Institute at Westchester County Medical Centre in New York. Goode has thoroughly reviewed the literature of QOL and shown the number of different areas in which QOL has been considered. Figure 12.2 shows the seven major areas. Goode's scheme of QOL concepts embraces social indicators, life domains, life events, psychological concepts, psycho-social concepts, the judgement of overall QOL, as well as behavioural outcomes (Figure 12.3).

In assessing QOL attention must be given to both objective and subjective indicators. Thus mortality/morbidity in a society, income, even a social network, may all be objectively assessed and shown to bear on QOL.

In contrast, subjective indicators are responses made by an individual bearing on her or his own judgements. They would include the global

Social indicators	Life domain	Life events	Psychological concepts	Psycho-social concepts	Overall QOL	Behaviour outcome
Community						
Mortality/ morbidity	Family life Neighbourhood	Divorce Illness	Coping Self-esteem	Social contact Social supports: – emotional concerns or caring – instrumental aid – informational aid – appraisal aid	Self-assessment of overall life satisfaction Satisfaction by life domain	Social interaction Community involvement Environmental control
Standard of living	Leisure activities	Marriage Retirement	Frequency and intensity of positive and negative affect			Independence
	Religious faith	Moving	Negative affect – restlessness – loneliness – boredom – depression – anxiety	Stress Social supports	Satisfaction by life concerns	Productivity
Individual						
Income	Education			Positive social interaction	Cognitive assessment of the importance of various life domains or concerns	Community integration
Health status	Social contact					
Marital status	Friendship		Positive affect – excitement – pride			

Figure 12.2 Scheme of concepts related to quality of life

Social indicators

Community	*Individual*
Physicians per thousand	Age
No hospital beds	Gender
Emloyment rate	Race
Mortality/morbidity	Income
Rate of violent crime	Education
Standard of living	Religion
Size of city	Health status
	Marital status

Life domain

Housing	Self
Income	Community organisations
Family life	Aggression
Neighbourhood	Social contact
National government	Friendship
Job/employment	Mobility
Leisure activities	Transportation
Religious faith	Financial security
Education	Food/eating
Health	Sleep
Safety	Beauty
Independence	Clothing
Natural environment	Affluence
Standard of living	Activity
	Freedom

Life events

New job	Birth/death of a child
Divorce	Retirement
Illness	Moving
Marriage	

Psychological concepts

Coping
Problem-solving capabilities
Assertiveness
Performance of role domains
Self-esteem
Frequency and intensity of positive and negative affect

Negative affect	– restlessness
	– loneliness
	– boredom
	– depression
	– anxiety
Positive affect	– excitement
	– pride

Anxiety
Depression

Figure 12.3 Concepts related to quality of life (*cont. overleaf*)

Control of others
Mental status   – self-esteem
                               – sense of purpose
                               – personal involvement
                               – insecurity

Psycho-social concepts

Social contact
Social supports   – emotional concerns or
                                 caring
                               – instrumental aid
                               – informational aid
                               – appraisal aid
Self-assessments of performance capabilities,
role demands, individual needs and aspirations
Stress   – role ambiguity
                               – negative life events
                               – social conflict
Social supports   Material aid
                               Behavioural assistance
                               Intimate interaction
                               Guidance
                               Feedback
                               Positive social
                               interaction
                               – control over one's life
                               – control others have
                                 over one's life
                               – performance in
                                 personal life

Overall quality of life

Self-assessment of overall life satisfaction
Satisfaction by life domain
Satisfaction by life concerns
Cognitive assessment of the importance of various
domains or concerns

Behaviour outcome

Social interaction   Independence
Community involvement   Productivity
Environmental control   Community integration

Figure 12.3 Concepts related to quality of life: social indicators; life domain; life events; psychological concepts; psycho-social concepts; overall quality of life; behaviour outcome

indicators under 'Overall quality of life', such as feelings of self-esteem, the expression of negative emotions and so forth. This idea of subjective indicators relates well to the growing emphasis on choice by service users and the contribution of their own aspirations to the development of services, whether through self-advocacy or other means. Goode integrates objective and subjective determinants of QOL within an ecological perspective in which the individual in interaction with the social and physical environment experiences a given level of QOL, with resulting behavioural outcomes. He characterises this model as 'client driven, ecological and consistent with the theoretical models'.

Such ecological models have been familiar in both the literature on disability and the lives of elderly people and are familiar in the diagrams of nested ecologies illustrated in Figure 12.4.

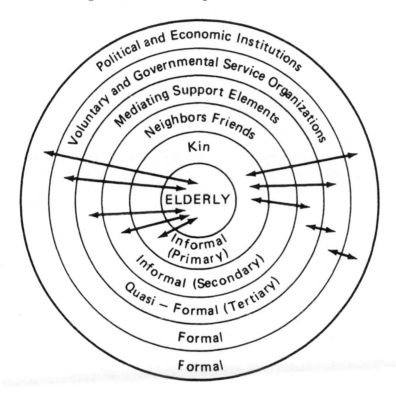

Figure 12.4 Nested ecology model: illustrating relationships with family, friends, services and wider societal factors
Source: Cantor and Little (1985)

Here relations with family and friends are clearly indicated, as are the service elements and indeed the wider societal factors that will condition the availability of resources. As Goode (1988) notes, QOL is intrinsically related to QOL of others within his or her environment, most immediately those in the family, but also friends and significant others.

As in Figure 12.3, Goode's own model places the service user's subjective perception of the resources and demands within the environment and the subjective perception of his/her personal needs. To describe in more detail this model is beyond the scope of this chapter, but I trust that the broad principles underlying the model are clear.

As Goode states: the achievement of a good QOL is 'experienced when a person's basic needs are met and when he or she has the opportunity to pursue and achieve goals in major life settings' (Goode, 1988).

QOL AND SERVICE PROVISION

For any given area of service provision – and here I am using 'service provision' to cover any form of statutory or voluntary service as well as financial support through benefits – we have to assess needs within the broad categories indicated. The emphasis will shift depending upon the needs involved in relation to a given area of service provision. To illustrate this, I am going to take the complex of activities which we refer to as day and leisure service and relate these to QOL assessments. We could consider other forms of service, e.g., residential provision, mental and physical health input and so on. However, my own immediate concerns have pointed me in the direction of such services.

The life domain relevant to day and leisure services will be broadly based and might include education, social contacts, religious activities and so on, i.e., the full spectrum of community involvement that goes beyond immediate family life. Assessment of need would be undertaken with respect to the person's expressed views in relation to a range of psychological and psycho-social concepts, notably their self-assessment of their own performance and capabilities and their needs and aspirations with respect to specific activities. Clearly stress and negative affect will suggest increased support or fundamental change in the person's life, while excitement and pride will provide us with pointers to future developments. Assessment may extend to mental health through psychological or psychiatric interviews with the individuals themselves or their carers. The techniques for relating mental health assessments to QOL evaluation as a means of assessing need are beginning to emerge (e.g. Moss and Patel, 1991) and point up the fact that many of the assessments implied in this model require the development of specific instruments relevant to local needs and expertise.

Goode (1988) has integrated the complex of concepts derived from QOL studies across the range of settings: home, community, school, care and medical, given that in some measure a person's home may be seen as the departure point for much leisure activity, and that the community will by and large embrace both leisure activities and day services, i.e. two elements from Goode's (1988) analysis.

I said earlier that Goode's integration of QOL concepts was essentially ecological. This implies, then, the matching of client needs to environmental resources across four domains defined by Goode, i.e., economic, social, political and cultural, implying the need for financial stability, supportive emotional relationships, political equity and cultural resources. In certain obvious ways, the content of the two environments, home and community, will be contrasted, e.g., the emphasis on living with family members in the one instance and peer interaction in the other. Prior to establishing such a match, it is first necessary to determine an individual's aspirations with respect to such resources and expose them to options if choice is to be meaningful and if the kind of engagement experienced is to offer fulfilment and progression.

Both objective and subjective assessment of needs will lead to the development of the overall day and leisure programme formulated by the case manager and will contribute to the reviews which permit monitoring. Outcome measures of the kind listed by Goode (1988) will also be employed to this end. As a psychologist, I am naturally particularly intrigued by the psychological dimensions of this process of need assessment and the expression of the views and feelings of those for whom services are being provided. While having a behavioural orientation I am quite comfortable with objective measurements of, for example, social engagement or improvements in adaptive behaviour. I also increasingly feel the need to begin to pose questions about the quality of the engagement people experience in their lives. At this point, therefore, I would like to focus down still further and consider the issues of choice and what I am going to call 'creative engagement'. What I mean by 'creative engagement' will become clearer in what follows. I am going to relate the idea particularly to leisure, but bear in mind that the ideas involved in considering engagement might be applicable to a wide range of day service activities and even to employment.

SOME PSYCHOLOGICAL DIMENSIONS OF QUALITY OF LIFE

It will be clear from the foregoing that the exercise of choice is crucial to the QOL model proposed by Goode (1988) and central to the assessment of needs required in the case management strategy. While many pay lip service to the right of people with intellectual disabilities to choose, the exercise of choice has increasingly raised major concerns for both service providers and parents, challenging them to respond to outcomes that may be practically and ethically inimical to them. Is choice an absolute right, even where certain choices are 'objectively' damaging to an individual or to others? Is there a point at which a limit on assumed responsibility is imposed and adults intervene with other adults whom they assume not to be exercising choice responsibly? In a recent paper by Bannerman *et al.* (1990) with the title 'Balancing the right to habilitation with the right to personal liberties: the rights of people with developmental disabilities to eat too many doughnuts and take a nap', the authors debate this vexed issue. Their conclusions are far from a 'yes' or 'no' answer to the question they have posed. They see choice in a more dynamic framework in which learning to exercise responsible choice becomes an inherent part of the overall curriculum or the service intervention available to a person. The activity of choosing becomes not a static absolute, but part of the process of societal and self-education.

In discussing choice we must also address the issue that conventional, verbal expressions of choice, or even voting with their feet, will not be an option for many people with severe and profound intellectual disabilities. Such people should not be excluded from the process of subjective QOL assessment because of communicative limitations, even though the balance may well tip decisively to 'objective' QOL assessment. Through the use of careful observation of their own idiosyncratic methods of communication, the provision of opportunities, and making time available for such people to respond, choice can be encouraged and services can be made responsive to those with even the most profound disabilities.

Let me turn from the issue of choice in relation to the assessment of needs and begin to consider how we view the quality of the engagement that people experience in a variety of pursuits. I am going to take my cue here from work in the field of leisure provision, but would reiterate – take what is to follow as a model that is applicable much more widely. In a recent book by Brown *et al.* (1989) concerned with the quality of life of adults with intellectual disabilities, the authors refer to the differential functions which can be served by leisure activities and which should provide a more differentiated context for assisting choice of a balanced and fulfilling pattern of leisure activity. These authors draw on Nash's (1953) *Philosophy of Recreation and Leisure*, a book that, while at times raising a smile, invites us to look more closely at the nature and challenge of the growing availability of leisure time in western society.

In an accompanying illustration, Nash shows a progression of leisure and occupation from negative pursuits – crime – and being a mere spectator, through performance of other people's creations and on to creative production and beyond. He also provides an abstract account of his scheme which is helpful and interesting, illustrated in Figure 12.5.

On the left of Figure 12.5 a scale runs from sub-zero, through zero up to 4 and on to infinity. He comments, 'A little of each above zero, depending on work patterns, may be good, but too many activities low on the scale are dulling and in the end progress and development of the individual and group are retarded' (Nash, 1953).

Acts performed against society form the lowest level. The examples Nash gives are ones which relate closely to some of the recent events in England, as he is talking about antisocial behaviour as a form of distorted leisure activity. He would certainly see the events in Blackbird Leys and Meadow Well and, more recently, Coventry, in this light. 'Hotting' may not be our idea of a leisure pursuit, but according to those who enjoy the activity, what is important is the 'buzz' it gives them in a life which lacks the opportunity for creative engagement in other fields, or where the opportunity for such engagement is not perceived.

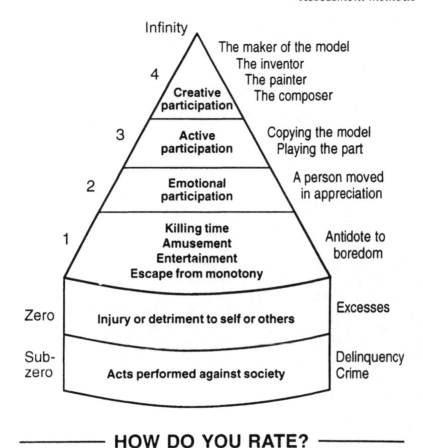

Infinity

The maker of the model
The inventor

4

The painter

Creative
participation

The composer

3

Active
participation

Copying the model
Playing the part

2

Emotional
participation

A person moved
in appreciation

1

Killing time
Amusement
Entertainment
Escape from monotony

Antidote to
boredom

Zero

Injury or detriment to self or others

Excesses

Sub-
zero

Acts performed against society

Delinquency
Crime

—————— HOW DO YOU RATE? ——————

Figure 12.5 Use of leisure time participation broadly interpreted
Source: Nash (1953)

If these sub-zero activities are very unlikely to be undertaken by people with severe and profound intellectual disability, not so Nash's zero level of 'Injury or detriment to self'. Emerson (1992) reports figures for self-injurious behaviour in institutional settings in the UK of up to 15 per cent, though lower figures for less restrictive settings. In the MENCAP PRMH Project survey (Hogg and Lambe, 1988) of people with profound and multiple disabilities, 22 per cent of adults' parents reported their son or daughter did 'physical violence to self'. The comparable figure for 'destruction to property' was 14 per cent. Also high on their lists were the self-stimulatory and stereotyped behaviours that act as a barrier to any kind of creative engagement with the world around, exhibited by over 40 per cent of adults with profound disabilities. While there is no one, simple, explanation for such behaviour, there can be little doubt that absence of stimulation from and interaction with the world do play their part in some cases.

Entertainment, amusement, escape from monotony, then, though forming only the above-ground base of Nash's (1953) pyramid, might well provide one such form of engagement. We know from several surveys that have been undertaken, that it is activities at this level that constitute the primary leisure pursuits for so many people with intellectual disabilities (Cheseldine and Jeffree, 1981). Watching television, or listening to music, invariably figure large in such reports. But such essentially passive activities also constitute a central part of use of free time for many of us. Nash has a sub-scale here that runs from 'killing time', to 'escape from monotony' to 'amusement' to 'entertainment'. The overall aim of all of these is an antidote to boredom. There is nothing inherently wrong with avoiding boredom. Certainly, if we can assist people with disabilities to develop strategies that avoid boredom, this would be a notable success, particularly if success were reflected in reduction or elimination of self-destructive behaviour.

In addition, we must take care to discriminate between psychological differences that may be detected in engagement in even the same activity, e.g., watching television. Argyle reports that in the wider population, people who watch a great deal of television emerge as a somewhat unsatisfied group of people, though those who watch soap operas seriously tend to be a much happier group. Argyle comments: 'People come to know the characters even though they are fictional. There is a tight supportive group and people feel they belong to this. It's like having a set of secondhand friends' (*Guardian*, 21 September 1991). The reality of *Neighbours*, let alone *Prisoner*, for many people with and without intellectual disabilities is apparent from the intensity and complexity with which events and personalities are discussed, episode by episode.

Psychologically, this point bears on what I believe Nash (1953) intended when he made the distinction between what is essentially passive enjoyment of 'entertainment' and active emotional participation while listening to music, going to the theatre, etc.

This distinction is crucially important in relation to leisure provision and creative occupation for people with intellectual disability. The last few years have seen exciting developments in the field of multi-sensory stimulation. What is urgently needed is a greater understanding of the kind of engagement in which people are involved when they enjoy such activities. There is no inherent reason why placing someone in a room which has cost tens of thousands of pounds to prepare, should be any more or less meaningful than sitting them in front of a television set. Only by understanding intimately the personality, the sensory strengths and the way in which the person communicates emotional experiences, can we begin to utilise these developments in a way which takes us from mere antidotes to boredom, to what Nash calls 'emotional participation'.

Such approaches are equally applicable when we move to Nash's (1953) active participation. Again, Argyle's work, cited above, has shown that people who do actively participate in leisure through sports, choirs, etc. are generally happier than those for whom there are only passive pursuits. There is nothing new in that finding. Particularly in the study of psychological and physical ageing, active involvement in leisure and social activities is one of the best predictors, along with good health and financial security, of successful ageing. Again I would suggest that we need to be sensitive to such contributions to the activity, and not overwhelm the person with excessive support that takes all the initiative from them. Similarly, sensitivity to progress is called for, with our making increasing, if sometimes minutely small, demands on the person.

From such active involvement, Nash (1953) moves to creative participation. Psychologists have traditionally proposed two varieties of creativity. One is creativity of the kind I think Nash has in mind, i.e. the artist or scientist innovator. We can all take our pick from our own personal first division of all time greats, whether it is Charlie Parker, Mozart, Jane Austen or whoever, people whose original work offers a new vision and serves as a model and influence for others. The second kind of creativity is not linked to the great names but suggests that each of us can be creative within a chosen sphere, doing things which for us are original and involve new perceptions. In this sense much of life can be creative, perhaps particularly so when behaviour is in the early stages of development. In both senses of 'creative' I would suggest that there is nothing to indicate that intellectual disability *per se* precludes such originality or expressivity. There is now a growing body of literature and works by people with intellectual disabilities that endorses such a view.

Helpful though Nash's scheme is, it might usefully be revised to a more democratic model which is non-hierarchical and which acknowledges that non-adaptive behaviour may in varying degrees be a consequence of any level of activity. Figure 12.6 illustrates a suggested revision.

The hierarchical structure has been removed, though Nash's four areas of activity are retained. Movement between them, however, is within a single plane reflecting that we can move between any pair and that all areas will contribute to our overall pattern of leisure time. I have increased the area of the circle as we move round it, with creative participation given greater weight than killing time, etc. The lower circle is intended to indicate that any of the categories of engagement can have detrimental consequences. Even creative participation is not entirely dissociated in some instances from self-destructive behaviour, whether through excessive drug and alcohol intake by a Charlie Parker or a Chet Atkins, or destruction of the nasal passages through paint fumes by the painter Paul Klee. However, the probability of such maladaptive behaviour is greatest in the 'Killing time' category, as reflected in the difference between the upper and lower circles, and is least in the case of creative participation.

In assisting people to plan both their obligated and non-obligated time, I would like to suggest that such a scheme could provide a useful heuristic for professionals in a number of ways with respect to development of a range of

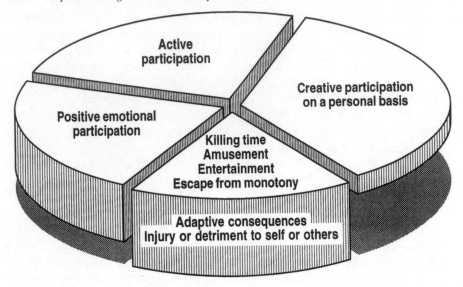

Figure 12.6 Use and significance of leisure time

day and leisure services. First, how does the range we identify potentially provide for experiences at the different levels of engagement described by Nash? By exposing adults with intellectual disabilities to such a wide repertoire of activities they will be in a position to make informed choices which have significant psychological consequences for them.

Second, evaluation of the significance of leisure activities for individuals can be undertaken on a psychologically and socially more meaningful level. Bear in mind the psychological concepts selected from Goode's (1988) QOL conceptual scheme earlier, i.e. self-esteem, and avoidance of negative affect, i.e. restlessness, loneliness, boredom, depression and anxiety and positive affect, i.e. excitement and pride. Recall, too, the psycho-social concepts of social contacts and support, stress and positive social interaction.

PROFESSIONAL DIRECTIONS

In relation to the professional context in which we now all work, our activities are inextricably bound up with the processes of case management. I began by noting the criticism that some will argue that this approach is excessively business orientated, and the human values that have led many into the field of human services are in danger of getting lost. This may well prove to be the case. Even at the level of business efficiency there are substantial studies questioning the success of the approach. Be this as it may, I have tried to suggest in this chapter where, in relation to assessment and monitoring, human values lie. I have dealt with the issue at two levels. First, I have considered the very rich and complex area of QOL and its many dimensions. I urged that we look at the psychological reality of choice and of the nature of creative engagement with their world by people with intellectual disabilities.

In Goode's (1988) final recommendations he addresses a number of issues that arise from the needs orientation underlying QOL assessment. I will take these as my starting point for considering professional directions that arise from QOL assessment in case management.

'The entire concept of service provision has to be redefined around individual needs and with QOL as a service outcome' (Goode, 1988)

This point clearly restates the requirement for needs-led, rather than service-led, provision. This implies the development of service models that at least minimise the inevitable pressure to service-led provision. What, for example, will be the consequence of the long-stay hospitals gaining trust status? Can such a development do other than accentuate this pressure? A recent social services proposal in the North West of England aimed to concentrate several hundred adults in a single day service facility. How could *this* lead to a needs-led service? And yet I will guarantee that whether a trust hospital or a mega-Adult Training Centre, the vast majority of service providers will claim that they are working in line with normalisation principles, believe in service users' choice, and are aiming to enhance quality of life. The implication of the conflict between service models and QOL values is clearly captured when Goode notes: 'Rather than adopting the notion of an ever more normal continuum of vocational and residential services, providers should aim at achieving a relatively stable, self-selected life style for consumers.' A further recommendation from Goode bears on attitudes and orientation:

'Providers need training in a QOL, value-based orientation to service delivery' (Goode, 1988)

The need here is to develop such training. Goode's QOL model could well provide suitable modules focusing on the various elements in the system that contribute to the assessment of needs. Such training should extend to managers. On some fronts work needs to be developed from a research base. The use of observational techniques to assess quality of life and response to services in non-verbal individuals with profound disabilities has a potential to contribute here. As a component of this research the use of such techniques by service providers is a central issue, and will in due course provide a wider assessment of QOL for this group. Such an approach could in time become one component of a wider training scheme. It is also related to a further recommendation by Goode, i.e.:

'A methodological approach should be taken to developing client-centred instruments and procedures to determine individual QOL needs' (Goode, 1988)

In the United States, Goode noted, such an approach awaits development. What is required here in the UK is a working party that could draw together the existing but fragmented approaches, integrate them, and evaluate them in field settings. Such an approach would need to be integrated into the wider case management system at both the assessment and monitoring levels. In due course such a system would feed back into the training of service providers envisaged above.

CONCLUDING COMMENT

I must point out that I have only scratched the service with respect to the complex of topics that emerge in Goode's recommendation from the Quality of Life Project. I have tried to select those that are of immediate relevance to professional development with respect to assessment and monitoring with regard to case management. I myself fluctuate between enthusiasm as to what might be achievable within this approach as informed by QOL concepts, and despair that the gap between what we know and the resources needed to implement QOL-orientated services is so great. On the more optimistic side, this orientation does have the potential to enable those who came into services with humanistic, person-centred intentions, to pursue such activities in a financially and managerially sound framework.

REFERENCES

Bannerman, D.J., Sheldon, J.B., Sherman, J.A. and Harchick, A.E. (1990) Balancing the right to habilitation with the right to personal liberties: The rights of people with developmental disabilities to eat too many doughnuts and take a nap, *Journal of Applied Behavior Analysis*, 23, 79–89.

Beardshaw, V. and Towell, D. (1990) *Assessment and Case Management*, King's Fund, London.

Brown, R.I., Bayer, M.B. and MacFarlane, C. (1989) *Rehabilitation Programmes: Performance and quality of life of adults with developmental disabilities*, Lugus, Toronto.

Cantor, M. and Little V. (1985) Aging and social care, in R.M. Binstock and E. Shanas (eds) *Handbook of Aging and Social Sciences, second edition*, Van Nostrand Reinhold, New York.

Cheseldine, S. and Jeffree, D. (1981) Mentally handicapped adolescents: Their use of leisure, *Journal of Mental Deficiency Research*, 25, 49–59.

Emerson, E. (1992) Self-injurious behaviour: an overview of recent trends in epidemiological and behavioural research, *Mental Handicap Research*, 5, 49–81.

Goode, D.A. (1988) *Quality of Life Persons with Disabilities: A review and synthesis of the literature*, The Mental Retardation Institute, Westchester County Medical Centre and New York Medical College, New York.

Goode, D.A. (1989) Quality of life and quality of work life, in W.E. Kiernan and

R.L. Schalock (eds) *Economics, Industry and Economy: A look ahead*, Paul H. Brookes, Baltimore.

Hogg, J. and Lambe, L. (1988) *Sons and Daughters with Profound Retardation and Multiple Handicaps Attending Schools and Social Education Centres: Final report*, MENCAP, London.

Jack, R. (1992) Case management and social services: Welfare or trade fare? *Journal of the British Society of Gerontology*, 2, 4–6.

Moss, S.C. and Patel, P. (1991) *Psychiatric and Physical Morbidity in Older People with Severe Mental Handicap*, Hester Adrian Research Centre, The University, Manchester.

Nash, J.B. (1953) *Philosophy of Recreation and Leisure*, C.V. Mosby, St. Louis.

National Development Team (1991) *The Andover Case Management Team*, National Development Team, London.

Scottish Department of Health Social Service Inspectorate and Scottish Office Social Work Services Group (1991) *Care Management and Assessment: Practitioners' Guide*, SSI and SWSG, Edinburgh.

Wolfsenberger, W. (1985) An overview of social role valorization and some reflections on elderly mentally retarded persons, in M.P. Janicki and H.M. Wisniewski (eds) *Aging and Developmental Disabilities: Issues and approaches*, Paul H. Brookes, Baltimore MD, pp. 61-76.

13 Community care plans: starting and finishing with individuals

Derek Thomas

INTRODUCTION

Community care planning process is a central mechanism in government proposals to improve community care. Responsibility for leading this is clearly located with local authority social services departments – in collaboration with other local authority departments and the health service.

What is important about community care planning is not just the preparation of public plans and strategy documents, but the development of a process of planning at a level that is integrated with, and arises from, our work with individuals. It is for this reason that I selected the title – 'Starting and Finishing with Individuals'.

There are five important questions:

1 Why is there an interest in user involvement at the present?
2 Why is it important/essential – what are the potential benefits?
3 How might this be done – what form could/should this involvement take?
4 What are we learning about this process?

WHY THE CURRENT INTEREST?

The Government's White Paper, *Caring for People* (1990) has provided extra legitimacy and impetus to the idea that those who use the services should have a say in their design and development and also in the maintenance and enhancement of quality.

These principles reflect various beliefs that developed during the 1970s and 1980s during a period of some growth. For example, beliefs that:

- more service did not necessarily mean better service . . . and that what was really needed was greater flexibility;
- public agencies were not sufficiently accountable for their use of public money and that those who used or might at some time use these services have a right to expect certain standards (in terms of quality and quantity). These have latterly been described as 'Charter Rights' and 'Charter Standards';

- the analysis of needs offered by professionals and their view of the services required could not be trusted;
- and a belief that many professionals were not prepared to listen to disabled people or properly involve them in key decisions about their lives or the services provided.

WHY IS IT ESSENTIAL?

Firstly, community care planning should be conceptualised as being not just about care services. It should instead be about the part to be played by public agencies in promoting participation in our communities by some people who have been seriously disadvantaged. This disadvantage initially took the form of marginalisation and exclusion. Latterly, the devaluation has taken the form of what has been called 'privileged charity' (arising in this country and elsewhere from the poor law).

Secondly, we have not yet learnt to distinguish person-to-person support from the buildings in which that support is provided. The latter should be viewed not as the service (look at the language we use: 'the Government has increased the number of ATCs or ATC places by . . .'; 'hostel places increased by . . .' – rather than 'we have increased this number of people in person-to-person support roles by . . .').

Key questions that arise from these viewpoints then become:

- How can people with learning disabilities 'in' services regain control of their lives?
- How can their differentness be celebrated and their contribution maximised?
- How can the major barriers to ordinary living, work and relationships be reduced and eventually removed?

These questions are important because only the users can know what he or she likes, what he or she wants less of and what he or she wants more of.

Our task as professionals or service providers is to listen and discover these things, to help identify and remove barriers, whether within the person or the environment: also to provide advice, technical assistance and where needed the necessary person-to-person support.

Therefore, whatever else, the community care plan is an essentially individual business. It should start, continue and finish with the individual.

HOW SHOULD THIS CONTRIBUTION BE MADE? WHAT ARE THE OPPORTUNITIES?

The first opportunities arise when services are being designed and redesigned. Those who use services should be the first to be asked what results or outcomes they want. The services have no justification in themselves. They are a means to an end and those ends are best defined by those who use the services.

But we can also ask what those who use the services like and don't like about existing services. The 'likes' give us clues about elements in the new service that should be retained: also if provided with additional information and/or experience, people can express preferences about new elements that could be incorporated in the new services.

This can take place as part of an individual planning process or as part of more general service design exercises involving groups of users. The world of qualitative market research regularly uses such approaches as part of the fact finding and analysis it offers to its clients.

The 'participation events' that are being organised in various parts of the country are providing important insights. But we need to ensure that this information and these views are fed back into general service planning.

Secondly users can and are getting involved in shaping policy agendas and in influencing policy direction. Many of the most powerful examples are to be found in North America and Canada – where self-advocacy is more developed, for example: the Canadian Association for Community Living demonstrated that users could influence their own agency's stand on sterilisation, on labels; they also influenced national policy statements by the Canadian Government and their approaches to dissemination/collaboration.

Amongst the examples of these important initiatives emerging in this country are:

- The development of People First groups;
- MENCAP's planned relaunch with new logo;
- North Western RHA – consultation with users on the Department of Health's latest policy drafts and the preparation of a video response.

People with learning disabilities are also now contributing to the selection of staff either indirectly, assisting with the preparation of job descriptions or more directly in the interview process. They are also making contributions to staff training.

Finally, examples are emerging of people contributing in various ways to the quality assurance process. Here are a number of possibilities:

- contribution to contract specification;
- contribution – on-going monitoring of services;
- contribution to external review teams.

Much of this need not be very costly in financial terms. However, there are practical and financial arrangements to be made in terms of salary/fees, travel, communication and personal support. The costs of not involving those who use our services are considerable. We will leave people locked in services – albeit 'community service' – locked in poverty.

Cost-efficiency judgements or value for money judgements will become meaningless because they are our judgements about value and effectiveness not theirs.

The potential benefits are immense. The process itself is – if done properly: EMPOWERING, SKILLING, VALUING OF INDIVIDUALS. It will, over time, reverse the processes of devaluation and discrimination that have been ever present. It is renewing and engaging for us as professionals in that it forces us to re-assess our beliefs, our values, our attitudes and our practices.

However, if the agency context is not right in terms of values, organisational culture, management style and resources and the process will become frustrating for users and their new enablers/advocates and may be attacked as 'idealistic', 'non-pragmatic' or 'too costly'.

WHAT ARE WE LEARNING?

We are learning that community care planning to date lacks connectedness with the views and lives of those who use services, and they are not being involved properly. The benefits – when planning is occurring – are considerable. The process is empowering, it helps users develop important skills and competences and it improves their sense of their own worth. It makes local plans and local strategy better.

It is not a highly expensive process, but there are financial costs for those who offer their time and expertise.

14 Caremanagement

Ann Richardson

INTRODUCTION

Caremanagement could be seen as the cornerstone of the new community care arrangements for people with learning disabilities, along with other priority groups, as established by the 1990 NHS and Community Care Act. But the idea of caremanagement did not first emerge at that time. It had already been introduced in a few areas of Britain, having been imported from the United States and Canada in the late 1980s. In the field of learning disabilities, perhaps the best-known example is the Wakefield Case Management Project, focused on the move of a number of individuals from long-stay hospital.[1] But there are also other early efforts to use a caremanagement approach in this context, including projects studied by researchers at the Personal Social Services Research Unit in Kent[2] and a project in Winchester for assisting people with learning disabilities in the community (National Development Team, 1991). Other writings on caremanagement also deserve attention (see Onyett, 1992; Pilling, 1992; Beardshaw and Towell, 1990).

This chapter is intended to provide some understanding of what caremanagement means in practice for both users and care managers. It explores in some detail what caremanagement *means*, considers the use of caremanagement in the context of people with learning disabilities and offers a few comments on the policy context.

It should be added here that the term initially in common use was 'case management', based on usage in the United States. In Britain, following arguments that the term was derogatory to service users by implying that they were 'cases to be managed', the confusingly similar term 'caremanagement' was introduced in its place. This term has been almost universally accepted since roughly 1990.

DEFINING CAREMANAGEMENT

A major problem in discussing caremanagement is the terminology used to define it. Most discussions begin with the *tasks*. In social work jargon, caremanagement is said to be about case finding, assessment, planning, co-ordination and monitoring and review. There are two regrettable effects of this language: it makes the process seem inherently mechanistic and it encourages people to dismiss it as nothing new. But caremanagement is far from mechanistic – it requires imagination and enthusiasm, encouraging professionals to really work *with* users. Furthermore, it is not simply new words for old work, but involves a new approach. This turns around the mind-set which says 'let us see what services are available for your needs' to 'let us see what can be arranged to meet your needs'.

In order to describe what caremanagement means in practice, it seemed sensible to devise a new terminology: a 'plain English guide to caremanagement'. First, however, it is important to identify the underlying *purpose* of the exercise. Caremanagement is the process of working with individuals to help them to obtain the services appropriate to their needs. It involves a set of independent but related tasks:

* identifying specific individuals for attention;
* seeking to understand their aims and aspirations;
* working out a plan of action to meet their needs;
* helping to get this plan put into effect; and
* keeping in touch to see how the plan is working (and making an appropriate response).

In addition to this process of working with individuals, a process of service development can (and should) accompany such activity to ensure that services are available to meet identified needs. This means working with agencies who might be able to provide such services for the individuals involved.

THE PROCESS OF CAREMANAGEMENT

A few short comments need to be added here on the five stages of caremanagement. The first is identifying those to whom it will be applied. This requires the development of some criteria for involvement and selecting individuals within these criteria. Both potential users and those who might provide advice to them need to know where to go to begin – or to inquire about – the process. This stage has particularly important implications for issues of *equity* – who receives and who does not receive the considerable attention entailed by a caremanagement approach.

The second stage involves determining individual needs and aspirations. This means working closely with users, talking to others (such as carers) where appropriate and producing a written statement of the user's needs and aspirations. A user-led approach means that decisions should arise as much as possible from users themselves and not be imposed from outside. This stage essentially sets the scene for all further work with each service user.

The third stage is making a plan for each individual, based on the written statement. The appropriate service response to the identified needs must be considered, options investigated and then costed to check that resources are available. The nature of the plan will differ according to the individual's needs; it may be highly complex or relatively simple. In some circumstances, there will be a need to assist the development of new services, in both the statutory sector and beyond.

The fourth stage is effecting change on the basis of the plan. Negotiations are required with service providers to obtain the necessary help and a contract set up on behalf of the individual user. Effecting such change is necessarily dependent on the services available and the response of providers to specific requests. The service development role is particularly crucial here.

The final stage of caremanagement entails checking that plans remain appropriate to the user's needs over time. Changes may be necessary either because of changes in the individual's own circumstances or because the service proved to be inappropriate in practice. This stage has often been omitted from service provision in the past and is important to ensure that people not only *receive* but *retain* services appropriate to their needs.

It can be seen that the process of caremanagement should be represented as a cycle, involving understanding users' needs, responding to them and then checking that services continue to be suitable. The two key elements of the process are that it is user-led (not service-led) and that one person is involved throughout. These need to be discussed in turn.

A USER-LED PROCESS

The term 'user-led' should mean starting with what users want (or are judged to need) and not with what services happen to be available. This is not an easy change for service providers to make; it is much easier to see what services are around and to fit people in to them, as has been traditional practice.

Providing a user-led service does *not* mean doing everything a user wants. Few people get exactly what they want in any service. Nor does it mean that there are no resource constraints – of course there are. But a user-led approach does mean starting with the user, genuinely listening to what is wanted and trying to think imaginatively about how this might be achieved. It also entails consulting the user about any decisions under consideration, using a process of trial and error to see what can be done and involving the user in working out any necessary compromise.

A key element in this process is an assumption of *uncertainty*. It may be very unclear at the outset what the best solution to a problem will be. Where work with users is service-led, there is no such uncertainty, because the 'solution' is where the worker begins. The one known part of the equation is the service available (a home help, a day centre place) and the central question is whether the user should be allocated it – and, if so, to what extent. But in a user-led process, the service may not exist at the time of planning and certainly is not part of the initial planning process. It is assumed, in short, that no one is clear about what the end point will be.

Coupled with this uncertainty is an assumption that there will need to be a process of *trial and error*. If there is uncertainty, there is a need to try out various options in order to assess whether or not they are appropriate. This may be just a matter of checking whether a wanted service exists and if so, whether it is available (for instance, that places are not all taken). There may also be a need to assess whether it is accessible (for instance, not too far away), provided at the right times and, of course, affordable. One cannot make any plans without a great deal of information.

This process is expressly what everyone goes through when looking to fill a need. When thinking of moving house, for example, most people start with a grand plan for a large house in a particularly desirable area. As they slowly gain information on what is possible within their budget, they frequently have to adjust their initial sights. If they cannot find something which meets their minimum standards, they do not move. What they do not have is someone saying: 'you can have House A or House B – take it or leave it'.

Or take another example of deciding to get some regular exercise. Many people start with ambitious plans for rising for an early morning jog. On the third day, they tend to find this is not quite so desirable and begin to explore alternatives. They may decide to swim in their lunch break or play squash with colleagues. One way or another, they work out an acceptable compromise to themselves or they decide not to do it. What they do not have is someone saying: 'you will go to the sports centre every Monday at 2 p.m. for a swim'.

Everyone likes some sense of choice, together with some involvement in finding the best solution for themselves. People have differing sets of needs and place differing weight on achieving them. Thus, in moving house, the compromise may concern its location, size or condition; in seeking exercise, the compromise may concern its timing, proximity or nature. The key question is *who* makes these decisions. A central point of caremanagement is that, as far as possible, it is the user who does so.

ONE POINT OF CONTACT

The second key aspect of caremanagement is that one person has responsibility for managing a user's case from beginning to end. (Hence, the original term 'case management'.) This is to ensure that someone is clearly accountable for obtaining the necessary services for each user. The care manager is expected to gain a full insight into what a user needs (traditionally called 'assessment'), to assist the process of meeting that need ('planning' and 'co-ordination') and keep in touch to ensure that services remain appropriate ('monitoring and review').

What care managers do not do, generally speaking, is provide services themselves – other than the 'service' of caremanagement with all the help and advice that entails. The care manager should be outside the service provision system, so that there is no conflict of interest when determining what the best arrangement for a user will be. It is felt that, in the absence of such a system, a care manager who was also a social worker might be inclined to urge a lot of social work help onto a user, especially where budgets were involved. This would not necessarily follow, of course, but the aim is to avoid any potential bias. It is part of the wider move to separate the 'purchaser' and 'provider' roles within statutory agencies.

It might be added in passing that there are some exceptions to all these 'rules'. In some areas, the process of assessment is separated from the process of caremanagement, so that there is not a single person responsible for each user. In some areas, care managers are also service providers. Indeed, in some areas, the user-led principle is not held to be paramount. In short, it is difficult to generalise fully.

THE SERVICE DEVELOPMENT ROLE

It is important to call attention to the often neglected service development role, a fundamental part of any caremanagement arrangement. This is essential to ensure that services are available to meet assessed need. The caremanagement process should serve as the 'eyes and ears' of those who plan services in the area, both statutory and beyond to the voluntary and private sectors. This means aggregating information on users' needs, so that subsequent planning can be built around them.

The service development role means working both with providers of existing services to help them to ensure that they provide what users want and with new providers to get new services off the ground. Such changes may be major or relatively minor – setting up some new arrangement altogether or urging minor adjustments to make services more responsive to user need. In the absence of such activity, if the appropriate service cannot be found, all a user will obtain is a sensitive assessment.

Service development activity requires the application of considerable entrepreneurial skill. It is not always easy to work out who might best provide a service and encourage that person or agency to take it forward. Simply attracting new providers to an area is a complex business. It also requires great political sensitivity. Local politicians may be sensitive to any sugges-tion that their own services are inappropriate – and in some areas may be outraged at the idea that traditional statutory services are to be provided by private agencies. Professionals of all kinds often have very strong views about the nature of services which users will need. Such developmental activity is also not always successful, which may mean frustration for everyone concerned.

CAREMANAGEMENT IS A PROCESS

Caremanagement is a *process*, a way of approaching care. In itself, it contains no assumptions about the kind of services people should want, in other words, *outcomes*. Nor does it presuppose a certain level of service or certain standards regarding quality. Caremanagement is often proposed alongside a set of other values about what should be provided. Users may sometimes make decisions which the care manager finds unacceptable or simply wrong. The care manager may advise them differently, but in the end, it is the user, wherever possible, who should decide.

This is not an issue limited to this context. Everyone tends to hold strong values concerning *both* process and content in managing their everyday affairs. There is often an uneasy relationship between them. For example, most people deeply value the democratic process as well as supporting the views of one particular political party. If the outcome of an election is not the party they support, they may well be disappointed, but such outcomes are accepted as part of having that process. The same is true for caremanagement; if users are to be genuinely asked about their preferences, then care managers should understand that their job is to help them to make choices – not to anticipate or determine what such choices should be.

It is likely, of course, that certain aims will prove to be held in common; for instance, a concern to maximise independence. But such aims are *not* built into the successful operation of caremanagement. For example, some people may wish to disengage from independent living for reasons of age or frailty and it is the job of the care manager to respect this wish. But such aims are not built into the caremanagement process and their achievement is not the basis on which caremanagement should be assessed. It is the good functioning of the process which is at issue. This is not widely understood and needs to be made clear to those introducing – and working within – a caremanagement system.

CAREMANAGEMENT FOR PEOPLE WITH LEARNING DISABILITIES

Caremanagement is not easy for any client group, but it may be particularly difficult for people with learning disabilities. There are issues of users' ability to articulate their needs clearly, their knowledge of what is possible, together with the tradition of a dependency relationship. Extra complexities may be added by the need to involve relatives, with all the potential conflicts of interest that this may entail. But this does not mean that caremanagement is inappropriate in this context. A few issues might be highlighted here.

There is no question that understanding what people with learning disabilities want may be difficult in some circumstances. Care managers need to help them to explore what is possible and to try out different situations. This may require some imagination in how to present them with new ideas. In addition, it may be necessary to think carefully about what they are expressing; a man in the Wakefield project who said he wanted to go swimming, for instance, just wanted to get out of the hospital setting by any known means. People with learning disabilities may not immediately understand what it would mean to move from hospital to the community or from the parental home – nor the implications of attending a local college or other facility. It may also be difficult to enable them to understand what the role of the care manager is.

There are also other problems. Costing may well prove an issue here. Care managers may need particular caution to ensure that they are not imposing their own views on the user. Caremanagement may also imply the co-operation of others, for instance hospital staff, in order to undertake outings with people with challenging behaviour, with all the resource implications that this entails. There will also be a need for considerable negotiation with existing providers about what is possible for this group. They may be reluctant to see people with learning disabilities becoming involved in local generic services, such as adult education or sports facilities. (There is nothing special about caremanagement here, but such conflicts may be more likely to arise in this context.) There may be particular difficulties with the service development role and few new service providers attracted to an area.

Overall, caremanagement in the case of people with learning disabilities is likely to require more time, more help from others (staff, volunteers and family) and more financial resources to meet needs. It has been found to be particularly problematic when moving people from hospital into the community, because of the complex nature of the services which need to be established. But it should be stressed that, overall, there is nothing inherently different about caremanagement for this group.

THE POLICY CONTEXT

For those who wish to understand the policy history of caremanagement in the UK, a few comments can be appended here. The NHS and Community Care Act 1990 does not make direct reference to caremanagement, but it does refer to the need for assessment. Section 47 (1), states that:

> where it appears to a local authority that any person for whom they may provide or arrange for the provision of community care services may be in need of any such services, the authority –
> (a) shall carry out an assessment of this need for those services and
> (b) having regard to the results of that assessment, shall then decide whether his needs call for the provision by them of any such services.

Where the assessment suggests the need for services from a district health authority or local authority housing department, the Act suggests that such services may also be sought.

The background to these provisions can be seen in the Department of Health's White Paper, *Caring for People*, published one year earlier. Here, it was argued that 'people whose needs extend beyond health care to include social care and support, e.g. for mobility, personal care, domestic tasks, financial affairs, accommodation, leisure and employment, which they cannot arrange for themselves' (Department of Health, 1989, sections 3.2.1–2) should be given an assessment by their social service department. This would not comprise everyone needing some form of care in the community. People with relatively slight needs for social care might be helped by the simple provision of advice or information and people with exclusively health care needs would continue to receive their care from community and primary health services.

The White Paper further commented on the nature of this assessment. Its aim should be 'to determine the best way to help the individual' and it should focus 'positively on what the individual can and cannot do, and could be expected to achieve, taking account of his or her personal and social relationships' (ibid, section 3.2.3).' Assessments should not focus solely on an individual's suitability for a particular service. They should review the individual's potential for living independently in the community, either at home or in residential accommodation. Assessments should take account of the wishes of the individual and his or her carer. Following an assessment, the social services department was given responsibility to design appropriate care arrangements, within available resources.

In discussing organisational arrangements for assessments, the White Paper proposed that a single individual 'should be responsible for ensuring that each case is dealt with effectively' (ibid, section 3.2.7). The term 'case manager' was reserved for those cases where 'an individual's needs are complex or significant resources are involved' (ibid, section 3.3.2) and in such circumstances, it was suggested that a case manager should be appointed to review the services provided and manage the resources, providing a single point of contact. That person might have some delegated budgetary responsibility for the service user. It was not required that this person be employed by the social services department nor be the person making the initial assessment.

Subsequent policy guidance spelled out in more detail the processes of what had by then come to be known as caremanagement and assessment. It was argued that these processes were intended to ensure that resources were used effectively, to enable people to live independently in the community wherever possible, to minimise the effects of disability, to treat service users with respect, to promote individual choice and build on existing strengths and to promote partnership between users, carers and providers in all sectors. Caremanagement systems were to 'respond flexibly and sensitively to the needs of users and their carers, allow a range of options, intervene no more than is necessary to foster independence, prevent deterioration and concentrate on those with the greatest needs' (ibid, section 3.5).

It might be noted that the role and purpose of caremanagement was well articulated in all these documents, except for one fundamental point. There appears to be some confusion about the neutrality regarding outcomes that is an essential part of pressing for the implementation of any *process*. Government guidance assumes that the purpose of caremanagement is both to achieve or retain independent living and to provide flexibility and choice. This is akin to arguing that the purpose of the democratic system in Britain is both to achieve a Labour government and to maintain electoral choice! This is not a dry academic argument in the context of caremanagement; those involved with the Wakefield Case Management Project found themselves in considerable difficulties over exactly this point. Initially set up with the dual purposes of working with a set of individuals using a case management approach *and* moving them out of a long-stay hospital, the inherent tension between them did not become evident until it was well under way.[3]

CONCLUSIONS

Caremanagement represents a fundamental shift. There may be much which is familiar – derived from existing best practice – and it should not be seen as altogether new. But the proposed emphasis on the *user* of services is not a negligible change. It will require a deep change in the organisational and professional culture of local and health authorities. Attitudes will need to alter at all levels – especially among those working directly with users. Care management is not primarily about introducing different models or engaging in new activities. It is about looking at work with users in a new way. This was well summed up by one Wakefield case manager: 'Case management is not *one* thing – but an approach and a set of values which makes you look at how best you can work with one individual and empower that person.'

AUTHOR'S NOTE

Research on the Wakefield Case Management Project was funded by the Joseph Rowntree Foundation, Yorkshire Regional Health Authority and the CMP itself. The material presented here represents the findings of the author, not necessarily those of the Foundation or the other funders.

ACKNOWLEDGEMENT

I would like to thank Ray Higgins for his assistance in preparing this chapter. A shorter version was published in N. Malin (ed.) *Community Care for People with Learning Difficulties*, Report on CCETSW Conference Series, Sheffield: School of Health and Community Studies, Sheffield Hallam University, 1993.

NOTES

1 There are three Working Papers from research directed by the author on this project: *Case Management in Practice*, NIHSS Working Paper 1, 1990; *Doing Case Management*, NIHSS Working Paper 4, 1991; and *The Limits of Case Management*, NIHSS Working Paper 5, 1992. All are written by Ann Richardson

and Ray Higgins and are available from the Publications Department, Nuffield Institute for Health, Fairbairn House, 71–75 Clarendon Road, Leeds LS2 9PL; tel: (0532) 459034. There is also a summary of the project's findings, published by the Joseph Rowntree Foundation in its *Findings* series, available from the JRF, the Homestead, 40 Water End, York YO3 6LP; tel: (0904) 629241.

3 The Personal Social Services Research Unit has published a number of writings on caremanagement. The most recent book is M. Knapp *et al.*, *Care in the Community: Challenge and Demonstration*, Aldershot: Gower, 1992.

3 See Ann Richardson and Ray Higgins, Working Papers 1 and 5, op. cit.

REFERENCES

Beardshaw, V. and Towell, D. (1990) *Assessment and Care Management: implications for the implementation of 'Caring for People'*, Briefing Paper no. 10, London: King's Fund Institute.

Department of Health (1989) *Caring for People: community care in the next decade and beyond*, Cm 849, London, HMSO.

National Development Team (1991) *The Andover Case Management Project*, London: National Development Team.

Onyett, S. (1992) *Case Management in Mental Health*, London, Chapman and Hall.

Pilling, D. (1992) *Approaches to Case Management for People with Disabilities*, London: Jessica Kingsley.

15 Quality assurance and inspection

Ian Sinclair and John Brown

INTRODUCTION

Since the passing by Parliament of the NHS and Community Care Act, 1990, the local agenda drawn up by social services, health and the independent sector has addressed a wide range of issues. Prominent among these have been questions about quality and inspection. Although social services did not acquire formal lead responsibility for community care services until April 1993 they began to tackle the relationship between community care provision, quality and inspection soon after the passing of the 1990 legislation.

The relationship has been symbolically marked by the creation of 'arms-length' inspection units and the search for measures that can be used to monitor a wide range of environments. The literature on quality assurance has burgeoned. Yet it is not at all clear whether this activity, which has built up a considerable momentum, will necessarily lead to the high-quality services that it is intended to deliver. In this chapter the case for quality assurance in the field of community care is outlined along with the logic behind the approach. This is followed by considering some of the difficulties involved in applying this logic and draws upon examples taken from services for the elderly and people with learning disabilities. The chapter ends with some speculative thoughts on the way these difficulties may be overcome and the benefits realised.

THE CASE FOR QUALITY ASSURANCE

The case for quality assurance and inspection in this field rests on four main planks.

First, there is the vulnerability of the clientele. They are commonly poor, badly provided with powerful connections and inhibited by their own handicaps from taking action on their own behalf. It is essential to ensure that they are not exploited.

Second, there is the nature of the market in care. There is commonly little choice of provision, those who make the decisions (social workers or relatives, for example) are not those who have the service, and relatives and users are frequently not in a good position to judge the quality of the service offered. Something other than 'market forces' is required to ensure that a high standard of service is provided.

Third, there is the fact that public money is involved. It is unacceptable that this is spent with no guarantee of the quality of the product.

Fourth, there is the pressure from politicians and professionals on all sides. Quality is a key focus of the new managerial revolution, it is a necessary concern in the new mixed economy of care if the only concern is not to be cost, and it fits the 'consumerist' rhetoric of professionals and politicians alike. Furthermore an increase in inspectors is as natural a response to scandals as an increase in the police is to a rise in crime.

There may well be other compelling reasons for quality assurance and inspection, but these four are surely enough to suggest that the approach they embody is both necessary and inevitable.

THE LOGIC OF INSPECTION

A further attractive feature of quality assurance and inspection is the logical way in which the approach has been developed. A study of the Social Services Inspectorate reports provides as good a starting point as any for surveying this logic, which seems to apply in much the same way to large entities such as departments or home help services as to small ones such as private old people's homes.

Basically the approach begins with a specification of the values which should underpin the service being delivered. These can include both basic values such as the need to respect the privacy and dignity of users and to do so irrespective of race, beliefs or gender, and 'service values' such as the need to prevent unnecessary admissions to residential care.

The inspector then looks for a strategy for implementing these values. The search is likely to cover both the 'mission statement', 'brochure', 'community care plan' or other means of setting out what the service is supposed to do *and* the means whereby the overall strategy was derived (what consultation processes were involved, were users consulted, what about the involvement of voluntary groups, what epidemiological information was sought and so on).

Having satisfied themselves that aims exist and have been properly endorsed, inspectors are likely to turn to the degree to which these aims have been worked out in detail. Thus they may look for the existence of goals and targets (numbers of people to be served, type of clientele to be accepted into the home), priorities and types of service to be provided. They will then assess the degree to which these goals are compatible with the resources (staffing, plant, transport, finance planned to be available). Is the home equipped for the disabilities of the clientele for whom it is intended, have the staff received appropriate training and so on? A similar audit is then undertaken on the procedures involved. Is there a clear structure of accountability? Is there a business plan (if relevant), a budgeting cycle which ties into other forms of planning, a plan for training and personnel, manuals of practice guidance?

The next step is to see how this combination of aims, plan, resources and procedures works out in practice. The methods used are various (e.g. inspection visits, surveys, intensive study of selected users). In general, however, this step is likely to involve observation (e.g. of staff practices in a home), talking to staff (e.g. to find out if they are aware of the precepts included in the practice manuals) and talking to users and their relatives to find their experience. The inspector may also use performance measures (e.g. waiting times, occupancy rates, absconding rates).

Finally inspectors are likely to be concerned with the degree to which the service is able to get feedback on its own behaviour and take action in the light of what it learns. They are therefore likely to be concerned with:

1 Criteria – the degree to which there are specified targets, rights, standards against which the service can be assessed.
2 Means and measures for assessing the criteria (e.g. through surveys, management information, audit, advocacy, self-assessment, scrutiny by line management).
3 Watchdogs – the degree to which there exist means for involving councillors, voluntary bodies, inspection units and so on in scrutinising the operation of the service.
4 A system for regular review of the service.
5 A procedure for responding to the reviews, typically with an identified individual responsible for the response.
6 The existence of sanctions (de-registration, termination of contracts, etc.) with evidence that these might be used.
7 The existence of supports (training, supervision, etc.) through which performance can be reviewed.

This approach has an impressive internal logic and can, as already stated, be applied in a wide variety of circumstances. Although overtly top down, it nevertheless emphasises the need for quality to be 'owned' at all levels of an organisation. Moreover, it relies on and emphasises feedback from the grass roots. There seems at first sight little that could be wrong with a system so logical and so in keeping with the spirit of the age.

PROBLEMS AND DIFFICULTIES

Despite its logic, promise and inevitability there are doubts over the effectiveness of inspection and suspicions are perhaps first raised by the occasions on which inspection has not worked.

An early example of such a failure is provided by the English nunneries in the late middle ages. These places had explicit rules setting the standards against which they were to be judged, and it might be expected that these rules were 'owned' at all levels of the organisation. In theory, therefore, the bishops whose job it was to inspect the nunneries should have had an easy task. In practice, however, according to Trevelyan the inspections were largely ineffective, with the nuns on occasion pursuing the bishop off the premises, while passing scornful comments on his Bull (Trevelyan, 1951, p.69).

Trevelyan's examples suffer from the fact that they may be more striking than representative – for history may record unusual scandal more than routine success. Nevertheless a casual scanning of the news repeatedly throws up examples of inspections which have not achieved their intended purpose. The bank BCCI was inspected in numerous countries throughout the world but continued nevertheless to its spectacular disaster. Britain's beaches are supposed to meet a European standard, which on monitoring by an independent organisation they are found to fail; the undesirable practices in prisons and special hospitals seem on occasion to have been both flagrant and proof against improvement by inspection; nearer home Pindown and the other scandals of residential life seem more often to have been highlighted by residents or the public than by the efforts of inspectors. As early as 1971 a study of probation hostels found that despite at least annual inspections by both the then Children's and Probation Inspectorates, they varied massively in their effects on the absconding and offence rates of their residents. Repeated inspection was insufficient to ensure uniformly high performance, or even to weed out appalling practice (Sinclair, 1975).

Perversely, however, there is also a danger that while inspections may be ineffective in improving performance they may on occasion be effective in lowering it. This could occur because the inspectors' need to concentrate on the measurable encourages service providers to focus on the irrelevant or even to adopt harmful practices. For example, if inspectors are known to be concerned with occupancy rates in old people's homes this may encourage a somewhat uncritical use of homes and subversion of the purposes of community care. Others may feel that inspectors give the wrong message about what matters in residential care.

> I think I was expecting the registration officer to be a kind of home's supervisor and I was hoping to have a discussion at a professional level. I had not expected her to go round turning taps on and off, flushing lavatories and looking inside the cups in the cupboard.
>
> (Sinclair I., 1988)

These difficulties of inspection are compounded or explained by a number of problems at a more detailed level. These involve:

1 Conflicts in the values which are supposed to underpin inspection. For example, the wish to give choice to consumers may conflict at a detailed level with a wish to get value for money and concentrate services on the most dependent.
2 Resource issues – a major part of the difficulties of community care has to do with lack of resources and yet this is something which may be seen as political and outside the purview of the inspector.

3 Invisibility – much poor practice goes on where it is not easily seen by the inspector and the greater the reign of terror the greater the fear of users who might inform.

4 Measurability – American, Australian and British research all points to the major difficulty of getting reliable measures of quality in inspections of old people's homes (the area in which most work has been done) (Braithwaite *et al.*, 1991; Day and Klein, 1987; Gibbs and Sinclair, 1992, Gustafson *et al.*; 1982, Spector *et al.*, 1987).

5 Indeterminacy – structural factors (e.g. staffing ratios) in services are notoriously weakly related to outcomes, so that it is hard to be certain that insistence on particular structural characteristics will produce good outcomes.

6 Difficulties in taking action – cases of poor practice are hard to prove, inspectors may be in doubt over whether they could make them stick before a tribunal, over the time that it would take to get a result, over the possibility that those inspected may simply take their business elsewhere, and over the issue of what should then happen to those who have been receiving a service.

These difficulties have to be faced in a situation where inspection units are being rapidly formed, are having new duties put upon them by the Children Act 1989, may be expected to combine a variety of duties (e.g. responsibility for complaints procedures) and are having to work out their role in the face of potentially differing expectations.

And if the difficulties cannot be overcome the consequences would not be negligible. It is costly to provide inspections and to prepare for them and meet the regulations they involve. The need to satisfy inspections may also distort the provision of care, favouring bureaucratic large organisations at the expense of small voluntary organisations, (including those setting out to serve black people).

Underlying possibilities such as these are fundamental issues surrounding the relationship between values, resources and outcomes. Quality and inspection are an integral part of the contractual process and these issues have to be placed within a set of parameters increasingly influenced by commissioning agencies. The way this can impinge upon the debate over values and resources is illustrated by developments within learning disabilities.

DEVELOPMENTS IN LEARNING DISABILITIES

Within the area of learning disabilities there has been a long debate over the role of inspection that goes back over two decades. When the first hospital inquiry report was published in 1969 (DHSS, 1969) the government's immediate response was to set up the Hospital Advisory Service (HAS). The emphasis was very much upon offering 'advice' to health authorities who invited the group in to comment upon the quality of the facilities along with the nature of the environment provided and how this promoted respect for the privacy and dignity of residents.

Over the next few years the work of the HAS expanded to encompass the range of residents/patients to be found in the long-stay sector. In 1975 the work of the HAS was broken down into client groups with a new group, the National Development Team (NDT), acquiring responsibility for people with learning disabilities. The remit remained still one of advice although, in certain limited circumstances, e.g. after a specific allegation, the group could initiate a request for a visit. The powers of inspection have, therefore, been limited.

The difficulty has been in taking action. With outside inspection being tightly circumscribed, there has been an emphasis very much upon generating checklists for the organisation to apply themselves. Among the first was one published by the NDT in 1978 and many examples have been published since then the latest, on meeting residential needs, being released by SSI at the beginning of 1993 (NDT, 1978; DoH/SSI, 1993).

Such checklists have taken the principles of normalisation (Wolfensberger, 1973) as the value-base from which to develop the items to focus upon when carrying out an inspection to identify quality. Yet the adoption of normalisation as a philosophy underpinning service provision has created its own difficulties for inspection. The widespread adoption of an approach incorporating the principles of normalisation, and an 'ordinary life', led to the impetus for small, community-based units providing accommodation for often no more than four residents (King's Fund, 1981). This contributed very much to the 'invisibility' of provision as large hospitals were run down to be replaced by provision scattered throughout neighbouring communities.

The emphasis upon an ordinary life, however, made it difficult at times to distinguish between process and outcome. It was all too easy to assume that an ordinary life could be achieved with ordinary skills and that specialist skills were not required. Although evidence has accumulated that to achieve an ordinary life can often require an extraordinary input (DoH, 1989; Sines, 1988; Thompson and Mathias 1992) there is the problem of how to assess appropriately the specialist input needed in any situation. This is especially the case in challenging behaviour where stopping an incident that occurs can be less appropriate as an indicator than anticipating and preventing it occuring in the first place (DoH, 1993).

Discussion of factors such as these has taken place amidst a conflict over values reflected in the long-standing debate over hospital versus community provision and in particular nurse versus social worker (Chief Nursing Officers of the United Kingdom, 1991). This conflict has persisted, and been reinforced to some extent by the government talking about health and social care which has polarised debate over responsibilities for developing services (DoH, 1991). At the same time, the context in which services are developing has tended to place the emphasis upon simple measures of efficiency and effectiveness as well as quality. This is due in no small part to the widespread adoption of the general management function throughout the National Health Service, and increasingly local government, which has emphasised the need for accessible measures of quality when evaluating both services and individuals (DoH, 1991). More than any other development this highlights the frequent tension between values and resources.

When Griffiths submitted his first report in the early 1980s on NHS management (Griffiths, 1983) he was preparing the ground for a rapid decline in hospital provision as the basis for residential care for people with a learning disability. In its penultimate report before being disbanded the Social Services Select Committee in 1990 illustrated the dramatic switch in provision from the hospital to independent sectors for people with learning disabilities (Social Services Select Committee, 1990). This switch, which halved the number of hospital beds from 52,000 to 27,000, has been attributed in no small part to managers seeking to achieve specific goals on hospital closure without necessarily having to be responsible for the result of their actions (Korman and Glennerster, 1990). The regular media exposure to stories of a 'discharged and dumped' nature indicate the problems.

As the introduction of the general management function has gained momentum it has become an integral part of a situation where the emergence of a contract culture has directly influenced the development of patterns of service provision and associated changes in organisational structures and administrative responsibilities. This has involved increasing emphasis upon local initiatives and responsibilities with, at the same time, corresponding emphasis upon local ownership (DOE, 1991). The issues this raises about comparability between settings and the role of national standards, however determined, goes to the heart of the debate over quality and inspection.

IMPLICATIONS AND CONCLUSION

There seems then to be a dilemma. Inspection is essential. It has not been as effective as might have been expected, and it is not too difficult to see why. Nevertheless there is no need to despair since progress may be made by tackling the problems outlined above.

The first set of issues concerns conflicts in values and lack of resources. The important thing here is, perhaps, that these should not be ignored in inspections. Inspectors need to develop the analytical acumen to note where conflicts of value are simply being pushed down to front-line providers, or where the latter lack the resources to undertake the jobs they are expected to do. The Audit Commission and the Inspector of Prisons, for example, have both done much to dispel the belief that they are simply tools of management by pointing to the difficulties facing staff and the consequences for the job they do. In this way inspection can become not simply a means of keeping the troops in line but also of challenging the generals over their management of the campaign.

The second set of issues concerns the technical problems of inspections (difficulties over measurement, and in observing malpractice). These difficulties need to be taken seriously.

In relation to malpractice, there needs, perhaps, to be an emphasis on 'whistle-blowing' (e.g. through the provision of confidential complaint lines, distribution to staff, relatives, and users of information on what should be expected and how to complain, making sure users know how to contact inspectors and what their function is) and on the identification of 'hard' indicators (staff turnover and sickness, absconding rates, occupancy rates) which may serve as early warning signs. Unheralded inspections are also advocated although there is no evidence one way or the other on their efficacy. Lessons need perhaps to be drawn from the field of child abuse on the ease with which warning signs can be noted by someone but nevertheless lost in the system so that a full picture is not drawn together.

In relation to measurability there is encouraging evidence from Australia (Braithwaite *et al.*, 1991) that reliable measures can be developed provided that a determined effort is made to do so. This study was concerned with homes for elderly people and the key ingredients for reliable measures seemed to be that these were few and rather general and that considerable effort was put into ensuring that inspectors had adequate training in their use. The Australian study concentrated on ratings made as a result of observation but, in principle, these could be complemented by questionnaires to users and hard information (e.g. on staff turnover), thus tackling the problem of measurement in different ways and, hopefully, increasing the validity of the judgements made.

The third set of problems relates to the difficulty of specifying structural characteristics (e.g. qualifications of head of home, proportion of single rooms) with clear relationships to outcome. Here, it has perhaps to be recognised that no structural characteristic determines a good service, and that insistence on too many structural characteristics as conditions of registration will simply raise costs and make it difficult for many good homes to compete. Nevertheless it is important that research is undertaken to try and identify the characteristics of homes that do *on average* matter. By insisting on these characteristics (e.g. proportion of single rooms or staff with certain levels of training) inspectors will be able to raise the standard of sets of homes, even if in this respect their effect on individual homes is likely to be small.

The last set of problems concerns the difficulties of taking action. The ease of taking drastic action (e.g. deregistration) should be enhanced by some of the steps outlined above but such action is never going to be common and the threat of it may be more important than the reality. In this situation it is important to consider the range of measures which can be used to enhance the effectiveness of inspections. These include the steps taken to ensure that the criteria used in inspections are publicised and as far as possible agreed, that there is a coherence between these criteria and those informing complaints procedures, registration, contracting and self-regulation, that the procedures to be followed after inspections is agreed, that there is clarity on the publicity to be given to the results of inspections (e.g. if care managers are to be informed), that inspectors are skilled in agreeing timetables with those inspected for improvement, that resources (training, supervision, etc.) are available to enable improvement, that improvement is seen as something which needs to take place over time so that repeated failures to meet standards are grounds for more serious actions than a first time 'offence' and no doubt much else.

In all this it has to be acknowledged that inspection units are feeling their way. Inevitably they will build on work that is currently in hand – inspection in the field of residential care, reviews of particular services, the developing practice of units monitoring themselves, the growth of management information. Work on domiciliary care, preventive work with children and so on will follow later. Inevitably development will be incremental, informed, one would hope, by research. Hopefully, too, allowance will be made for the need not to distort the market in care. Social services departments need to deal with agencies which are stable and bureaucratic and thus appropriate subjects for the standard inspection. They also need agencies which are less bureaucratic, smaller and perhaps maverick. They have to ensure that both kinds of agency continue to exist and that their inspection procedures do not drive out the one and leave the other.

So we would conclude that although much evidence suggests that inspection is very difficult, nothing suggests that it is impossible. Given goodwill and an open acknowledgement of the difficulties inspection should yet fulfil its promise.

REFERENCES

Braithwaite, J., Braithwaite, V., Gibson, D., Landau M., and Makkai, T. (1991) *The Reliability and Validity of Nursing Home Standards*, Canberra, The Department of Health, Housing and Community Services.
Chief Nursing Officers of the United Kingdom (1991) *Caring for People – Mental Handicap Nursing* (Cullen Report), PL/CNO(91)5, London, Department of Health.
Day, P. and Klein, R. (1987) 'The Regulation of Nursing Homes: a Comparative Perspective', *The Millbank Quarterly* 65 (3) pp. 303–47.
Department of Environment (1991) *The Internal Management of Local Authorities: a consultation paper*, London: Department of Environment.
Department of Health and Social Security (1969) *Report of the Committee of Inquiry into Allegations of Ill-treatment of Patients and other Irregularities at the Ely Hospital, Cardiff*, Cmnd 3975, London: HMSO.
Department of Health (1989) *Caring for People: community care for the next decade and beyond*, Cm 849, London: HMSO.
Department of Health (1993) *Services for People with Learning Disabilities and Challenging Behaviour or Mental Health Needs* (Mansell Report), London: HMSO.
Department of Health/Social Services Inspectorate (1993) *Guidance on Standards for the Residential Care Needs of People with Learning Disabilities/Mental Handicap*, London: HMSO.
Gibbs, I. and Sinclair I.A.C. (1992) 'Consistency: a prerequisite for inspecting old people's homes?' *British Journal of Social Work*, 22, 535–50.

Griffiths, R. (1983) *NHS Management Inquiry*, London: DHSS.
Gustafson, D., Peterson, R., Casper, S., Macco, A., Can Koningsveld, R. and Kopetsky, E. (1982) *The Impact of the Wisconsin Quality Assurance Project: A Field Evaluation*, Madison: University of Wisconsin.
King's Fund (1981) *An Ordinary Life*, Project Paper No. 40, London: King's Fund.
Korman, N. and Glennerster, H. (1990) *Hospital Closure*, Milton Keynes: Open University Press
National Development Team (1978) *A Checklist of Standards*, London: DHSS.
Sines, D. (ed.) (1988) *Towards Integration: Comprehensive services for people with mental handicaps*, London: Harper & Row.
Sinclair, I.A.C. (1975) 'Influence of wardens and matrons on probation hostels: a study of a quasi-family institution', in J., Tizard, I.A.C. Sinclair, and R.V.S. Clarke *Variation of Residential Experiences*, London: Routledge & Kegan Paul.
Social Services Select Committee (1990) *Community Care: Services for People with a Mental Handicap and People with a Mental Illness*, HCX 664, London: HMSO.
Spector, W., Takada, A., Durgovich, M., Laliberte, L. and Tucker, R. (1987) *PaCS Evaluation: Final Report*, Baltimore: Health Care Financing Bureau.
Thompson, T. and Mathias, P. (eds) (1992) *Standards in Mental Handicap: Keys to Competence*, London: Bailliere Tindall.
Trevelyan, G.M. (1951) *Illustrated English Social History*, Vol. 1, London: Longmans Green.
Wolfensberger, W. (1973) *Normalization*, London: MENCAP, Imprint.

16 The survival of collaboration and co-operation

John Hattersley

INTRODUCTION

It is well known that the individuals who come into contact with the many services set up to provide care, treatment and support, and which lead, where possible, to independence, good health and an acceptable life in society, have complex and changing needs. This means that no single part of an organisation, or even one organisation in total, is likely to meet all of the needs of any individual. Society has imposed a series of structures on the way that services are resourced and delivered, and each person requiring help or treatment has to negotiate his or her way through these complicated structures in the hope that specific, individual needs can be assessed, planned for and met. In this complex world the individual 'client' is often dependent on collaboration and co-operation between and within services to ensure that his or her needs are comprehensively met in a high-quality way. This chapter sets out to describe some of the issues that surround the issue of collaboration based upon the author's personal experience and drawing upon the discussions in the professional journal of one of the professions, *Clinical Psychology*, which has a key interest in teamwork and collaboration.

Although this chapter is designed to provide insights into services for people with learning disabilities, the issues raised and the proposed solutions have implications for a wide range of client groups. In the following discussions the difficulty of deciding how to refer to individuals with learning disabilities who require some form of service has been resolved by using the generic term 'client' as a shorthand.

One definition of co-operation is 'working together to the same end' while collaboration is defined as 'working jointly' (*The Concise Oxford English Dictionary*). Each of these can be interpreted to suggest that the people co-operating or collaborating must know the end to which they are working and must be prepared to work together towards this end. This chapter will assume these as working definitions. It is perhaps worth noting, without further comment, that, according to the same dictionary, collaboration can also be used to mean 'to co-operate traitorously with the enemy'. The term collaboration will be used throughout.

Collaboration must occur at a number of levels if services are to be planned and delivered effectively. In the first place, the authorities which determine and control strategy and policy must collaborate. This has not proved to be easy in the past and the many changes that are being introduced following recent legislation may not improve this position (NHS and Community Care Act, 1990). The two main public bodies which are required to collaborate are the health and local authorities.

Health authorities have been given an explicit purchasing role and have been removed from having any direct responsibility for the management and delivery of services. They have also been reconstituted to include a relatively small number of board members; five executive and five appointed members. In moving towards a competitive and market-driven system of health care, the appointed membership is now concentrated on key, local people who can bring experience from business and industry, which is now seen to be more relevant than other experience which has been valued in the past. The influences exerted previously by a membership which included local politicians, representatives of voluntary agencies, local people with a knowledge of health care and even trades union officers, have been removed. It is likely that, with these changes, the potential to view collaboration as important and desirable will be reduced.

In turn, local authorities are determined by their own special organisation and processes. At authority level they are made up of locally elected councillors who are driven by a range of political imperatives, working within structures which are often remote from the executive officers and the employees who deliver the services. The apparent closeness to, and dependence on, the people living in local communities who elect them does not guarantee that they will recognise and respond appropriately to the needs of these individuals. The vastly differing cultures between the two authorities can severely hamper the opportunity for meaningful collaboration, particularly where the political 'colour' of the two organisations is disparate.

In practice, informed strategic planning is usually delegated to specialists who may not be executive members of the authorities. These individuals are regularly left to find ways of achieving collaboration between the authorities within the imperatives and guidelines laid down by legislation, central bodies and their own organisations. It would seem logical that these planners should set themselves an agenda which allows them to analyse the complexity and structure of their organisations to see if these are a necessary part of the mechanisms required to manage and control the services they deliver. In practice, many organisations evolve gradually, without explicit review, and the resulting 'monsters' can often establish their own demands for collaboration which exist only because of the unnecessary divisions and barriers which have developed. This has been recognised at the highest level in views such as those expressed by Sir Roy Griffiths in his assessment of community care. He favoured making collaboration a necessary part of service delivery at all levels and would have preferred to see a joint purchasing organisation, incorporating the relevant parts of the current Health and Social Services (Griffiths Report, 1988).

Even without this joint purchasing authority, the purchaser–provider relationship offers a potentially strong basis for encouraging collaboration. If the purchaser can become skilled at determining when collaboration is necessary and then specify services to include the right level of collaboration with designated resources, then there should be a much higher probability that it will actually occur. To help this process purchasers will have to be much clearer about service outcomes, be able to determine if collaboration is genuinely required to achieve these outcomes, state who it should be between and then indicate what systems will be needed to guarantee delivery. At present, however, purchasers have a logical reluctance to becoming closely involved in the details of service provision. This reluctance must not be allowed to undermine the provision of crucial elements of a service such as collaboration. By definition collaboration requires a partnership in service delivery and the purchaser can provide a major incentive for independent NHS Trusts to collaborate with each other and with other organisations. Without this incentive, providers are more likely to compete to provide that part of the overall service not currently controlled by them. The word survival is used in the title because, although it is clear that collaboration is occurring between many individuals in different parts of the services, the changes in climate which have been introduced appear to have the potential to lead to its eventual extinction.

THE CLIMATE OR SETTING CONDITIONS

There are a number of important factors which set the scene within which collaboration is expected to occur:

1 The Government has passed a series of pieces of legislation, including the NHS and Community Care Act, the Children Act and the Mental Health Act, which impose responsibilities and constraints upon public services.
2 The Government has set out to introduce new management cultures and practices into public services which, in the past, have been driven by a wide range of factors and which have often remained poorly planned and specified. This new culture involves services having a much clearer view of what is being done and where the service is going, culminating in the production of business plans which not only specify the organisation's strengths and weakness, but set a strategy with clear targets to take the service forward.
3 Services are expected to become more business-like and to introduce annual efficiency savings. These savings can involve providing the same level of service for less money or providing more services for the same money, depending on whether a cash release is required.
4 Services are expected to improve their quality in a variety of ways, in

particular by listening to what consumers or customers want and value. The Government is setting out explicit quality targets and statements in documents such as the Patient's Charter, and public services are expected to achieve these quality standards.

5 A contract culture, set within a system which is to be driven by 'market forces', has been introduced into the whole of the National Health Service and, in turn, local authorities are being pushed down a similar road. Open competition to tender for a wide range of support services has been established for several years. Clear service specifications for areas such as catering and cleaning have been used to give much tighter quality, financial and management control in order to drive out what have been seen as restrictive and costly practices. Efficiency improvements have been achieved by increasing performance levels and reducing waste. Other key services, such as the provision of legal advice, are no longer provided in-house but are bought in from local firms.

6 The contract culture has been extended to the provision of clinical care and treatment. A clear distinction has been drawn between the purchasing and the provision of health services. Health authorities act on behalf of local populations to assess their health needs and then use the resources provided by the Department of Health to purchase suitable services to meet these needs. As this process develops District Health Authorities and Family Health Services Authorities are no longer constrained to purchase their services locally, and independent providers, including the NHS Trusts, can compete on price and quality to deliver services which will meet the specifications determined by the health authorities. The approach will be pushed a significant step further with the introduction of the care-programming model into community care. This model relies on the release of funds currently tied up in the provision of residential care services through funding from the Department of Social Security which is available to individual clients and patients for the purchase of residential and nursing home care. In 1993 this funding was channelled through local authority social services departments to allow them to purchase packages of care services to meet the needs of individuals in a more flexible way. Social services departments now have the legal responsibility to assess the community care needs of individuals and to purchase, on behalf of the client, the agreed services from a mixed economy of providers. They are also expected to monitor the services to ensure their delivery to a specified level of quality. All of this occurs within a limited envelope of resources which was never designed to meet all of the needs of every individual. It is hoped that this new model of resource allocation will improve the appropriateness of what is purchased, and thus its quality, for the individual.

7 Service planners are expected to consult and collaborate in the preparation of strategic plans. This consultation should include the consumers and the voluntary sector, with the intention of making sure that the services

purchased take into account a wide range of views and desires. Local authorities are expected to collaborate actively with health authorities in the development and implementation of their plans. Community Care Plans must now be published and made public each year, with the first plans published in April 1992.

ADVANTAGES OF COLLABORATION

There are many potential advantages to be gained from groups of staff and clients collaborating together:

1 With good collaboration crucial information can be more easily shared. This can help inform the range of people involved with each client by ensuring that they have knowledge of the client's relevant history, the part currently being played by each person helping the client, the possible help that each profession might offer and the availability of specific skills.

2 Communication between the various professionals and between the client and the professionals can be enhanced by making it more accurate, by sharing client records and through regular meetings. Where a range of people, including the client, advocate and carers, are involved, communication is crucial but can be particularly difficult. Professionals often develop technical languages of their own designed to provide accurate information to one another. Great care is required to prevent team members from being isolated from important information.

3 True collaboration provides many opportunities to learn from others. The collaborators can learn to share each others' values and to share skills across professional boundaries. The importance of the underlying value systems of individual team members has been described by Tollinton who points out that 'where team members came from different agencies, each with different aims, training, organizational structures and expectations, the differences in value systems and the implications of unacknowledged differences were easy to see. (For example, team members at times used the same words, such as "helping", "assessing", "team membership", but each member used the word to mean something slightly different)' (Tollinton, 1992, p. 25). Learning may occur from each other through the explicit sharing of skills or through less direct methods such as modelling appropriate behaviour.

4 Regular working together provides a venue and a mechanism for people to deal with that behaviour of others, including their attitudes, which causes problems or leads to regular conflicts within the team.

5 Where collaboration works, clients can have easier access to a wider range of therapists, skills and therapeutic approaches. Additional benefits can accrue to the client through the combination of therapeutic approaches and the sharing of new knowledge gained from single-profession research.

6 Work in helping people with 'problems' can be extremely demanding and

stressful. Collaborators who have a common understanding of the area and the specific client can provide continuing support for each other through difficult times. Many professional groups and service managers are becoming increasingly aware of the value of providing staff with supervision or mentoring to help them explore and deal with their own reactions and to enhance staff development.

FACTORS WHICH CAN INHIBIT COLLABORATION

There are many factors which can affect collaboration adversely:

1 Differences in the values and philosophy held by professional staff or organisations can make it difficult for staff to work together. This is a special problem where the values of individuals are not explicit or clear to those who have to work together. Under these circumstances any lack of collaboration is more easily attributed to 'personality differences' with the potential for scapegoating individuals.

2 Differences in pay and conditions of service can lead collaborators to resist working together. This can be exacerbated where one of the less-well-paid professionals feels that they carry an extra burden of responsibility. For example, nurses often feel they are the only ones who have a 24-hour, 7-day a week responsibility, with other professionals being paid more yet working fixed hours within a 'normal' working week.

3 Some professional staff view themselves as having a 'consultancy' role and do not expect to carry a caseload. This can lead to tensions when collaboration demands regular teamwork. Clinical psychologists have often argued that the most appropriate role for their profession, which is relatively small in number, is a consultative one which would make best use of their skills and academic training. In one district service psychologists were allocated as core members of teams and, within the agreed 'democratic' ethos, came to be treated as 'generic' mental health workers. As a result 'the "consultative" role for psychologists became difficult to achieve, because often other professions did not see psychologists as having specialist knowledge or skills . . . Moreover, being seen as one of many generic mental health workers meant that certain profession-specific "rights" were lost, for example, time for further study and for research, and an office' (Anciano and Kirkpatrick, 1990, p. 11).

4 Collaboration requires special skills and additional effort. It also takes time to develop trust and methods of working together. Some staff seem unwilling or unable to make this extra investment.

5 Individual characteristics and the interpersonal skills of individuals become far more important when staff are expected to collaborate. For example, where a number of staff are strongly competitive, struggles can develop over issues such as team leadership or the choice of treatment for clients, and this can undermine collaboration.

6 Collaboration can be damaged by high staff turnover and recruitment problems. The development of trust and team building take time and the regular involvement of individuals getting to know each other and sharing both their strengths and weaknesses. In this exercise there is no substitute for availability and access to each other.

7 There are strong pressures from the professions and from external forces to introduce improved quality control procedures. Such procedures can expose the practices of specific professional groups and this exposure can lead them to become more protective of their own positions, making them less likely to take risks in collaborative work (Alexander, 1992, p. 16; Searle, 1991, p. 16).

TEAMS AND TEAMWORK

Collaboration is particularly important where people have to work together in formal teams which set out to improve the delivery of services to a group of clients. There are several models which can be applied to teams and Ovretveit (1985) has described three of these. In the first, a narrow range of professionals with a high degree of interdependence collaborate together to provide services. The second type of team has a membership which is dependent on each other only at the administrative level. Finally, a team may be based on both the professional and administrative interdependence of the team members. In practice many of the teams referred to in the literature are of the first type and depend on agreement to collaborate reached at the level of the professionals who make up the team.

Many factors can cause problems for the smooth operation of such teams:

1 There may be uncertainty about the role of the team within the overall strategies of the parent authorities. This can lead to a lack of an agreed operational policy for the team, leaving individual staff struggling to determine their own roles. Many team problems arise from a situation where multi-disciplinary teams are created in isolation and then retrospectively address the needs of the client group. Some teams have been set up after clear planning (Lam and von Abendorff, 1988, p. 6), while others seem to have emerged locally without explicit plans (Reiman, 1989, p. 19). Teams need to establish at the outset 'what is the *nature* of the team, what is the *client group* and how (they) can define the *core problems* of that client group' (Clydesdale, 1990, p. 6). With this information it should be possible to determine who are the key team members and to reach agreement with the team and their managers on roles and an operational policy.

2 Where one member of the team is a doctor the concept and excessive practice of 'medical responsibility' can undermine trust and leave some people feeling devalued. Some doctors feel they must take responsibility for the work of every member of the team, regardless of the training and

experience of the other team members. Watson described the team of which she was a member by saying ' The climate among members seemed to me initially to be characterized by suspicion, especially of the role and power of the consultant psychiatrist . . . Referrals were brought to the team meetings in the main by the consultant' (Watson, 1990, p. 27). This can become particularly divisive where the doctor has little or no knowledge of the area of expertise of the other professionals.

3 If the senior line managers of the team members do not understand the work of the team, they may interfere with the practice of their staff to the detriment of the team and its operation. In some cases the professional line manager can exert too much control over what is viewed to be professional practice, possibly forcing individual team members to behave in ways which can inhibit collaboration with team members from a different profession. As teams become more established roles can become blurred and 'the idea of the generic worker (can reign) supreme along with the idea that a team is made up of equal individuals who are equally capable of doing the same thing' (Clydesdale, 1990, p. 7). This can threaten the whole team and Clydesdale is led to consider not only whether clinical psychologists should be in a child psychiatric team but whether such a team should exist at all. He concludes that the needs of children would be better met by a team of clinical psychologists who would then network with other professions as required. This sort of analysis supports an earlier suggestion that, before attempting to obtain collaboration, the need for it should be properly assessed.

4 Many teams have members who are relatively junior and are not in a position to commit their agency to the team's strategy and plans. Neither can they commit the resources of their agency to meet the needs of individual clients as they are identified by the team. Under these circumstances, support from the line manager who actually controls the resources is essential.

5 Teams without clear leadership or an operational policy can experience difficulty in setting, agreeing and taking action on priorities within the limited resource base. The difficulties in agreeing a team leader may be a result of differences in opinions over the appropriate background and training required. There may also be conflict in relation to the tension that seems to exist between team leadership and the exercise of professional autonomy (Dickinson 1989, p. 16). Team leadership will usually require the individual to take on a co-ordinating role without the power to instruct other team members to carry out tasks, and it is clear that 'Leadership styles to avoid are autocratic reigns of terror or compulsive hoarding of knowledge, power and credit for team success' (Onyett and Malone 1990, p. 17). These authors also suggest a useful list of tasks to be undertaken by the team leader including caseload allocation and monitoring, conflict resolution, review of team policy and practice and representing team

matters to general management. Without committed support from team members such tasks are virtually impossible.

6 Teams need clear agreements about how clients and their families or carers are to be involved in the processes of needs assessment, the choice of appropriate services and in helping with the delivery of these services to the client.

7 The maintenance of case records is crucial to the delivery of a service over an extended time period. Teams must reach agreement on confidentiality, access and whether or not all team members are prepared to use a single set of notes.

8 There should be explicit agreement within the team on the co-ordination of work with individual clients and 'clarity over the respective responsi-bilities of case managers and other agencies is needed. It is also important to be clear about accountability for service shortfalls, routes of information for quality assurance, and arrangements for the management of direct-care staff working in teams' (Onyett, 1992, p. 23). There is always the possibility of poor liaison with others involved in a case and for the mechanisms for review and case closure to fail. In addition, a well-developed allocation and review process can help avoid an uneven or unfair distribution of workload. Where individuals carry high caseloads they are unlikely to find time to explore new developments and to update their own professional skills and knowledge.

9 It is unlikely that any group of people collaborating to deliver services to a range of clients, often with complex problems and needs, will avoid some conflict. Team members who have developed a process for dealing with conflicts will probably be able to work together with greater success. Dickinson describes the occupational stress which can result where a team cannot reach consensus and points out that 'This sort of dissatisfaction has to be recognised by line managers and a safe mechanism for expressing and negotiating unresolved conflict is necessary. One such forum is staff support groups' (Dickinson, 1989, p. 16).

HELPING COLLABORATION SURVIVE

It is clear that collaboration will not happen by accident and will require considerable effort from a range of people. The following suggestions are put forward as ways to help collaboration occur and thrive, once it has been decided that it is necessary:

1 An obvious way to help collaboration to survive is to minimise the need for collaboration. There are many situations in which collaboration is sought, without a clear understanding of why it is necessary. It is possible to reduce the failures that occur by avoiding the expectation of col-laboration between organisations and professionals whose roles and ways of operating make collaboration unnecessary or extremely difficult.

Wherever it is possible, managers should make the responsibilities of organisations and professionals clear and public. They should encourage professionals who specialise, to have clear criteria for referrals into and out of their services and to establish explicit processes for communicating with, and linking to, other services.

2 Managers and professionals should define clearly what collaboration is needed, and where and how it is to occur. At the level of an individual patient this is often difficult to do and may only become clear following a detailed assessment of the individual, their problems and needs. At the level of organisations it may be possible to be much clearer at the stage of planning and implementing a specific service, particularly as the process of service specification becomes more sophisticated and practised.

3 Where it is possible to specify that collaboration is needed and what it should involve, it should be built into service contracts. To help improve the probability that people will collaborate it should be possible to find ways to make collaboration meet some of the self-interests of all parties to the contract. This approach will only be possible if there is an explicit definition of collaboration, and people at all levels have ownership of both the need for this collaboration and the processes to be implemented to achieve it.

4 If staff are to implement collaborative ventures, then the training received by all professions should include the requirement for collaboration and should teach the skills and knowledge to implement it. The inclusion of the skills necessary to ensure participation and collaboration is particularly important during the pre-qualification education phase for all professionals. Foundation training should occur together wherever topics make it achievable. The curricula for all professional groups should include specific training designed to increase the chances of fruitful collaboration. At the level of post-qualification training, efforts should be made to bring staff together in multi-disciplinary, multi-agency groups and collaboration should feature as an essential topic in as many courses as possible. Such training, however, must be properly funded and supported as part of the 'rights' of staff who are expected to work in this way.

5 Training should also be incorporated into the induction period of teams, with a specific focus on helping integration into the team. 'The content should include specific training in communication skills, including team identity, agreeing roles and problem solving' (Dickinson, 1989, p. 16).

6 Managers and professional advisers can help by ensuring that job descriptions and the objectives set during the process of staff appraisal include collaboration where it is agreed to be necessary. An important part of objective setting within appraisal is to ensure that targets are clear and achievable. In a well-run appraisal system the individual being appraised will have the opportunity to help set the objectives and should find it much easier to have personal ownership of the final outcomes. It

is particularly important for senior managers to include appropriate collaboration in the appraisal targets both for themselves and for the staff for whom they are responsible.

7 At the planning stage the role of each team member should be defined particularly with reference to other members. Where professions have already established particular contractual rights designed to enable them to carry out their specialist roles, these should be understood and agreed with the team and its managers (Anciano and Kirkpatrick, 1990, p. 11).

8 Services should endeavour to provide the necessary support for each client to enable and empower them to insist on collaboration and co-operation where it is required to meet their individual needs. The advent of the Patient's Charter and the much clearer focus by managers on quality audit and quality control should begin to make both managers and the staff delivering the service much more sensitive to the need to listen to the individual receiving the service. For people with learning disabilities a great deal of careful and unbiased advocacy will be required. This could come from many sources but whoever provides the advocacy must place the issue of 'necessary collaboration' near the top of their priority list of targets to be achieved.

9 The line management accountability of staff who are expected to collaborate must be clear. Where a range of professional staff are expected to work together to deliver services there is often a major problem when they have different line managers who can be based a long way apart and rarely meet. There are clear advantages to having a common line manager or having managers who themselves operate as a team. This can help in dealing with inter-professional disputes and can ensure a genuine commitment to supporting the operational team. Where management and professional accountability are separated there must be clear rules about dealing with conflicts that arise. The actual solutions will need to be determined locally. The important step is to make sure the issues are actively addressed at the time that teams are established.

10 It is necessary to set out to minimise fragmentation of every type. Bob Hudson in Chapter 17 in this book has given us some helpful insights into the nature and types of fragmentation which can occur. Whether this fragmentation is organisational, cultural, professional or budgetary, it is clear that it is the enemy of collaboration. At the very least managers should recognise it and minimise its effects but, where possible, it should be removed.

11 The central pressure for collaboration should be used actively and wisely. Many government departments, including the Department of Health and the Department for Education, continue to place great emphasis on improving collaboration both within and across service and professional boundaries. This is clear in relation to the area of planning at the level of both service provision and care planning for individual clients. There are circulars, requests, guidance, legislation and orders which can be used

positively and productively to enhance the probability of collaboration occurring. Other bodies such as the Central Council for Education and Training in Social Work (CCETSW) have become increasingly insistent on collaboration between education and service providers within the delivery of training for social workers. As yet their main focus has been on partnerships between the employers and the education providers but it may be possible to extend this to collaboration with other groups.

12 It should be possible to build on the strengths of people who already collaborate. Some individuals seem to be natural collaborators, others learn to collaborate while some others appear almost unable to work together, even on simple, well-defined tasks. Where collaboration is already valued, it is important to build on it even if the people who work together do not immediately fit the ideal model of the team envisaged by the manager. If collaboration is an essential ingredient of service delivery it may be better to retain it and support it where it exists and then gradually re-shape the form and function of the team rather than risk losing it. Watson in her deliberately positive article concludes that 'clinical psychologists (should) try to avoid the radical path as teams get off the ground, opting instead for a more organic development which would allow for mistakes to be recognized and rectified, and which would maintain the flexibility to change direction in the light of changing circumstances' (Watson, 1990, p. 28).

13 Where a team has been formed, then any new appointments should ensure that the skills and willingness to collaborate are present in the candidate before the post is offered. This will mean that the team should have an active part in the selection and appointment process. This can be difficult in multi-disciplinary and multi-agency teams but will pay dividends in the longer term.

CONCLUSIONS

Many professions have embraced with enthusiasm the introduction of collaboration and the growth of formal teams because this has allowed them to obtain resources from general managers to expand their numbers. In practice, however, collaboration is beginning to be viewed by some professions as undermining their own expertise and even their own existence. Historically, clinical psychologists have taken on a therapy role which has regularly led them into conflict with the medical profession. This conflict has often been dealt with by avoiding it, perhaps through the practice of taking direct referrals from general practitioners and social workers. In making this point Alexander suggests that 'Perhaps such a strategy was inevitable, considering the relative powerlessness of psychology when compared to the medical profession' (Alexander, 1992, p. 15). This has been mirrored in the development of other professional groups such as community nurses. As a result individual practitioners have 'become relatively unaccustomed to working in teams, to working jointly with other professions and to displaying publicly (their) working practice and skills' (Alexander, 1992, p. 16) and in some clinical specialities the value and use of multi-disciplinary teams has been very directly questioned (Clydesdale, 1990, p. 7).

In a similarly critical paper, Searle looked at the operation of a multi-disciplinary team built around community nurses, an occupational therapist and a clinical psychologist. Her data led her to conclude that 'Putting people together in "teams" is little better, from the consumers' viewpoint, than operating as separate departments who do home visits. What actually happens is that referrals are arbitrarily allocated to individuals according to no real system, with no consideration of what is best for the client, and very little joint working' (Searle, 1991, p. 17).

Within this climate of doubt about the value of teamwork, some of the more recent changes which have taken place within the NHS have resulted in direct changes in the contracts of clinical staff, with many staff believing that there has been no true consultation and negotiation on these changes. This can lead to staff feeling that they have lost control over their professional lives. Some of the specific changes which might contribute to this feeling have been described by Tollinton as 'possible alterations in the previously recognized career structure and reward system; the new lines of accountability and responsibility which may be emerging; and the changes in the activities around which the clinical psychologist is given authority to function' (Tollinton, 1992, p. 24). The loss of control can lead to decreases in self-esteem and motivation which not only affect team operation but may lead some professionals to withdraw from the system which has imposed the changes on them. Other writers have concluded that they 'need to accept and make creative the tension between professional and team management and to retain multidisciplinary work even at some cost to professional control' (Jones *et al.*, 1990, p. 31).

This chapter has set out some of the issues surrounding collaboration and has offered some suggestions designed to help it survive. Achieving collaboration will require active and committed individuals to drive the initiatives, people to carry it through the difficult times and, above all, people who are prepared to take risks. The topic must be placed high on the agenda of every client, their advocates, their carers and all of those who work with them or contribute to the planning, purchasing and provision of their services. Collaboration cannot be left to chance and, where it is agreed to be a necessary part of the successful delivery of high-quality services, the training and performance of individuals must do everything possible to ensure that it will occur.

REFERENCES

Alexander, P. (1992) 'Psychology, clinical practice and community mental health teams', *Clinical Psychology Forum*, February: 15–18.

Anciano, D. and Kirkpatrick, A. (1990) 'CMHTs and clinical psychology: the death of a profession', *Clinical Psychology Forum*, April: 9–12.

Clydesdale, J. K. (1990) 'Psychologists and teams: has death already occurred?' *Clinical Psychology Forum*, December: 6–7.

Dickinson, D. (1989) 'Leadership, teamwork and morale within a neighbourhood resource centre', *Clinical Psychology Forum*, 24: 15–17.

Griffiths Report (1988) *Community Care: Agenda for Action*, London: HMSO.

Jones, A., Corke, R. and Childs, D. (1990) 'Working for whom? The NHS Bill and its implications for action', *Clinical Psychology Forum*, June: 28–31.

Lam, D. and von Abendorff, R. (1988) 'Community teams for elderly people: some issues on the planning and working of multidisciplinary teams', *Clinical Psychology Forum*, 18: 6–8.

Onyett, S. (1992) 'Not another paper about models of case management', *Clinical Psychology Forum*, May: 20–4.

Onyett, S. and Malone,S. (1990) 'Making the teamwork work', *Clinical Psychology Forum*, August: 16–18.

Ovretveit, S. (1985) *Organizational Issues in Multi-Disciplinary Teams*, Brunel Institute of Organization and Social Studies, Health Services Centre working paper, Brunel University.

Reiman, S. (1989) 'Multidisciplinary teamwork in a community setting: a discussion paper', *Clinical Psychology Forum*: 18–21.

Searle, R. T. (1991) 'Community mental health teams: fact or fiction?', *Clinical Psychology Forum*, February: 15–17.

Tollinton, G. (1992) 'Some reflections on the organizational changes in the NHS', *Clinical Psychology Forum*, August: 24–6.

Watson, C. (1990) 'Another perspective on CMHTs and clinical psychology', *Clinical Psychology Forum*, October: 27–8.

17 Is a co-ordinated service attainable?

Bob Hudson

The prime goal facing health and social care agencies in the learning disability field is to focus upon the unique needs of each individual and flexibly deploy services from a range of agencies to meet those needs. There is no single established way of doing this, but it is clear that the established system does not do it well. Exhortations to organisations, professions and other provider interests to work together more closely litter the policy landscape, but the reality is too often a jumble of services fractionalised by professional, cultural and organisational boundaries, as well as by tiers of governance (Webb, 1991).

This chapter will briefly look at the nature of fragmentation in service delivery and at different levels of collaboration. The experience of collaborative working in the 1980s in the field of special needs education and community mental handicap teams will be considered. Finally, the prospects of achieving some measure of unity through the introduction of caremanagement in the 1990s will be examined.

FRAGMENTATION AND COLLABORATION: THE CONCEPTUAL DEBATE

Service fragmentation can appear in a range of inter-related ways. *Resource* fragmentation exists when responsibility for a particular domain of activity is divided between more than one budget holder. This has long been the position in relation to learning disability, where 60 per cent of the combined health and personal social services budget is locked into hospital care for a small and diminishing number of residents (Audit Commission, 1986). Taking a wider perspective, the resource fragmentation dilemma is compounded by the fact that community care monies come from a number of budgets spread across different government departments, including the hospital and community health services budget, the personal social services budget, joint funding from the Department of Health, housing and recreation from the Department of the Environment, education from the DFE, employment from the Department of Employment and social security from the DSS. Resource fragmentation becomes especially problematic when no mechanism exists to significantly transfer budgets between cost centres to effect a shift in strategy. This is the current position in relation to learning disability.

Organisational fragmentation refers to the inability of organisations with a shared interest in a domain of activity to develop a complementary or co-ordinated strategy. This goes beyond problems of budget transfers. Rather it focuses upon the dynamics of organisational life and the ways in which they serve organisational interests rather than user interests. In relation to learning disability, the Audit Commission (1989) conducted a survey of fifty local authorities and reported a 'lack of sufficient trust or common purpose' between health and local authorities – 20 per cent exhibited insufficient commitment to joint planning and 60 per cent had not agreed joint strategies for the resettlement of hospital residents. The community care white paper (Department of Health, 1989) acknowledged that joint finance and Joint Consultative Committees had been ineffective, and the Audit Commission (1989) reported difficulties with the 'dowry system'.

Cultural fragmentation refers to the impact of distinct occupational social-isation processes resulting in conflicting perceived professional interests and professional stereotyping. This has contributed to services being insensitive, inefficient and ineffective, as professionals stick to their own cultural and organisational enclaves. The world of learning disability has its own version of this fragmentation. The cultural fragmentation between medical, nursing and social care interests was starkly revealed in the aftermath of the Jay Report (1979) and has not been seriously addressed since that time. The legacy is such issues as the uncertain status of those with an RNMH qualification in the post-hospital setting and the unclear relationship between community mental handicap nurses and social workers.

This initial review of the nature of fragmentation suggests the need to be realistic about the attainability of a 'seamless' service. Collaboration has no qualities of spontaneous growth or self-perpetuation (Hudson, 1987), and in general, professions and organisations strive to maintain their autonomy. From an agency's viewpoint, collaboration raises two main difficulties. First, it loses some of its freedom to act independently. Second, it must invest scarce resources and energy in developing and maintaining relationships with other agencies, when the returns on this investment are often unclear and intangible. Booth terms this the 'realistic stance' on collaboration and identifies five dimensions to it:

- collaboration is a self-interested process in which organisations will participate only if it suits them;
- the spirit of collaboration cannot be invoked by an appeal to the public interest;
- the success of collaboration will be determined by the balance of incentives and constraints bearing on each of the main parties;
- the pursuit of narrow organisational interest is rational in terms of the agency's survival and the security of its members;

- organisations will generally seek to maximise autonomy and minimise dependency.

(Booth, 1988)

Notwithstanding this, *Caring for People* and the subsequent policy and practice guidance have placed a huge emphasis upon improved collaboration as the key to the community care reforms. It serves as an illustration of Rein's argument (Rein, 1983) that collaboration is seen as both problem and remedy, and that it is one of the paradoxes of social policy that calls for better collaboration are met with accounts of failed attempts to achieve it. Can a less pessimistic message be found in relation to learning disability? What can be learned from the experience of the 1980s to inform the prospects for the 1990s?

LEARNING FROM THE 1980s: SPECIAL EDUCATIONAL NEEDS

The publication of the Warnock Report (1978) created a momentum in the field of special needs education towards greater interprofessional collaboration in the identification, assessment of, and provision for, special needs pupils. The close co-ordination of medical, educational and psychological professionals in these processes was a major recommendation of the report, and was duly translated into the Education Act 1981. Such an approach is based upon the premise that the quality of service ultimately delivered is dependent upon the ability of professionals to surrender their self-interest and place the needs of service users at the forefront. In effect, the 1981 Act gave collaboration a legal imperative and might have been expected to give a huge boost to a seamless approach to service delivery.

Some of the major evaluations of the implementation of the 1981 Act carry a more circumspect message. In her classic study on the basis upon which children with 'mild educational subnormality' are referred, assessed and admitted to special schools, Tomlinson (1988) queried the epistemological status of the concept 'educationally subnormal' and took as her starting point the premise that the category is socially constructed by the judgements and decisions made by professionals about children. She reported a lack of professional consensus and collaboration on the assessment, with teachers, psychologists, health staff and others using different accounts to define their social construction of the 'slow learning pupil'. Her conclusion, confirmed in a subsequent consideration of the impact of the 1981 Act (Tomlinson, 1988) was that professional collaboration was little more than a power struggle to control access to resources for special educational needs, with educational psychologists emerging as the dominant professional group. In a recent study in Scotland, Thomson *et al.* (1991) arrive at broadly similar conclusions, reporting that multi-professional assessment teams operate successfully in only a minority of areas. Again, there was resentment of psychologists' domination.

These interprofessional divisions are mirrored at interorganisational level. In their major evaluation of the 1981 Act, Goacher *et al.* (1989) distinguish between three approaches to policy making: 'collaborative' approaches, involving genuine multi-disciplinary discussion between health, education and social services personnel, to achieve a consensus of approach and a co-ordinated structure; a 'consultative' approach in which the LEA invited representatives of services onto a working party which formed the forum for the LEA to promote its own proposals for change; and a 'coercive' approach, where the LEA decided upon its new procedure and informed health and social services agencies of its requirements. Goacher *et al.* found that decisions regarding 'statements' and provision were mainly taken by the LEA officers – only one example of multi-service decision making was uncovered – and conclude that 'despite frequent contact between services, the gulf in understanding between them still appears to be wide'.

The consequence of this LEA hegemony has been to leave other participants marginalised and confused about their role in relation to the 1981 Act procedures. Goacher and his colleagues found that social services departments had no clear idea of their role in the statementing process, and often simply did not know how to respond to an LEA notification on assessment of a child. A report from the National Association of Health Authorities (1988) makes a similar point in relation to the health contribution, suggesting that 'health authority staff tend to feel both undervalued and frustrated that the exclusion of their views results in the child and family receiving less than optimum support'. The procedures established in the wake of the 1981 Act exhibit several of the characteristics of the caremanagement process – screening, multi-disciplinary assessment and individual care planning – and the evidence would suggest that caremanagement will not find it easy to resolve the legacy of fragmentation.

LEARNING FROM THE 1980s: COMMUNITY MENTAL HANDICAP TEAMS

The *raison d'être* of community mental handicap teams (CMHTs) has been to 'confront head on those concerns . . . that care provision for people with a mental handicap was fragmented, that services were inaccessible, and that organisational and professional boundaries prevented continuity of care' (Brown and Wistow, 1990). The experience of CMHTs therefore constitutes a useful test of the extent to which the established system of care provision could develop a collaborative strategy. The idea of CMHTs was first promoted by the National Development Group in the mid-1970s and most local areas now boast a CMHT of some sort. A related development at the time was a response to the proposal in the Court Report (1976) for district handicap teams covering all disabled children. Indeed, over the years, such multi-disciplinary teams have been seen as an appropriate model for a wide range of groups, including elderly people, those with mental health problems, drug users and children at risk.

Probably the most noticeable feature of CMHTs is their variation in size, membership and function. An early survey by Plank (1982) on size, found a range from two to eleven, with most on the small side. This has been confirmed by the more recent survey of English CMHTs by Brown (1990) which found two-thirds to have less than four members. Size variation is reflected in membership variation. Plank's (1982) survey found that 18 per cent had no social services representation, 20 per cent no community mental handicap nurse, 50 per cent no psychologist or consultant in mental handicap and 80 per cent no therapists. The English CMHT survey suggests that since then there has been an increase in the membership of CMHTs and in the involvement of clinical psychologists. The analysis of CMHTs in Wales puts forward a fourfold typology of staff teams:

- 'basic team' (16 per cent) consisting solely of social workers and nurses;
- 'professional oriented team' (29 per cent) which included members of additional professions;
- 'service oriented team' (42 per cent) comprising social workers, nurses and service organisers;
- 'integrated team' (13 per cent) of social workers, nurses, other professionals and service organisers.

(McGrath and Humphreys, 1988)

The Welsh evidence suggested an encouraging degree of multi-professional membership, but the All Wales Strategy on Mental Handicap does give a central role to CMHTs and generally offers a more coherent and progressive model for service delivery than anything yet attempted elsewhere in the UK.

This variation in size and membership is reflected in the variation in functions of CMHTs. Mansell (1990) distinguishes between three functions of CMHTs. First, a 'gatekeeping' or co-ordinating role, primarily concerned with direct 'routine family maintenance', which fills a gap in service provision. Second a 'service development' role, to build up a range of residential and support services within the community, and which could involve little or no direct work with clients. And finally a 'direct service delivery' role – a logical extension of the service development role, in which the CMHT becomes a managerial team appointing and employing basic grade direct care staff.

How successful has this exercise been in collaborative activity? Those involved in the two major surveys (in England and Wales, respectively) do make encouraging noises. Brown and Wistow suggest that the CMHT contribution has been to provide:

- a mechanism for establishing a substantial, specialist fieldwork resource, and one which is ring-fenced against competition;
- a vehicle for strengthening cooperation between health and social services authorities at field and (more limitedly) management and planning levels;

- an organisational framework for the growing number of health service staff working outside traditional hospital settings.

(Brown and Wistow, 1990)

The Welsh evaluation (McGrath and Humphreys, 1988) concludes that the main achievement has been 'the implied conceptual shift involved in recognising that planning must start from the needs of the handicapped person and the family, with a mechanism that allows them to participate in discussions'. More soberly, it is also acknowledged that the very existence of multi-disciplinary mechanisms is no small achievement, given the considerable pressures on professionals to retain their separate identities and ways of working.

Notwithstanding these achievements, it remains the case that CMHTs have been far from an unblemished success. Three particular difficulties are identifiable: the persistence of role ambiguity; problems in securing a co-ordinated response, and confusion over organisational accountability.

1 *Role ambiguity*

Given the lack of clarity about the original idea of CMHTs, it is un-surprising that many of them lack operational policies – Brown's (1990) study of the West Midlands, for example, found that only a quarter had been provided with a framework of operational objectives. The conse-quence has been that conflict and uncertainty, rather than consensus and rationality, are the characteristics of policy making and implementation. In these circumstances, a process of bargaining and negotiation takes place between team members (and between them and their respective employers) about roles and emphases. The outcome may be institutionalised as operational procedures, but Brown and Wistow (1990) argue that organ-isational solutions cannot be regarded as sufficient to resolve the complex interactional problems which shape relationships between health and social services agencies and professional groupings.

This process of negotiation is not confined to the internal organisation of CMHTs, for they must also find a niche in the local service-providing environment. In this case study of 'the Borough', Brown (1990) found the CMHT inhabiting an environment made up of established parts of the service system (such as hospitals, day centres and hostels) within which they had to 'find a niche' to develop their own work. This is not an easy process, especially when others (such as District Handicap Teams) may be engaged in a similar activity. He suggests that the shortcomings of much current practice can be laid at the failure to address such matters in the design of teams.

2 *Securing a co-ordinated response*

It might be expected that one outcome of this complex role negotion would be that CMHT members secure more co-ordinated patterns of working. The Welsh survey did indeed find that 'teams in general exhibited a high degree of commitment, mutual trust and support' but also concluded that: 'The various professions have different methods of working, value systems and priorities, and frequently show a lack of knowledge and understanding of other professions, and a tendency to stereotype them' (McGrath and Humphreys).

Both the English and Welsh surveys saw the relationship between social workers and community mental handicap nurses as particularly difficult. 'Case ownership' tended to be on an individual basis, with cases acquired through the separate networks with which they were associated. From then on, members worked with considerable independence from each other, despite appearing to perform much the same tasks. This 'role assimilation' differs sharply from the 'role complementarity' model which constitutes the rationale for multi-disciplinary teams. Even where team policies have been established on joint working, there may be little more than peer group pressure to exert over recalcitrant members.

3 *Organisational accountability*

The management structure within which the CMHT operates is a crucial factor in its effectiveness, and since multi-disciplinary working also requires multi-agency co-operation, the environment is complex. The Wales survey found CMHTs in difficulty where management support to the team as a unit was weak, with no over-arching system at middle management level to mirror the multi-agency nature of the teams. Organisation is not a peripheral issue for CMHTs but is central to their existence. The mistake which is often made is that there is no formal review point where the team and higher management agree and specify details, and this is often because there is no structure and process for team accountability.

This confusion over accountability is also seen in the tension between CMHT's developing custom-built 'care packages' and traditional bureaucratic planning and administrative systems with an emphasis upon 'macro' service development. The Welsh survey found that managers experienced dual loyalty, but that even where they were sympathetic to team aims 'remarkably few indications were given of how teams could be helped to overcome the constraints that impeded their work'. Indeed, McGrath and Humphreys (1988) concluded that: 'We sensed that senior managers all too often perceived CMHTs as something which denuded their power and influence, rather than as a proper attempt to empower consumers and their families.'

What the CMHT experience tells us is that the multi-disciplinary team, planning individual care packages on a 'bottom up' basis requires clear lines of support if it is to survive, let alone flourish. In particular, it needs:

- a clear statement of support from the centre;
- a clear statement of a local role;
- a clear system of management support;
- a clear indication of how to relate to other local services.

LOOKING TO THE 1990S: COLLABORATION AND CAREMANAGEMENT

The government is putting considerable faith in caremanagement as a fresh means of attaining a co-ordinated approach to service assessment and delivery. Caremanagement programmes may differ markedly in goals, settings and target populations, and although there may not be a widely accepted definition of the term, there is some consensus about the components of the process. Kane *et al.* see these as:

- Screening: procedures to identify those in the target population who need care management;
- Assessment: typically a comprehensive, multidimensional, functionally oriented evaluation of an applicant's needs and situations;
- Care Planning: using the assessment information to drive a plan for care;
- Implementation: either through 'brokering' or purchase of service;
- Monitoring: this covers both the user's progress and the adequacy of the provider;
- Reassessment at fixed intervals.

(Kane *et al.*, 1991)

The call for enhanced collaborative activity lies at the heart of several concerns critical to caremanagement: the recognition that boundaries between professionals, service and agencies militate against user-sensitive responses; the existence of some overlap and duplication of service coverage; and a feeling that services may even be pulling in different directions. These difficulties have been fully acknowledged by the Department of Health, and an ambitious agenda of co-ordinated activity has been laid at the door of caremanagement in respect of assessment, care plans and service development. The key to believing that care managers might be able to act as orchestrators of diverse services combined to respond flexibly to individual needs lies in the notion of the purchase/provider split. The intention is that in some form, budget-holding will be devolved to a 'micro contracting' level close to the user, and that provider organisations in the new 'quasi market' will play to the tune of the purchasing care manager.

It is still too early to make a judgement on caremanagement. The early projects funded by the care-in-the-community initiative and evaluated by the PSSRU at the University of Kent were optimistic in their findings, but more recent evaluations have been less sanguine. In the learning disability field, most interest has been generated by the Nuffield Institute evaluation of the Wakefield Care Management Project (Richardson and Higgins, 1990, 1991, 1992). On the particular issue of caremanagement and collaboration, the Wakefield studies throw up three problem areas: organisational and professional fragmentation; organisational disinterest; and organisational inertia. Each of these diminishes the power of the care manager to effect collaboration through the purchasing function.

The Wakefield CMP was established to effect the transfer of residents from hospital to the community, and it soon fell foul of the organisational and professional fragmentation described earlier in this chapter. Care managers found difficulties in their relations with hospital staff who had a more traditional approach to residents, felt some prior ownership of the residents, held deep reservations about the ability of residents to move away, and saw the CMP as a threat to their security. Hospital consultants are key actors in the decision-making process, and they tended to be sceptical about the project, as well as resentful of the threat to their authority to determine client futures posed by the introduction of caremanagement.

Organisational disinterest represents a different kind of threat. Whereas organisational and professional fragmentation destroys collaboration because of a disputation over domain legitimacy, organisational disinterest destroys it through simple neglect. The Wakefield Project found this to be especially true of the local authority housing department, which is described as 'an embarrassment to the project'. The principal service required of the hospital leavers was housing, and the user-led nature of caremanagement led to the expectation that clients would move to individual houses and flats tailored to their particular needs. In practice, the housing department simply did not respond, other than to offer 'miscellaneous' properties – large or unusual properties of limited interest to families on the ordinary waiting list, and traditionally seen as 'special needs' housing.

Organisational inertia refers to the unwillingness or inability of existing services providers to respond to change. Service development is an inherently political task, and requires trying to interest those already working in an authority in developing new services and providing incentives to do so. The Wakefield CMP seemed to be in a good position to do this, since it had funds waiting to be put to work, but it found its own organisation to be unresponsive. Richardson and Higgins argue that bureaucracies are simply geared to 'more of the same', and conclude that 'the real problem encountered was an organisational resistance to take on anything new'.

It would be wrong to build too much upon the Wakefield experience, for the project was concerned with a particularly complex task and was in business some time before the Department of Health gave an official imperative to the caremanagement process. However, it does suggest that it would be premature to regard caremanagement as the solution to the fragmentation dilemma. Given the pessimism of much previous experience, the realistic option would seem to be to continue experimenting with different models of caremanagement in particular places and with different objectives. This should surely encompass a more serious attempt to introduce and evaluate a range of pilot projects on the radical model of caremanagement – service brokerage. Salisbury (1987) describes service brokerage as having three elements: individualised funding, calculated according to personal strengths, needs and service requirements and then attached to those individuals on an ongoing basis; personal networks of family and friends which are recognised as having status, and in the case of a user with communication difficulties might have a decision-making role in purchasing and contracting services; and a 'broker', accountable to individuals and personal networks, to help develop personalised plans and arrangements for community living.

The strength of the model is that it reasserts the position of service users as the *raison d'être* of any service-providing configuration, with the broker's involvement at the discretion of the individual or the personal network. In effect, then, the task of developing a coherent user-sensitive service is laid upon the user or the user's personal network. Despite much talk of user involvement in the past few years, no significant attempt has been made in Britain to introduce a pilot brokerage system. Part of the problem is that it would require a change in the law to allow local authorities to make cash payments to clients, but the real obstacle is the implied transfer of power from bureaucracies and professionals to users – a move usually dismissed as unrealistic. However, a recent review of the experience of clients of the Independent Living Fund (Kestenbaum, 1992) suggests that severely disabled clients are often well able to make financial decisions about their own needs with some guidance from advocates, personal networks and professionals.

CONCLUSION

This review has not been optimistic about the attainability of a seamless service in the field of learning disability. It has identified some of the problems encountered in past experiences and has cautioned against unrealistic expectations of current and new initiatives. Some progress may well be possible, but this is likely to be incremental and adapted to local circumstances. However, the wider canvass must not be ignored. Given a diversity of interests and values, the rational-altruistic model of collaboration across professional and organisational boundaries has several prerequisites:

- at least some set of common goals;
- a system-wide view of needs and problems;
- some consensus about the nature of these needs and problems;
- agreement on how to tackle the problem;
- agreement on the priority to be accorded to each potential claim.

It is a challenge which we have scarcely begun to address.

REFERENCES

Audit Commission (1986), *Making a Reality of Community Care* (HMSO), London.
Audit Commission (1989), *Developing Community Care for Adults with a Mental Handicap*, Occasional Paper 9 (HMSO), London.
Booth, T. (1988), *Developing Policy Research* (Gower), Aldershot.
Brown, S. (1990), Finding a Niche in the System: the case of the Community Mental Handicap Team, in Brown, S. and Wistow, G. (eds) *The Roles and Task of Community Mental Handicap Teams* (Avebury), Aldershot.

Brown, S. and Wistow, G. (eds) (1990), *The Roles and Task of Community Mental Handicap Teams* (Avebury), Aldershot.

Court Report (1976) *Fit for the Future: the Report of the Committee on Child Health Services*, Cmnd 6684 (HMSO), London.

Department of Health (1989), *Caring for People: Community Care in the Next Decade and Beyond*, Cm 849 (HMSO), London.

Goacher, B., Evans, J., Welton, J. and Wedell, K. (1989), *Policy and Provision for Special Educational Needs: Implementing the 1981 Education Act* (Cassell), London.

Hudson, B. (1987), Collaboration in Social Welfare: A Framework for Analysis, *Policy and Politics*, Vol. 15, No. 3, 175–83.

Jay Report (1979), *Report of the Committee of Enquiry into Mental Handicap Nursing and Care*, Cmnd 7468 (HMSO), London.

Kane, R., Penrod, J., Davidson, G., Moscovice, I. and Rich, E. (1991), What cost case management in long term care?, *Social Service Review*, June, 281–303.

Kestanbaum, A. (1992), *Cash for Care*, Independent Living Fund, London.

Mansell, J. (1990), The Natural History of the Community Mental Handicap Team, in Brown, S. and Wistow, G. (eds) *The Roles and Task of Community Mental Handicap Teams* (Avebury), Aldershot.

McGrath, M. and Humphreys, S. (1988), *The All Wales CMHT Survey* (University College of North Wales), Cardiff.

National Association of Health Authorities (1988), *Health Authorities Concerns for Children with Special Needs* (National Association of Health Authorities), Birmingham.

Plank, M. (1982), *Teams for Mentally Handicapped People* (Campaign for Mentally Handicapped People), London.

Rein, M. (1983), *From Policy to Practice* (Macmillan), London.

Richardson, A. and Higgins, R. (1990), *Case Management in Practice: Reflections on the Wakefield Case Managment Projects*, Working Paper, No. 1 (Nuffield Institute for Health Service Studies), Leeds.

Richardson, A. and Higgins, R. (1991), *Doing Care Management: Learning from the Wakefield Case Management Project*, Working Paper, No. 4 (Nuffield Institute for Health Service Studies), Leeds.

Richardson, A. and Higgins, R. (1992), *The Limits of Case Management: Lessons from the Wakefield Case Management Project*, Working Paper, No. 5 (Nuffield Institute for Health Service Studies), Leeds.

Salisbury, B. (1987), *Service Brokerage* (G. Allan Roeher Institute, Canada).

Thomson, G., Riddell, S. and Dyer, S. (1991), Interprofessional Collaboration and the Implementation of the Education (Scotland) Act 1981, *Journal of Educational Policy*, Vol. 6, No. 1, 47–62.

Tomlinson, S. (1988), *Educational Subnormality: A Study in Decision Making* (Routledge and Kegan Paul), London.

Tomlinson, S. (1988), Why Johnny Can't Read: Critical Theory and Special Education, *European Journal of Special Needs Education*, Vol. 3, No. 1, 45–58.

Warnock Report (1978), Special Educational Needs (HMSO), London.

Webb, A. (1991), Coordination: A Problem in Public Sector Management, *Policy and Politics*, Vol. 19, No. 4, 229–42.

Author index

Subject index